CARDIOLOGY RESEARCH AND CLINICAL DEVELOPMENTS

CONGENITAL HEART DISEASES

AN UPDATED APPROACH TO SOME IMPORTANT ISSUES

CARDIOLOGY RESEARCH AND CLINICAL DEVELOPMENTS

Additional books in this series can be found on Nova's website
under the Series tab.

Additional e-books in this series can be found on Nova's website
under the e-book tab.

CARDIOLOGY RESEARCH AND CLINICAL DEVELOPMENTS

CONGENITAL HEART DISEASES

AN UPDATED APPROACH TO SOME IMPORTANT ISSUES

RAÚL CAYRÉ, M.D., PH.D.
AND
JOSÉ MILEI, M.D., PH.D.
EDITORS

NOVA BIOMEDICAL

New York

Library of Congress Cataloging-in-Publication Data

ISBN: 978-1-61122-003-2

Library of Congress Control Number: 2014946528

Published by Nova Science Publishers, Inc. † New York

Contents

Preface

Congenital heart diseases are of the utmost importance in modern cardiology. This is a book that deals with essential matters which are developed by experienced researchers in their respective fields. An updated approach to these issues was largely sought after. The authors share their own papers and experience with the enthusiastic professionals reading their work all throughout the chapters in an easy-to-read format.

Modern medical practice demands continuous research on specific topics. Thereafter, this book is devoted to the development of the coronary arteries facing the fact that coronary artery disease is the most common cause of mortality in the developed world. The the role of the estrogen receptor and transforming growth factors in coronary intimal hyperplasia and thorough descriptions of new diagnostic techniques in congenital heart diseases are also displayed (severe congenital heart defects are generally diagnosed during pregnancy or soon after birth while less severe defects often are not diagnosed until children are older). Accordingly, complex malformations of the heart, fetal arrhythmias and pulmonary hypertension are also included.

In as much as other specific subjects are relevant as well, topics like an etiological overview of intrauterine ductus arteriosus constriction, restrictive cardiomyopathy in children or hybrid procedures for congenital heart disease, namely palliation of hypoplastic left heart syndrome, closure of muscular ventricular septal defect and stenting of branch pulmonary arteries are developed as well.

Last but not least, the long-term outcomes of congenital heart diseases, including medical, interventional and emergency treatments, are examined.

Chapter 1 – The embryological development of the coronary arteries in humans is still controversial. It is unclear whether there is a dual process of angiogenesis and vasculogenesis or a single process of vasculogenesis. Objective: This chapter examines the development of the coronary arteries in human embryos within the context of recent experimental findings. Methods: Of 131 human embryos and fetuses, 22 between stages XIII (27±2 days) and XVIII (48±1 day) were studied. Results: Islands of angioblastic cells appeared in stage XIII. By stage XV two distinct subepicardial vascular networks were seen which connected to the aorta by stages XVII-XVIII. Endothelial indentations were seen in stages XV and XVI only in the region of the aorta just above the developing aortic sigmoid valves; no direct connections could be confirmed to the subepicardial vascular network therefore we cannot conclude that these are involved in the formation of the proximal coronary trunks as has been previously proposed. Compaction of the ventricular myocardium began in stage XV at the base of the heart and extended towards the apex. Conclusion: The coronary arteries in the human embryo seem to develop through vasculogenesis with the appearance of islands of angioblastic cells which coalesced to form two subepicardial capillary networks; these were clearly distinct by stage XV. The connection of both vascular networks via coronary channels to the aorta was invariably present by stage XVIII.

Chapter 2 – Congenital heart defects (CHD) and/ or their repair process lead to an increased risk for adult cardiovascular disease compared with the general population.

Intimal hyperplasia is a pre-atherosclerotic lesion that may be produced as a consequence of the activation of transforming growth factor beta-1 (TGF-β_1) pathway or ERα inhibition.

This chapter deals with the authors recent findings in this regard and comments in their latest results in connection with relevant reports from other authors.

The authors examined the coronary arteries from a pediatric population with CHD and evaluated the possible relationship between the frequency of intimal hyperplasia and the magnitude of TGF-β_1 in order to enlighten the possible role of TGF-β_1 in the genesis of these lesions. The coronary arteries of 10 control patients and 98 CHD patients (54% cyanotic type, 32% surgically repaired) were stained and assessed for the presence and degree of intimal thickening. The expression of TGF-β_1 and ERα was determined by immunohistochemical examination.

The frequency of coronary intimal hyperplasia did not depend on the group, i.e.: cyanotic CHD group (66%) and non-cyanotic CHD group (64%). However, the frequency of coronary intimal hyperplasia was higher in patients with surgically repaired CHD than in patients without surgical intervention (80% vs. 47% respectively, $p=0.0002$).

The degree of positive immunostaining for TGF-β_1 or ERα did not depend on the group. i.e.: cyanotic and non-cyanotic type. On the other hand, examination of the intimal layer showed that TGF-ß$_1$ expression was higher and expression of ERα was smaller in patients with surgically repaired CHD compared with those without surgery.

The relationship between the frequency of intimal hyperplasia and the expression of TGF-β_1 and ERα in arteries from 98 pediatric patients with congenital heart defects indicated that: 1) intimal hyperplasia was a common finding in the coronary tree of these patients, 2) both TGF-β_1 and ERα seemed to play a major role in this phenomenon and 3) surgical correction of CHD was associated with further coronary vascular remodeling.

Chapter 3 – New diagnostic techniques can help to understand the myocardial function in congenital heart disease. Echocardiography is a reliable, noninvasive tool to evaluate heart structure and contractile function of the left and right ventricle in children and adults. 2D color Doppler imaging of the myocardium enables rapid qualitative assessment of wall dynamics, providing a good spatial resolution to differentiate between velocity profiles of subendocardial and subepicardial layers, and allows simultaneous analysis of various myocardial regions. Tissue Doppler velocity imaging (TDI) offers a different approach, as it does not rely on geometric assumptions. Possibly, the best option for the evaluation ventricular function is the combination of different methods: TAPSE, TDI and index of myocardial performance. Two-Dimensional (2D) Speckle-Tracking Echocardiography (STE) is a relatively new, angle independent technique that is used for the evaluation of global and segmental myocardial function. Myocardial strain values regional ventricular deformation. Myocardial strain rate (SR) is a time derivative of strain and has shown to correlate linearly with left ventricle (LV) peak elastance, which is a load-independent global measure of ventricular systolic function.

Conclusion: New echo technology can identify early left and right ventricular dysfunction. This may allow earlier intervention and help to avoid irreversible damage to the myocardium in congenital heart disease.

Chapter 4 – Coronary artery anomalies are some of the most confusing, neglected topics in cardiology. The occurrence of coronary artery abnormalities is reported to be approximately 0.2% to 5,6 %. These anomalies are usually not symptomatic and have no clinical significance, although in some particular cases can be fatal. Recently Coronary Computed Tomography Angiography, replaces the method of choice, coronary invasive angiography, for detecting coronary anomalies, based on its ability to accurately depict the anatomy of the heart and thorax. A useful classification it is very important to understand the complex topic of coronary artery anomalies (CAAs). There are four types: Anomalies of origination and course, anomalies of intrinsic coronary arterial anatomy, anomalies of coronary termination and anomalous collateral vessels. Each tipe has differents items that are shown in correlative figures in this chapter. The Malignant type, it is also reported as anomalous origination of a coronary artery from the opposite sinus (ACAOS) with intussusception of the ectopic proximal vessel, which is the subgroup of CAAs that has the most potential for clinical repercussions, specifically sudden death in the Young. It is very important the adequate knowledge of these anomalies in order to achieve an appropriate and accurate diagnosis, that can be the key for the good prognosis of this group of patients.

Chapter 5 – The ductus arteriosus plays a fundamental role in directing 80–85% of the right ventricular output arising from the superior vena cava, coronary sinus, and a small part from the inferior vena cava to the descending aorta. Its histological structure is predominantly made up by a thick muscular layer, different from the aorta and the pulmonary artery, which increases with gestational age. The fibers have a circumferential orientation, especially at the external layers, facilitating and making effective ductal constriction. These factors may generate lumen alterations, which may cause fetal and neonatal complications, such as heart failure, hydrops, neonatal pulmonary hypertension, and even death. Classically, maternal administration of indomethacin and/or other anti-inflammatory drugs interfere in prostaglandins metabolism, causing ductal constriction. However, many cases of fetal ductal constriction, as well as of persistent neonatal pulmonary artery hypertension, remain without an established etiology, being referred as "idiopathic." In recent years, a growing body of evidence has shown that herbs, fruits, nuts, and a wide diversity of substances commonly used in daily diets have definitive effects upon the metabolic pathway of inflammation, with consequent inhibition of prostaglandins synthesis. This anti-inflammatory action, especially of polyphenols, when ingested during the third trimester of pregnancy, may influence the dynamics of fetal ductus arteriosus flow. The aim of this review is to present these new observations and findings, which may influence dietary orientation during pregnancy.

Chapter 6 – Fetal cardiac arrhythmias (FCAs) detected during a routine clinical obstetric or ultrasonography examination constitute, in our experience, a relatively frequent finding and generate a marked anxiety in the family and the obstetrician. At least 2% of all pregnancies this problem is presented.

In our 25-year experience (1988-2013) a total 203 FCAs was detected. 8 patients (p) (3,9%) with premature ventricular contractions; 53p (26,1%) with flutter or atrial fibrillation; 66p (32,5%) with supraventricular tachycardia; and only 2p (0.98%) with ventricular tachycardia; 5p (4,5%) sustained sinusal bradycardia; 1p (0,5%) second-degree heart block and 68p (33,5%) with complete atrioventricular block (CAVB).

They manifest at any gestational age, as early as 13th week of gestation until the term.

The association with cardiac malformations was more frequently in patients with complete congenital heart block 31 of 68 p (45.5%). The tachycardias they found were associated in 6 of 129p (4, 6%).

The aim of the present chapter is to help to recognize the different FACs, carry out a correct analysis, perform an adequate diagnosis and choose the best therapeutic behavior and follow-up. The authors will therefore describe the different methods of analysis of the fetal cardiac rhythm (FCR), revise their disorder patterns, and describe their therapeutic options and responses.

Conclusion: FCAs impose an emergency for the cardiologist since they generate a marked anxiety in both the family and the obstetrician. In flutter and fibrillation as well as in SVT the association of hydrops and/or cardiac malformation does not imply a bad prognosis sign. Hospital admission should be limited to the presence of hydrops or prematurity before 26th week of gestation according to our criteria.

In CAVB, the presence of hydrops, FCF< 50 bpm and/or the association to cardiopathies are of very bad prognosis. In the cases without malformation with maternal positive antibodies, the treatment with corticoids must be performed promptly after maternal blood extraction.

Fetal-maternal Doppler of umbilical and middle cerebral arteries gives us the possibility of ruling out hypoxic component, and it must only be taken into account that cerebral/umbilical resistance index relation must be >1 whatever the gestational age.

Doppler of ductus venosus, suprahepatic veins and umbilical veins must be controlled since they may allow distinguishing fetuses with higher risk of developing hydrops.

Chapter 7 – This chapter is an actualized review of different aspects related to pulmonary hypertension associated with congenital heart disease. The main message that they try to convey to the readers is the importance of early diagnosis and treatment of congenital heart disease, to avoid pulmonary vascular disease; this means, the importance of prevention of pulmonary vascular disease. Considering that left to right shunts are the more frequent congenital heart disease associated with pulmonary hypertension, this topic is analyzed in wide form, from physiopathology until treatment, emphasizing the importance of a clinical approach for early detection of Congenital Heart Disease. I propose a pyramidal approach to the diagnosis and treatment of congenital heart disease associated with pulmonary hypertension.

The authors emphasize that it is not correct to extrapolate the result of studies made in adults and apply it to children. I mention that the Dana Point Classification (with the Update of Nice) is difficult to apply to children; for this reason I see that it is more applicable to use in pediatric patients the, Panama Classification: Classification of pulmonary vascular disease in children.

I give special importance to two topics: The adult with congenital heart disease and Pulmonary Hypertension, including the Eisenmenger Syndrome, and pulmonary hypertension associated with congenital heart disease at altitude. This last topic is very important, considering that a great population lives at high altitudes (more than 140,000,000 people); on the other hand, hypobaric hypoxia gives a special characteristic to pulmonary hypertension at high altitude, which influences biopathogenesis, clinical aspects, diagnostic approach and treatment.

Chapter 8 – The term "functionally univentricular heart" embraces heterogeneous categories of complex cardiac malformations that, in the context of congenital heart diseases, exemplify one of the most challenging objectives of the study. The management of patients with an anatomical or functional "single ventricle" represents an unlimited task in the pediatric cardiology and surgical field. The vision of this matter in this "undone chapter" can be summarized in three stages: the prelude, the epic and the future. In the early 1940s, the preface era, an experimental work inspired what is named nowadays as the Fontan/Kreutzer operation – the total right ventricular bypass was first reported in humans in the early 1970s. In the following 40 years several modifications and refinements of the initial surgical design, improved perioperative care and management of algorithms-based protocols produced a drastic increase in perioperative survivors – the heroic epic. However, when patients grew into adulthood, coping with a complete univentricular circulation as a result of the palliative procedures, they faced numerous complications and multi-organ system difficulties that seriously limited their quality of life. Continuous research and multidisciplinary efforts in several directions are needed to answer the future of Fontan failure patients. Perhaps this would include the expected potential clinical application of a mechanical "new neo subpulmonary ventricle" compatible with a normal life span similar to people with a normal biventricular circulation.

Chapter 9 – Restrictive cardiomyopathy is a rare disease in childhood characterized by ventricular diastolic dysfunction usually with preserved systolic function, with a progressive clinical course and poor outcome. This chapter reviews the definition, epidemiology, genetics, natural history, clinical presentation, role of diagnostic tools, outcome, and current management of pediatric populations with this uncommon disease based on our clinical experience and literature studies. Restrictive cardiomyopathy in childhood is a rare entity with high mortality rates that still arises controversy around its definition and treatment. The stratification of risk factors for sudden death, cardiac failure, thromboembolic events and increase in pulmonary vascular resistance requires prospective longitudinal studies with large pediatric populations in order to acquire better knowledge of the course and outcome of this disease. The identification of specific genetic mutations is paving the way for a better understanding of the molecular pathology of restrictive disorders. This line of research will most probably lead to the design of new therapies that can delay or reduce the need for heart transplant.

Chapter 10 – TRANSCATHETER CLOSURE OF ASDs- PFOs: The type, size, and shape of atrial septal defects (ASDs) can vary greatly. Ostium secundum (OS) are the most common ASDs, are present in the region of the fossa ovalis, and account for 75% of all ASDs. The position and size of the ASDs, number of defects, distance between the defects, type of defects, and relationship with other structures must be determined to result in a successful procedure. ASDs that are not suitable for trans-catheter device closure are sinus venous defects (4-11%) and ostium primum ASDs (15-20%).

TRANSCATHETER CLOSURE OF VENTRICULAR SEPTAL DEFECTS (VSD): Common congenital heart disease (20%). Indications for VSD closure are: symptoms of heart failure; signs of volume overload in left heart chambers; history of endocarditis; and post-operatory residual VSD with volume overload. The procedure is not recommended in absence of the crista since this type of VSD has a deficient aortic and pulmonary margin. The risk factors for complications are age (<5 months) and weight (<5 kg), which are associated with a higher risk of early complications. The localization of the defect: pm VSD has an increased risk of complete cAVB after device implantation. The success rate was very high, as closure was successfully achieved in 95.3% of subjects in the follow-up.

AORTIC COARCTATION: Occurs in about 0.04% of live births and comprises about 7% of known congenital heart disease. Surgery is the best option in native coarctation in patients <25 kg and covered stent in patients >45 years old, to avoid morbidity. In postsurgical residual gradient, the best option is angioplasty or stent, depending on age, type of defect, elasticity of the wall and other complications. If the aorta must be expanded to adult size, or when the initial measure requires a final diameter 3 times greater, covered stent is preferred.

Conclusion: Therapeutic intervention helps in congenital heart disease by solving an increasing number of pathologies and is complementary to other surgical lesions.

Chapter 11 – Evolving surgical and catheter-based techniques and a collaboration environment between surgeons and interventionalists resulted in the advent of the so-called hybrid procedures in congenital heart disease. Although the hybrid approach starts with a collaborative effort between surgeons and interventionalists, it continues with careful planning among different subspecialties such as imaging, intensive care and anesthesia. The goals of hybrid therapies include reduction of morbidity and mortality in patients with more complex diseases, mitigation of the negative cumulative effects of multiple procedures, improvement in quality of life and delivery of a more cost-efficient care. Also the hybrid environment encourages the sharing of expertise, ideas, equipment and techniques, which is crucial to introduce novel therapies for challenging patients. These procedures have significantly expanded the therapeutic options for several patients with complex congenital heart disease in the last 10 years. In this chapter the authors will discuss the application of the hybrid approach in the management of hypoplastic left heart syndrome, muscular ventricular septal defects and pulmonary artery stenosis.

Chapter 12 – The surgical management of transposition of the great arteries with ventricular septal defect and left ventricle outflow tract obstruction is a true challenge in congenital heart surgery. Different surgical techniques such as the Rastelli procedure, "Reparation a` l'Etage ventriculaire", the Metras modification, Nikaidoh operation and its modifications were defined.

Although the Rastelli operation has been the most widely performed surgical procedure over the past decades, several studies have shown suboptimal long-term prognosis after its practice. A newer operation described by Bex and Nikaidoh has been performed with promising outcomes. The anatomical characteristics usually enable biventricular repair, though in some hearts univentricular palliation may be the only surgical option.

Chapter 13 – Major advances and refinement in the diagnosis and surgical treatment of congenital heart defect in the last four decades has resulted in an increasing number of adult survivors.

The incidence of congenital heart diseases is around 1%. Nearly 6000 children are born with one congenital heart defect in Argentina per year. Two thirds of them require surgical treatment mostly within the first year of life. Fortunately, surgical mortality has been reduced to low single figures in the last 20 years and 90% of the operated patients are expected to reach adulthood. It is noteworthy that congenital heart surgery is "reparative" and not curative. Except for the ligated patent ductus arteriosus in the first months of life, all congenital heart lesions whether operated on or not will require lifelong control. Even the

Atrial Septal Defect (ASD) operated upon in the first years of life may be exposed to the development of atrial fibrillation or sick sinus disease in the fourth decade.

Chapter 14 – Children with congenital heart disease require adequate clinical support. Intensive care units (neonatal and cardiovascular) and pediatric emergency departments have a vital role in the care of these patients. This chapter presents the key aspects for proper management of these children: early diagnosis, timely treatment, clinical support and prevention and treatment of complications.

In: Congenital Heart Diseases
Editor: Raúl Cayré and José Milei
ISBN: 978-1-61122-003-2

Chapter 1

Observations on the Development of the Coronary Arteries in the Human Embryo

Julio D. Civetta[1], Lilliam M. Valdes-Cruz[2] and Raúl O. Cayré[3,4]*

[1]Former Professor of Anatomy, School of Medicine, National University of Northeast, Corrientes, Argentina

[2]Director of Noninvasive Pediatric and Congenital Cardiac Imaging, Cardiac Care Center, Joe DiMaggio Children's Hospital Hollywood, Florida, US

[3]Head of Teaching and Research Department, Cordis Heart Institute, Resistencia, Chaco, Argentina

[4]Consultant of Cardiac Research Institute, Prof. Dr. Alberto C. Taquini, UBA-CONICET (ININCA). National University of Buenos Aires and National Council of Research, Science and Technology

Abstract

The embryological development of the coronary arteries in humans is still controversial. It is unclear whether there is a dual process of angiogenesis and vasculogenesis or a single process of vasculogenesis. Objective: This chapter examines the development of the coronary arteries in human embryos within the context of recent experimental findings. Methods: Of 131 human embryos and fetuses, 22 between stages XIII (27±2 days) and XVIII (48±1 day) were studied. Results: Islands of angioblastic cells appeared in stage XIII. By stage XV two distinct subepicardial vascular networks were seen which connected to the aorta by stages XVII-XVIII. Endothelial indentations were seen in stages XV and XVI only in the region of the aorta just above the developing aortic sigmoid valves; no direct connections could be confirmed to the subepicardial vascular network therefore we cannot conclude that these are involved in the formation of the proximal coronary trunks as has been previously proposed. Compaction of the ventricular myocardium began in stage XV at the base of the heart and extended towards

* E-mail: raul.cayre@gmail.com.

the apex. Conclusion: The coronary arteries in the human embryo seem to develop through vasculogenesis with the appearance of islands of angioblastic cells which coalesced to form two subepicardial capillary networks; these were clearly distinct by stage XV. The connection of both vascular networks via coronary channels to the aorta was invariably present by stage XVIII.

Keywords: Coronary arteries, human coronary embryogenesis, coronary arterial development

Introduction

The embryological development of the coronary arteries in humans continues to be controversial. Descriptive studies in human embryos have considered it to be a dual process of angiogenesis, that is the sprouting of new vessels from the aorta, and of vasculogenesis, the organization of a vascular plexus from the *de novo* differentiation of angioblastic cells located in the epicardial region which later remodel into definitive vessels. [1-5] This dual morphologic mechanism has also been proposed in descriptive and experimental studies in various animal species such as rabbit [6, 7], pig [8], rat [9] and chick. [10, 11]

However, other descriptive studies in human and rat embryos [12, 13] and experimental studies performed on quail, chick and chicken-quail chimeras [14-25] questioned this dual origin of the coronary arteries. Instead, these authors postulated a single process of vasculogenesis through which pericardial vessels penetrate the wall of the aorta by ingrowth from the peritruncal ring thereby establishing a connection with its lumen.

In a recent review of the latest studies on the origin and development of the coronary arteries, Silva-Junior, et al. summarize the current understanding of the process as a series of temporally regulated events including vasculogenesis, angiogenesis, arteriogenesis and remodeling. [26]

In this chapter we reexamine data on the development of the coronary arteries in human embryos within the context of these recent experimental findings.

Material and Methods

The authors had access to a collection of 131 human embryos and fetuses all products of spontaneous abortions or ectopic pregnancies. Of these, 22 embryos were found to be between stage XIII (27±2 days) and stage XVIII (48±1 day) according to Streeter GL [27] y Pineau H [28], having a crown-rump (CR) length between 4.5-18 mm. These constitute the material selected.

The younger embryos were fixed in 10% formaldehyde and the older ones in Bouin solution. They were embedded in paraffin and serially sectioned in axial cuts (20 embryos) or in sagittal cuts (2 embryos). The thickness of the serial histologic sections ranged from 7um to 20um. Those in stages XIII-XVI were stained with hematoxylin and eosin and those in stages XVII-XVIII with either Mallory Heindenheim or hematoxylin and eosin. They were analyzed with biological photomicroscopes Olympus CX 40 and Nikon Eclipse E200 and photographed with an Olympus SC 35 Type 12 camera and with a Nikon Coolpix 5000 digital camera. Two wax reconstructions following the method of Born [29] were made from one embryo measuring 18mm CR length: one of the entire heart and another of the lumina of the coronary arteries connected to the lumen of the aorta.

Results

Table 1 summarizes the data on the 22 embryos examined. As previously reported by Hutchins, et al [30], some morphologic findings were found abruptly in one stage, while others appeared more gradually over two or even three stages in individual human embryos. For this reason we report our observations as the sequence of events observed in the various stages.

Table 1. Summary of embryos analyzed

N	Embryo	Stage	Length CR (in mm)	Age in days	Cut Planes	Histological Stain
1	MAM-1	XIII	4,5	27 ± 2	Axial	Hematoxylin-eosin
2	PAU-3	XIV	5	28 ± 2	Axial	Hematoxylin-eosin
3	FCH	XIV	6,5	30 ± 2	Axial	Hematoxylin-eosin
4	TEMAR-2	XV	8	35 ± 1	Sagittal	Hematoxylin-eosin
5	BAC-1	XV	8	35 ± 1	Axial	Hematoxylin-eosin
6	PET-5	XV	8,5	36 ± 1	Axial	Hematoxylin-eosin
7	TEMAR	XVI	9,5	37,8 ± 1	Axial	Hematoxylin-eosin
8	EGG-1	XVI	9,5	37,8 ± 1	Sagittal	Hematoxylin-eosin
9	GIR-1	XVI	10,5	39,4 ± 1	Axial	Hematoxylin-eosin
10	SECL	XVI	11	40 ± 1	Axial	Hematoxylin-eosin
11	CIV-2	XVI	11,5	40,7±1	Axial	Hematoyilin-eosin
12	GV-1	XVII-	12	41,3±1	Axial	Hematoyilin-eosin
13	GT	XVII	13	42,5±1	Axial	Mallory Heindenheim
14	MM-1	XVII	13	42,5±1	Axial	Hematoxylin-eosin
15	TE-10	XVII	13,5	43,1±1	Axial	Hematoxyilin-eosin
16	BLU-3	XVII+	14	43,7±2	Axial	Hematoxylin-eosin
17	JU-4	XVII+	14,8	45 ± 2	Axial	Hematoxylin-eosin
18	MON-1	XVIII	15	46 ± 2	Axial	Mallory-Heindenheim
19	MO-1	XVIII	16	46 ± 2	Axial	Hematoxylin-eosin
20	BLU-2	XVIII	17	47 ± 2	Axial	Mallory-Heindenheim
21	VE	XVIII	17	47 ± 2	Axial	Hematoxylin-eosin
22	GON-2	XVIII	18	48 ± 1	Axial	Mallory Heindenheim

CR=crown-rump.

Stage XIII

Islands composed of angioblastic cells (erythroblasts or nucleated erythrocytes) were observed in the parietal pericardium in front of the conus and of the anterior wall of the primordium of the trabeculated portion of the left ventricle (Figure 1 A, B). Angioblastic cells were also found in the subepicardial space of the ventricular wall at the level of the anterior interventricular sulcus and in the diaphragmatic wall of the ventricular pouch (Figure 1C, D). These islands had no connection to each other or to the ventricular cavity. The ventricular myocardium had a spongy appearance particularly in the trabeculated pouch of the left ventricle (Figure 1C, D).

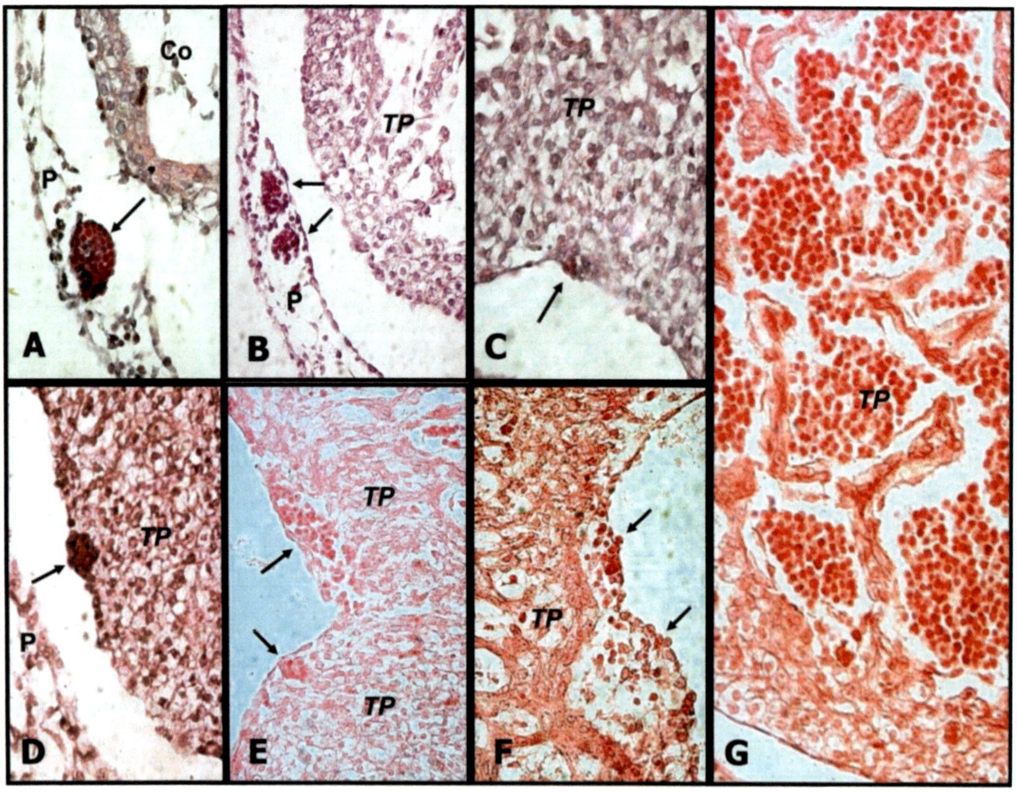

Figure 1. Microphotographs of axial cuts of a stage XIII 4.5 mm crown-rump (CR) length human embryo MAM-1 (Panels A–D) and of a stage XIV 5mm CR length human embryo PAU-3 (Panels E–G). A: Angioblastic cells (arrow) in the parietal pericardium in front of the conus. B: Angioblastic cells (arrows) in the parietal pericardium in front of the anterior wall of the primordium of the trabeculated portion the left ventricle. C: Angioblastic cells (arrow) in the anterior interventricular sulcus. D: Angioblastic cells (arrow) in the diaphragmatic wall of trabeculated pouch of the left ventricle. E: Blood islands (arrows) in the ventricular wall adjacent to the anterior interventricular sulcus. F: Primary capillary (arrows) in the ventricular wall at the level of the posterior interventricular sulcus. G: Spongy myocardium with numerous trabeculae and vascularization dependent on the ventricular cavity. (Hematoxylin-eosin stain). Co: conus; P: pericardium; TP: trabecular pouch.

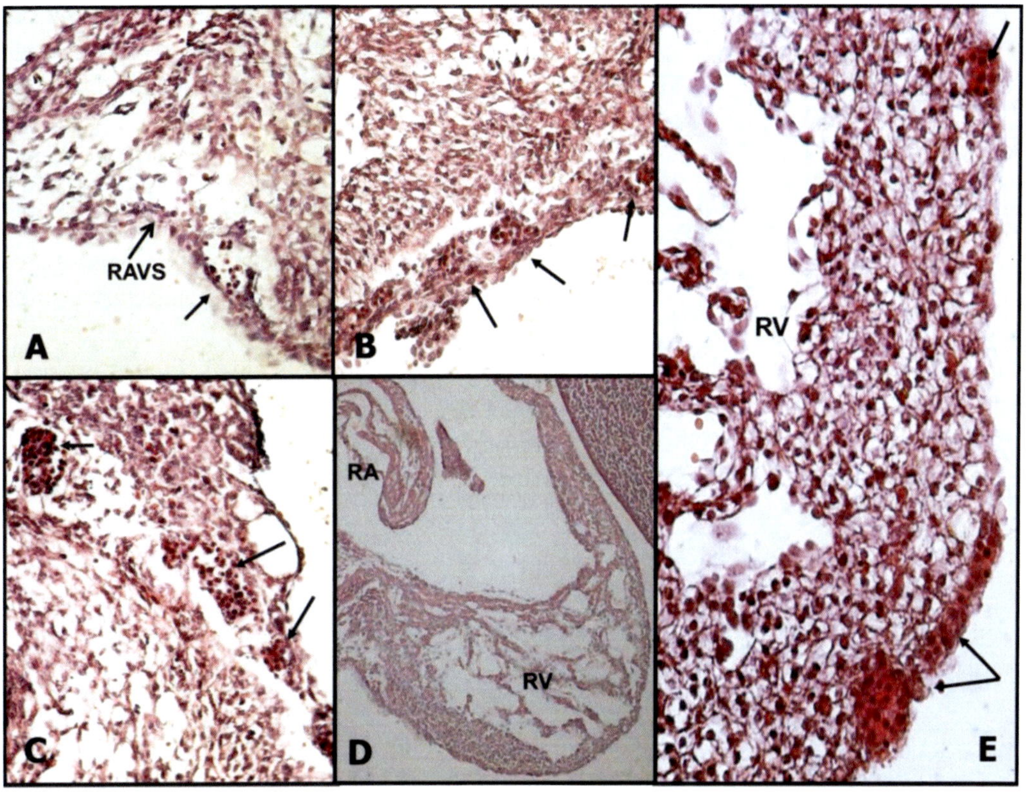

Figure 2. Microphotographs of sagittal cuts of stage XV 8mm CR length human embryo TEMAR-2. A: Subepicardial vascular network (arrow) along the right atrioventricular sulcus. B: Subepicardial vascular network (arrows) on the diaphragmatic wall of the ventricles. C: Subepicardial vascular network (arrows) on the anterior wall of the right ventricular outflow tract. D: Beginning of compaction of the ventricular myocardium along the base of the heart. E: Subepicardial vascular network (arrows) in the anterior wall of the right ventricle. (Hematoxylin-eosin stain). RA: right atrium; RAVS: right atrioventricular sulcus; RV: right ventricle.

Stage XIV

A larger number of blood islands were observed in the walls of both ventricles near the interventricular sulcus (Figure 1E, F). Some islands coalesced having the appearance of primary capillaries with nucleated erythrocytes forming a rudimentary subepicardial vascular network (Figure 1F). The ventricular myocardium had a more spongy appearance with numerous trabeculae and vascularization dependent on the ventricular cavity (Figure 1F, G).

Stage XV

More advanced development of the subepicardial vascular network was appreciated with two clearly distinct networks (Figures. 2, 3). The more developed one was located along the right atrioventricular sulcus (Figure 2A), the posterior interventricular sulcus, the diaphragmatic wall of both ventricles (Figure 2B) and the anterior wall and outflow tract of the right ventricle (Figure 2C, E). The less developed network was found in the anterior interventricular sulcus (Figure 3A), the adjacent areas of both ventricles (Figure 3B, C) and the left atrioventricular sulcus (Figure 3D). At this stage the vascular networks had not reached the peritruncal region.

In one embryo (TEMAR 2, stage XV), a blood island of nucleated erythrocytes was seen in the region of the sinus venosus adjacent to the right atrioventricular sulcus (Figure 3E).

In this stage we noted the start of the process of compaction of the ventricular myocardium at the base of the heart. The ventricular apex had a spongy, non compacted myocardium with trabeculae (Figure 2D). In some areas the lumen of the ventricular cavity almost reached the pericardium.

In this same stage we observed small indentations of the aortic endothelium in several areas of the aortic root, in the region of the developing aortic sigmoid valves. These indentations did not extend beyond the endothelial layer (Figure 3F).

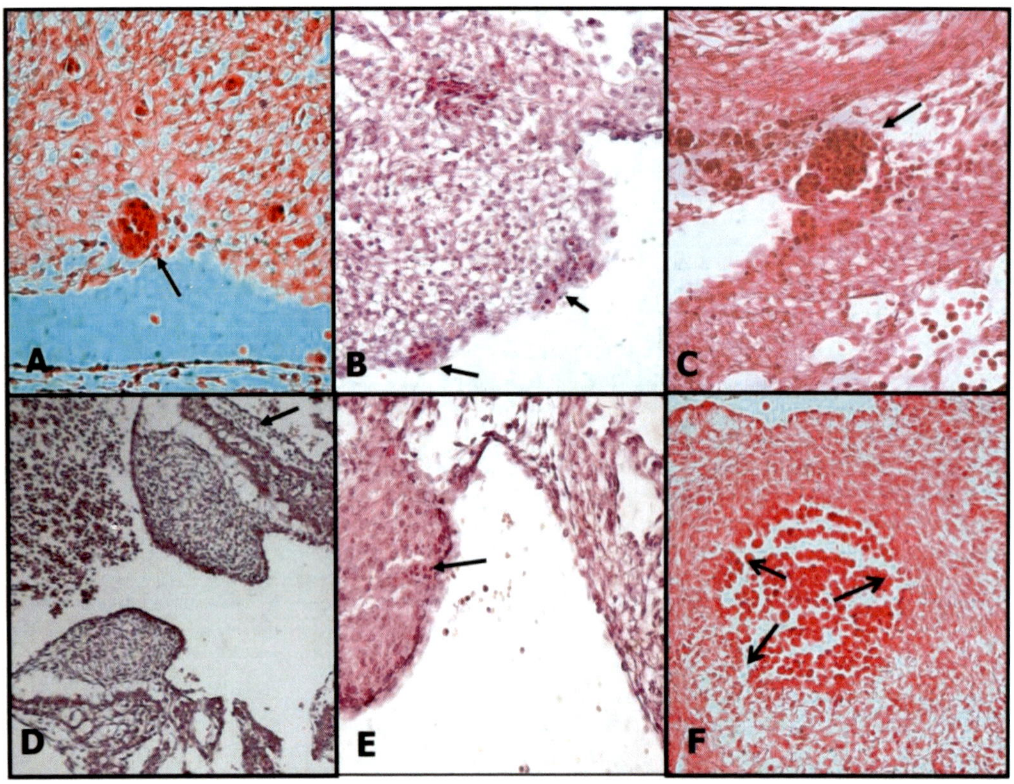

Figure 3. Microphotographs of histologic cuts of two stage XV human embryos: TEMAR-2 (Panels B, D, E) 8mm CR length sagittal cut and PET-5 (Panels A, C, F) 8.5mm CR length axial cut. A: Subepicardial vascular network (arrow) at the level of the anterior interventricular sulcus. B, C: Subepicardial vascular network (arrows) on the ventricular walls adjacent to the interventricular sulcus. D: Subepicardial vascular network (arrow) at the level of the left atrioventricular sulcus. E: Angioblastic cells (arrows) in the wall of the sinus venosus adjacent to the right atrioventricular sulcus F: Indentations of the aortic endothelium (arrows) adjacent to the developing aortic sigmoid valves. (Hematoxylin-eosin stain).

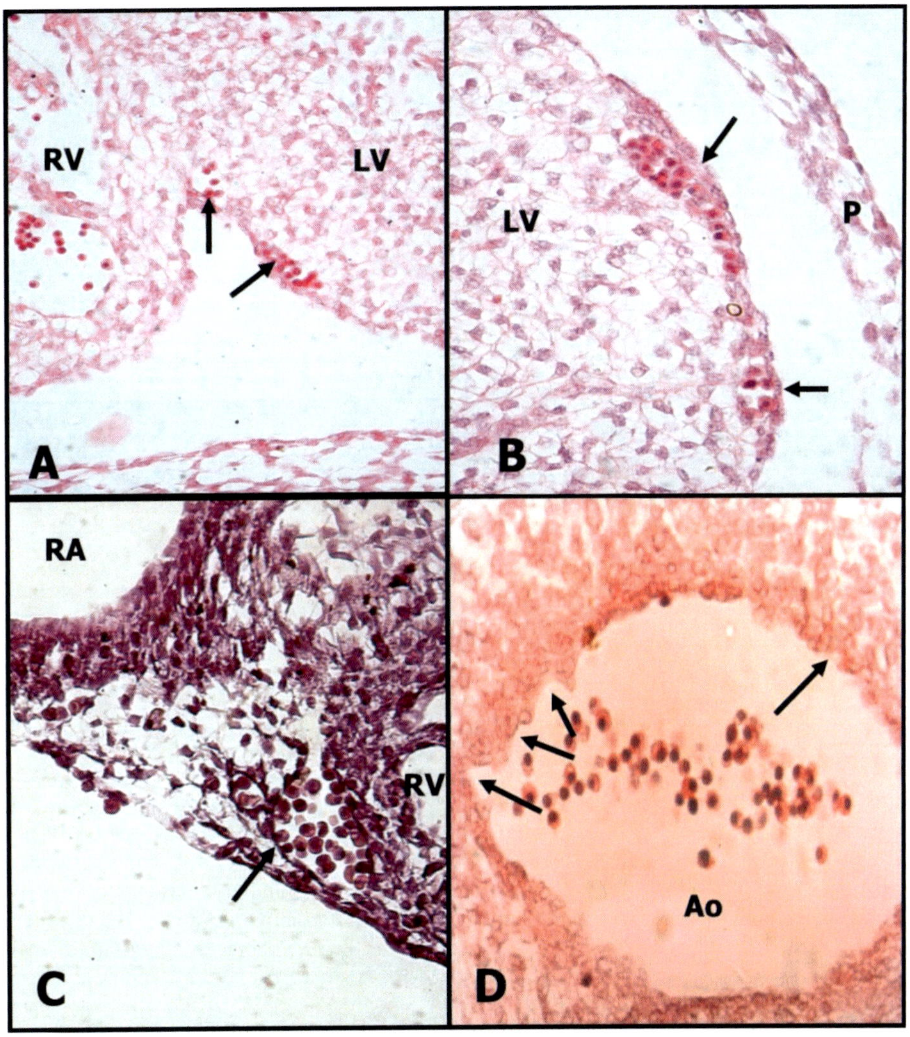

Figure 4. Microphotographs of histologic cuts of two stage XVI 9.5mm CR length human embryos: TEMAR (Panels A, B, D) axial cut and EGG-1 (Panel C) sagittal cut. A: Subepicardial vascular network (arrows) at the level of the anterior interventricular sulcus B: Subepicardial vascular network (arrows) along the lateral wall of the left ventricle. C: Subepicardial vascular network (arrow) at the level of the right atrioventricular sulcus. D: Indentations of the aortic endothelium (arrows) adjacent to the developing aortic sigmoid valves. (Hematoxylin-eosin stain). Ao: aorta; LV: left ventricle; P: pericardium RA: right atrium; RV: right ventricle.

Stage XVI

There was a more developed subepicardial vascular network (Figure 4A-C). The indentations of the aortic wall already seen in stage XV were again observed in this stage; these were not connected to the subepicardial vascular networks (Figure 4D). We also noted the presence of intercalated truncal swellings, the beginning of the formation of the aortic sigmoid valves.

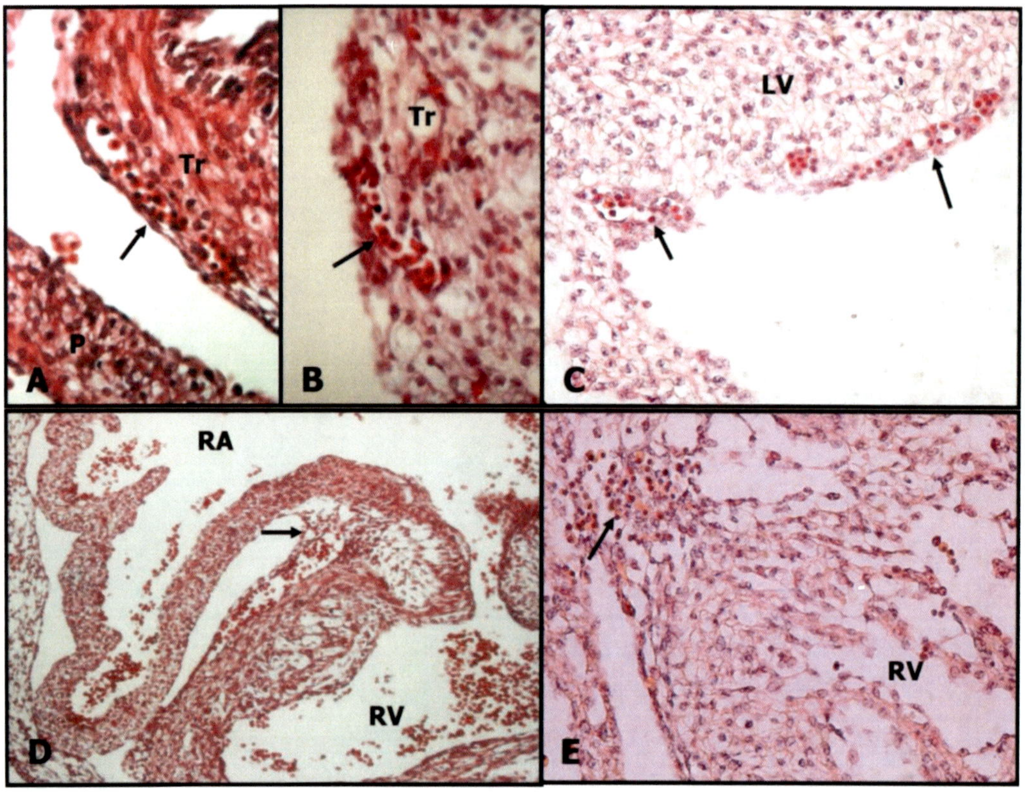

Figure 5. Microphotographs of axial cuts of two stage XVII human embryos: GV-1 (Panel A, B, D) 12mm CR length and TE-10 (Panels C, E) 13.5mm CR length. A: Subepicardial vascular network (arrow) at the level of the right lateral wall of the truncus. B: Subepicardial vascular network (arrow) at the level of the anterior wall of the truncus; C: Subepicardial vascular network (arrows) in the anterior wall of the left ventricle and the anterior interventricular sulcus. D, E: Subepicardial vascular network (arrows) along the right atrioventricular sulcus. (Hematoxylin-eosin stain). LV: left ventricle; RA: right atrium; RV: right ventricle; Tr: truncus.

Stage XVII

There was marked development of the subepicardial vascular networks (Figure 5) with appearance in the peritruncal region (Figure 5A, B).

The process of myocardial compaction was further developed and now was seen in the region of the cardiac apex (Figure 6A). In one embryo, TE-10, there were intramyocardial sinusoids which connected the subepicardial network with the ventricular cavity (Figure 6B, C).

In embryo JU-4, there was a left coronary channel connecting the subepicardial network to the aortic lumen, corresponding to the origin of the left coronary artery (Figure 7A-C). There was also a right coronary channel connecting the subepicardial network to the aortic lumen, corresponding to the origin of the right coronary artery (Figure 7D-F); this occupied a more cephalic position with respect to the left coronary channel.

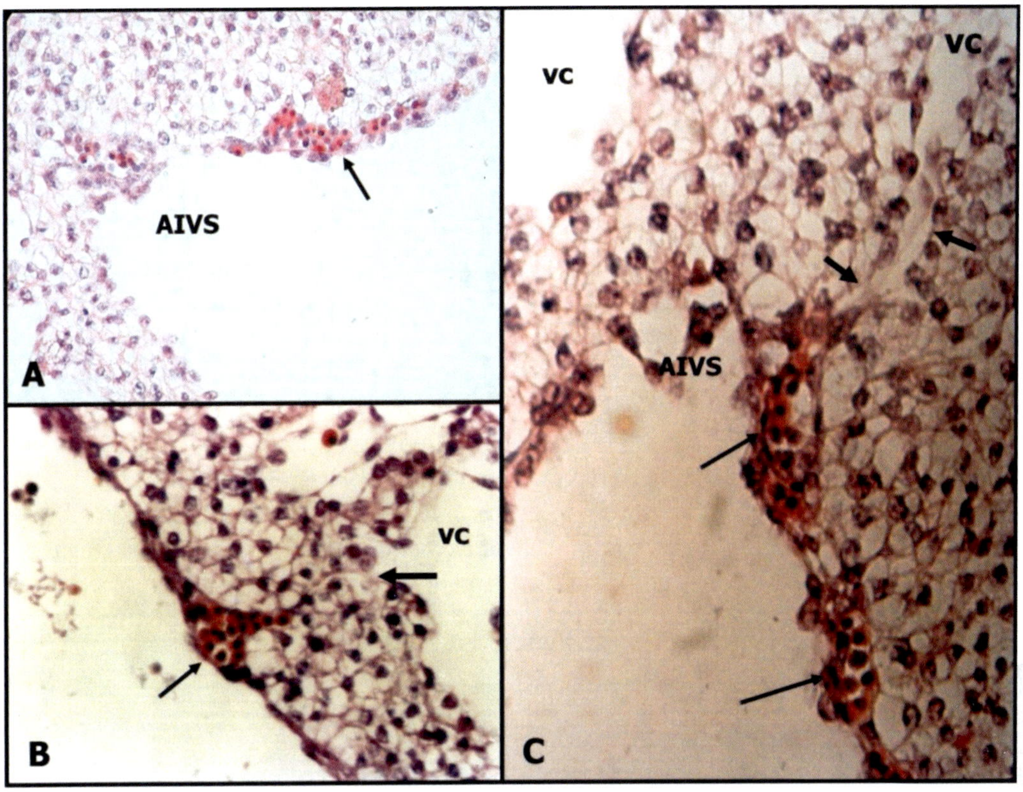

Figure 6. Microphotographs of axial cuts of stage XVII 13.5mm CR length human embryo TE-10. A: Left ventricular apex demonstrating the progress of myocardial compaction now present at this level. The arrow points to the subepicardial vascular network in the anterior wall of the left ventricular apex. B,C: Subepicardial vascular network penetrating the ventricular myocardium (thin arrows) and connecting with the ventricular cavity through an intramyocardial sinusoid (thick arrows). (Hematoxylin-eosin stain). AIVS: anterior interventricular sulcus; VC: ventricular cavity.

Stage XVIII

All embryos of this stage demonstrated the origins of the left and right coronary arteries and their respective connections to the corresponding subepicardial vascular network (Figure 8). The wax reconstruction of embryo GON-2 (Figure 8F) shows the origin of the right and left coronary arteries emerging from the aorta and the spatial position of the proximal segments with the right being in a more cephalic plane than the left.

Discussion

Our observations in 22 human embryos stages XIII-XVIII demonstrate that the first feature in the development of the coronary arteries is the appearance, through a process of vasculogenesis, of islands of angioblastic cells (erythroblasts) in the parietal pericardium in front of the conus, and of the anterior wall of the primordium of the trabeculated portion of the left ventricle, in the subepicardial space of the ventricular wall adjacent to the interventricular sulcus and near the cardiac apex (Figure 1A-D). To our knowledge, this is the first time these findings are described in a stage XIII human embryo. We documented the progression of the vasculogenetic process during stage XIV (Figure 1E, F) with the formation of subepicardial capillaries resulting from coalescence of the blood islands and the beginnings of a subepicardial capillary network. This has been previously reported in human embryos during stages XIV [3, 4, 30, 31], XV-XVI [12] and XVI-XIX [32]. A similar vasculogenetic process has been observed in chick embryos [10, 18-20] and in chicken-quail chimeras. [22]

By stage XV (Figures 2, 3), two clearly distinct subepicardial vascular networks were seen which have been previously reported as the origins of the right and left coronary arteries. [4] Distinct coronary channels were seen only in the regions corresponding to the right and left coronary arteries (Figure 7). The connection of the subepicardial vascular network to the aortic lumen was seen in one stage XVII embryo but was invariably present in all stage XVIII specimens (Figure 8). None of our stage XVII or XVIII embryos had an earlier origin of the left anterior coronary artery as has been reported by other authors. [3, 12, 13]

During stages XV and XVI we observed indentations of the aortic endothelium in several areas around the aortic root, in the region of the developing aortic sigmoid valves (Figures. 3F, 4D).

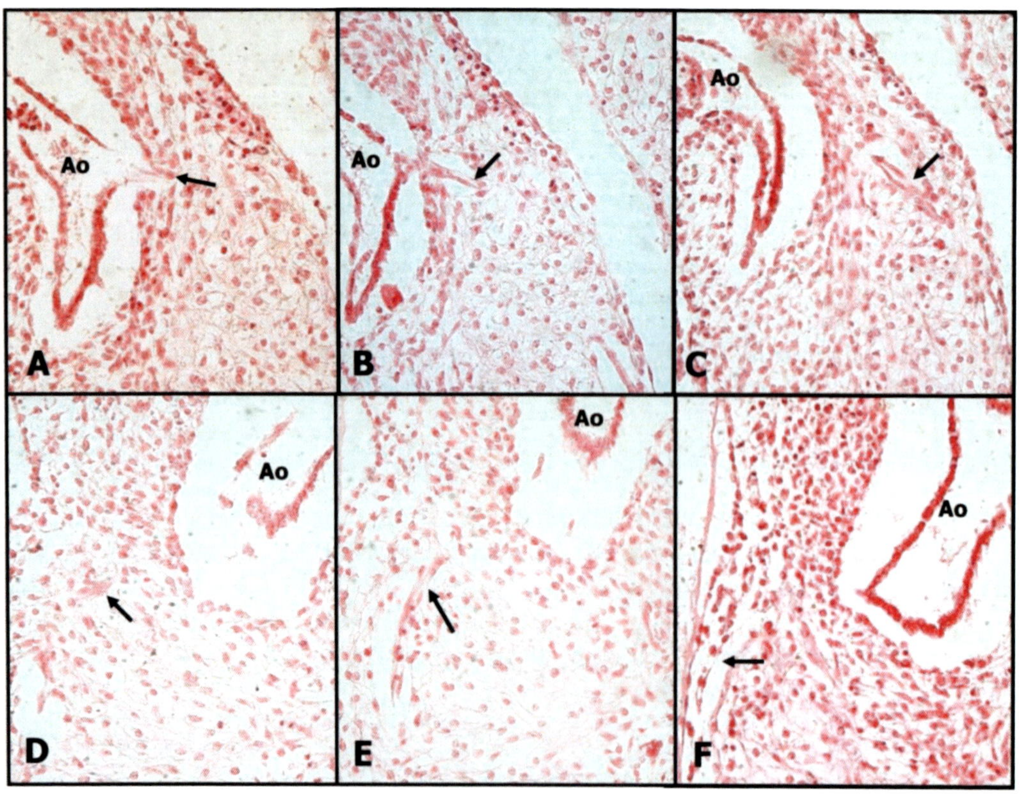

Figure 7. Microphotographs of axial cuts of stage XVII 14.8mm CR length human embryo JU-4. A, B: Left coronary channel (arrows). C: Subepicardial vascular network origin of the left coronary artery (arrow). D: Right coronary channel (arrow). E, F: Subepicardial vascular network origin of the right coronary artery (arrows). (Hematoxylin-eosin stain). Ao: aorta.

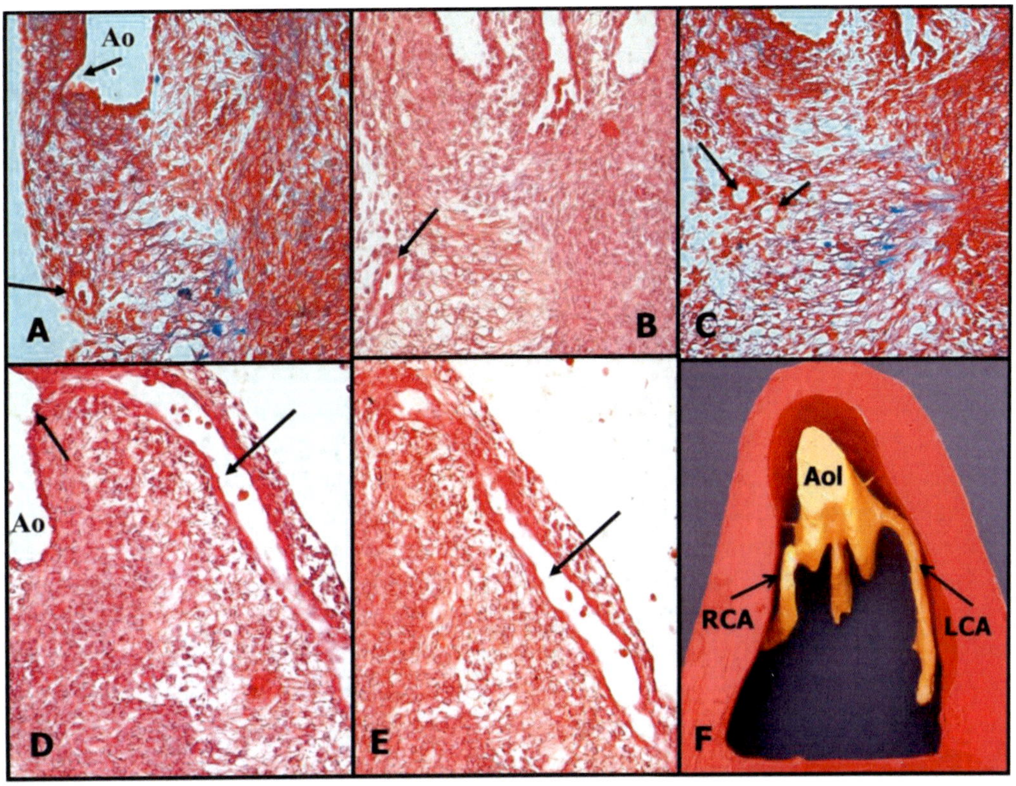

Figure 8. Microphotographs of axial cuts of stage XVIII 18mm CR length human embryo GON-2. Photograph of three-dimensional wax reconstruction of the same embryo. A: Ostium of the right coronary artery and distal section of same (arrows). B: Tangential section of the right coronary artery (arrow). C: Transverse section of the right coronary artery and one of its branches (arrows). D: Ostium of the left coronary artery and longitudinal section of same (arrows). E: Longitudinal section of the left coronary artery (arrow). F: Three-dimensional wax reconstruction of the area corresponding to the aortic sigmoid valves and proximal portions of the right and left coronary arteries (arrows). (Trichromic Mallory Heindenheim stain). Ao: aorta; Aol: aortic lumen; LCA: left coronary artery; RCA: right coronary artery.

These indentations were restricted to the endothelial layer of the aorta and we could never demonstrate direct connections to the subepicardial vascular network. Several authors have described indentations in the aortic endothelium just above the developing sigmoid valves in human embryos [1, 3-5, 32, 33], in embryos of rabbit [6, 7], rat [9], chick [10, 11] and pig [8] and have called them *aortic endothelial sprouts or coronary buds.* It has been speculated that these endothelial indentations represented the primitive coronary arterial system which later connected with the vascular network thereby concluding a dual process of angiogenesis and vasculogenesis. However, upon careful analysis of these publications we failed to find definitive evidence that the indentations shown either reached the media of the aortic wall or connected directly to the vascular network. In their study of human embryos, Hutchins, et al [30] mentioned the presence of small indentations of the endothelium into the arterial walls. They interpreted these as secondary changes possibly due to contraction of the vessels during histological preparation and specifically stated no clear evidence of endothelial sprouts or incipient coronary artery in any embryo. Nonetheless, they speculated that the coronary arteries do arise presumably from these attempts at endothelial outgrowths which are successful only at the points where the wall tension of the aorta is elevated. Conte and Pellegrini [4] also mention the presence of multiple coronary buds in the aortic wall as well as in the wall of the pulmonary artery. No embryo in our series had endothelial indentations in the pulmonary arterial wall. Since we did not find direct connections of the endothelial indentations to the subepicardial vascular network, we cannot conclude that they are involved in the formation of the proximal coronary trunks.

Our observation in a stage XVII embryo of coronary channels connecting the subepicardial networks with the aortic lumen, (Figure 7) would be consistent with a process of vasculogenesis starting from the subepicardial vascular network. Recent experimental embryology studies in different animal species have also denied the existence of coronary buds and negated a process of primary angiogenesis from the aorta. [12-15, 18] These authors concluded that, as a result of a process of vasculogenesis, the subepicardial vascular networks penetrate the wall of the aorta through coronary channels thereby establishing their connection to the aortic lumen, and not vice versa. Experimental studies conducted in chick, quail and chicken-quail chimeras have shown that the endothelial and smooth muscle cells of the coronary arteries have a different cell lineage from the endothelial and smooth muscle cells of the aortic walls. [16, 19-23, 25] These results would lend convincing evidence in favor of a single process of vasculogenesis. [34-36]

Recent experiments using retroviral tracers in chicken-quail chimeras have shown that the endothelial and smooth muscle cells of the coronary arteries originate from the epicardium. [19, 23] Experimental studies using monoclonal antibodies in quail embryos [16], retroviral cell tagging techniques in chick embryos [19, 21] and antiendothelial antibodies in chicken-quail chimeras [22] have suggested that the cells that will give rise to the epicardium originate from epithelium associated with the septum transversum. Later it becomes a structure composed by transient extracardiac mesothelial cell population which comes to lie between the liver and the sinus venosus and has been called the proepicardial organ (PEO). From there, cells migrate to the sinus venosus and later to the atrioventricular sulcus and the ventricular wall adjacent to the interventricular sulcus. To the best of our knowledge, the existence of a PEO has not been demonstrated in the human embryo. In fact, the early location of the precursors of the epicardium, myocardium and endocardium in the human embryo is still under debate. [37, 38] In this context, it is interesting to note that we observed in one embryo (TEMAR-2, stage XV) angioblastic cells in the region of the sinus venosus, adjacent to the right atrioventricular sulcus (Figure 3E) as well as angioblastic cells along the atrioventricular sulcus, the diaphragmatic wall of both ventricles and at either side of the interventricular sulcus (Figure 3B, D).

Recently, Ando, et al. [39], using double immunostaining and confocal microscopy in quail embryos concluded that the initial formation of the proximal coronary arteries consists of endothelial strands which penetrate the aortic wall at several sites. Only those at the facing sinuses fuse to form the proximal right and left coronary arteries and develop a medial layer thereby demarcating the definitive coronary arteries from the aortic media. They suggested that these strands are derived from mesenchymal cells, probably endothelial progenitors originating from the so-called proepicardial organ (PEO), as was already mentioned by other authors. [16, 21, 25]

More recently, Red-Horse et al. [40], using histological and clonal analysis in mice and cardiac organ culture, propose that coronary vessels have two sources of progenitors. The major source are differentiated venous endothelial cell originated from angiogenic sprouts of the sinus venosus, which proliferate and spread to form the coronary plexus, and subsequently redifferentiate and remodel into coronary arteries, capillaries and veins. The minor secondary source is the endocardium, from which cells separate to form blood islands and then join the coronary plexus near the interventricular septum.

Wu and colleagues [41] propose a major ventricular endocardial origin for coronary arteries. Using a NFATc1-Cre mouse line the authors trace ventricular endocardial cells to the forming vascular outline of the arterial portion of the coronary system with a few marked cells found in coronary veins. However, the authors do not exclude contributions from other sources, or distinct origins in other species such as chick.

Pires-Gomez and Perez-Pomares [42], point to a diverse origin of the coronary endothelium, where the arterial and venous systems have distinct origins at different morphological sites and in different stages of embryonic development. This will require further effort to clarify the origins and the pathways involved in the assembly of this tissue.

We noted that the process of compaction of the ventricular myocardium begins during stage XV at the base of the heart and extends towards the apex (Figure 2D). This is in agreement with the findings of Agmon, et al. [43] Rychter, et al. state that the appearance of the coronary arteries coincides with the start of the compaction of the myocardium. [44] However, in our study angioblastic cells, the primordia of the coronary arteries, were detected during stages XIII and XIV, *before* any ventricular compaction was appreciated.

In our series, the connection between the subepicardial vascular network and the left ventricular cavity through sinusoids was seen in one embryo stage XVII (Figure 6B, C). This connection has been described in human embryos of stage XV [4, 32, 45] as well as in chick embryos [10, 18] and chicken-quail chimeras. [22] Hutchins, et al. [30] found only indirect evidence of communication between epicardial vessels and the ventricular cavity. We postulate that the reason coronary-cameral communications are not always seen is due to the rapid regression of the intertrabecular spaces as the process of myocardial compaction progresses.

Conclusion

In the context of recent experimental findings, our observations offers the following insights into human coronary morphogenesis: 1) the coronary arteries in humans *seem to develop through an embryonic process of vasculogenesis with* the appearance of islands of angioblastic cells seen as early as stage XIII. The organization of a vascular plexus progressed with the coalescence of the blood islands to form a subepicardial capillary network. By stage XV there were two clearly distinct subepicardial vascular networks. The connection of both vascular networks via coronary channels to the aorta may be seen in stage XVII but was invariably present by stage XVIII. 2) Endothelial indentations, documented in stages XV and XVI, were seen only in the region of the aorta just above the site of the developing aortic sigmoid valves. No direct connections were confirmed to the subepicardial vascular network, therefore we cannot conclude that they are involved in the formation of the proximal coronary trunks as has been previously proposed. 3) Angioblastic cells were seen in the region of the sinus venosus in one embryo suggesting the possibility that these may originate from the *proepicardial organ.* 4) The process of compaction of the ventricular myocardium began during stage XV at the base of the heart and extended towards the apex. 5) Connection between the subepicardial vascular network and the left ventricular cavity through sinusoids was seen in one embryo stage XVII.

References

[1] Hackensellner HA. Akzessorische Kranzgefäßanlagen der Arteria pulmonalis unter 63 menschlichen Embryonen-serien mit einer größten Länge von 12 bis 36mm. *Z. Mikrosk. Anat. Forsch.* 1956; 62: 153-64.

[2] Licata RH. Coronary circulation: embryology. In: Abramson D, ed. Blood vessels and lymphatics. New York: Academic Press Inc, 1962: 258-61.

[3] Hirakow R. Development of the cardiac blood vessels in staged human embryos. *Acta Anat.* 1983; 115**:** 200-30.

[4] Conte G, Pellegrini A. On the development of the coronary arteries in human embryos, stages 14 -19. *Anat. Embryol.* 1984; 169: 209-18.

[5] O'Rahilly R, Muller F. The cardiovascular and lymphatic systems. In: O'Rahilly R, Muller F, eds. Human embryology & teratology. 2nd Edition. New York: Wiley-Liss, 1996: 159-206.

[6] Lewis FT. The question of the sinusoids. *Anat. Anz.* 1904; 25: 261-79.

[7] Grant RT. Development of the cardiac coronary vessels in the rabbit. *Heart* 1926; 13: 261-77.

[8] Bennett HS. The development of the blood supply to the heart in the embryo pig. *Am. J. Anat.* 1937; 60: 27-53.

[9] Dbaly J, Ostádal B, Rychter Z. Development of the coronary arteries in rat embryos. *Acta Anat.* 1968; 71: 209-22.

[10] Rychter Z, Ostádal B. Mechanism of the development of coronary arteries in chick embryo. *Folia Morphol. Prague* 1971; 19: 113-24.

[11] Aikawa E, Kawano J. Formation of coronary arteries sprouting from the primitive aortic sinus wall of the chick embryo. *Experientia* 1982; 38: 816-18.

[12] Bogers AJJC, Gittenberger-de Groot AC, Dubbeldam JA, Huysmans HA. The inadequacy of existing theories on development of the proximal coronary arteries and their connexions with the arterial trunks. *Int. J. Cardiol.* 1988; 20: 117-23.

[13] Bogers AJJC, Gittenberger-de Groot AC, Dubbeldam JA, Huysmans HA. Scanning electron microscopy substantiates histology in showing the inadequacy of the existing theories on the development of the proximal coronary arteries and their connexions with the arterial trunks. *Acta Morphol. Neerl. Scand.* 1988/89; 26**:** 225-37.

[14] Bogers AJJC, Gittenberger-de Groot AC, Poelmann RE, Peault BM, Huysmans HA. Development of the origin of the coronary arteries, a matter of ingrowth or outgrowth? *Anat. Embryol.* 1989; 180: 437-41.

[15] Gittenberger-de Groot AC, Bogers AJJC, Poelmann RE, Peault BM, Huysmans HA. Development of the coronary arterial orifices. *Ann. NY Acad. Sci.* 1990; 588: 377-79.

[16] Virágh S, Gittenberger-de Groot AC, Poelmann RE, Kalman F. Early development of quail heart epicardium and associated vascular and glandular structures. *Anat. Embryol.* 1993; 188: 381-93.

[17] Vrancken Peeters M-PFM, Gittenberger-de Groot AC, Mentink MMT, Hungerford JE, Little CD, Poelmann RE. Differences in development of coronary arteries and veins. *Cardiovasc. Res.* 1997; 36: 101-10.

[18] Waldo KL, Willner W, Kirby ML. Origin of the proximal coronary artery stems and a review of ventricular vascularization in the chick embryo. *Am. J. Anat.* 1990; 188: 109-20.

[19] Mikawa T, Fishman DA. Retroviral analysis of cardiac morphogenesis: discontinuous formation of coronary vessels. *Proc. Natl. Acad. Sci. USA* 1992; 89: 9504-08.

[20] Hood LC, Rosenquist TH. Coronary artery development in the chick: origin and deployment of smooth muscle cells, and the effects of neural crest ablation. *Anat. Rec.* 1992; 234: 291-300.

[21] Mikawa T, Gourdie RG. Pericardial mesoderm generates a population of coronary smooth muscle cells migrating into the heart along with ingrowth of the epicardial organ. *Dev. Biol.* 1996; 174: 221-32.

[22] Poelmann RE, Gittenberger-de Groot AC, Mentink MMT, Bokenkamp R, Hogers B. Development of the cardiac coronary vascular endothelium, studied with antiendothelial antobodies, in chicken-quail chimeras. *Circ. Res.* 1993; 73: 559-68.

[23] Dettman RW, Denetclaw W Jr, Ordahl CP, Bristow J. Common epicardial origin of coronary vascular smooth muscle, perivascular fibroblasts, and intermyocardial fibroblasts in the avian heart. *Dev. Biol.* 1998; 193: 169-81.

[24] Mark-Paul FM, Vrancken Peeters M-PFM, Gittenberger-de Groot AC, Mentink MMT, Poelmann RE. Smooth muscle cells and fibroblasts of the coronary arteries derive from epithelial-mesenchymal transformation of the epicardium. *Anat. Embryol.* 1999: 199: 367-78.

[25] Muñoz-Chapuli R, González-Iriarte M, Carmona R, Atencia G, Macias D, Perez-Pomares JM. Cellular precursors of the coronary arteries. *Tex. Heart Inst. J.* 2002; 29: 243-49.

[26] Silva-Junior GO, Miranda SWS, Mandarim-de-Lacerda CA. Origin and development of the coronary arteries. *Int. J. Morphol.* 2009; 27: 891-98.

[27] Streeter GL. Developmental horizons in human embryos. Description of age groups XI, 13 to 20 somites and age group XII, 21 to 29 somites. *Carnegie Contrib. Embryol.* 1942, 30: 211-45.

[28] Pineau H. La croissance et ses lois. Paris. Laboratoire d'Anatomie de la Faculte de Medecine de Paris 1966.

[29] Born G. Beitrage zur Entwicklungsgeschichte des Saugerhier herzens. *Arch. F. Mikr. Anat.* 1889; 44: 284-378.

[30] Hutchins GM, Kessler-Hanna A, Moore GW. Development of the coronary arteries in the embryonic human heart. *Circulation* 1988; 77: 1250-57.

[31] Obrucnik M, Malínsky J, Lichnovsky V. The early stages of differentiation of the vascular bed in the ventricular wall of the human embryonic heart as seen in the electron microscope. *Folia Morphol.* 1972; 20: 49-51.

[32] Licata RH. A continuation study of the development of the blood supply of the human heart. Part II: The deep or intramural circulation. *Anat. Rec.* 1956; 124: 326.

[33] Licata RH. The human embryonic heart in the ninth week. *Am. J. Anat.* 1954; 94: 73-125.

[34] Tomanek RJ. Formation of the coronary vasculature: a brief review. *Cardiovasc. Res.* 1996; 31: E46-E51.

[35] Markwald R. Coronary morphogenesis. *Tex. Heart Inst. J.* 2002; 29: 242.

[36] Baldwin HS. Early embryonic vascular development. *Cardiovasc. Res.* 1996; 31: E34-E45.

[37] Reese DE, Mikawa T, Bader DM. Development of the coronary vessel system. *Circ. Res.* 2002; 91: 761-68.

[38] Jörg Männer. Does the subepicardial mesenchyme contribute myocardioblasts to the myocardium of the chick embryo heart?. A quail-chick chimera study tracing the fate of the epicardial primordium. *Anatomical. Rec.* 1999; 255: 212-226.

[39] Ando K, Nakajima Y, Yamagishi T, Yamamoto S, Nakamura H. Development of the proximal coronary arteries in quail embryonic hearts. *Circ. Res.* 2004; 94: 346-52.

[40] Red-Horse K, Ueno H, Weissman IL, Krasnow MA. Coronary arteries form by developmental reprogramming of venous cells. *Nature* 2010; 464: 549-53.

[41] Wu B, Zhang Z, Lui W, Chen X, Wang Y, Chamberlain AA, Moreno-Rodriguez RA et al. Endocardial cells form the coronary arteries by angiogenesis through myocardial-endocardial VEGF signaling. *Cell* 2012; 151: 1083-96.

[42] Pires-Gomez AAS, Perez-Pomares JM. The epicardium and coronary artery formation. Review. *J. Dev. Biol.* (online). 2013; I: 186-02. Available at www.mdpi.com/journal/jdb/ DOI: 10.3390/jdb1030186, accesed October 27, 2013.

[43] Agmon Y, Connolly HM, Olson LJ, Khandheria BK, Seward JB. Noncompaction of the ventricular myocardium. *J. Am. Soc. Echocardiogr.* 1999; 12: 859-63.

[44] Rychter Z, Rychterova V. Angio-and myoarchitecture of the heart wall under normal and experimentally changed morphogenesis. In: Pexieder T, ed. Mechanisms of cardiac morphogenesis and teratogenesis. Perspectives in cardiovascular research. New York: Raven Press, 1981:431-452.

[45] Licata RH. The developmental basis of the blood supply to the human heart. *Anat. Rec.* 1955; 121: 330-31.

In: Congenital Heart Diseases
Editor: Raúl Cayré and José Milei
ISBN: 978-1-61122-003-2

Chapter 2

TGF-β_1 and Estrogen Receptor Alpha in Coronary Intimal Hyperplasia in Pediatric Patients with Congenital Heart Disease

Rocío Castilla[1], Matilde Otero-Losada[1], Angélica Müller[1], Francisco Azzato[1], Giuseppe Ambrosio[2] and José Milei*[1]
[1]Instituto de Investigaciones Cardiológicas "Prof. Dr. Alberto C. Taquini", ININCA-UBA-CONICET, Buenos Aires, Argentina
[2]Division of Cardiology, University of Perugia School of Medicine, Perugia, Italy

Abstract

Congenital heart defects (CHD) and/ or their repair process lead to an increased risk for adult cardiovascular disease compared with the general population.

Intimal hyperplasia is a pre-atherosclerotic lesion that may be produced as a consequence of the activation of transforming growth factor beta-1 (TGF-β_1) pathway or ERα inhibition.

This chapter deals with our recent findings in this regard and comments our latest results in connection with relevant reports from other authors.

We examined the coronary arteries from a pediatric population with CHD and evaluated the possible relationship between the frequency of intimal hyperplasia and the magnitude of TGF-β_1 in order to enlighten the possible role of TGF-β_1 in the genesis of these lesions. The coronary arteries of 10 control patients and 98 CHD patients (54% cyanotic type, 32% surgically repaired) were stained and assessed for the presence and degree of intimal thickening. The expression of TGF-β_1 and ERα was determined by immunohistochemical examination.

* Correspondence to: José Milei MD, PhD. Instituto de Investigaciones Cardiológicas "Prof. Dr. Alberto C. Taquini" ININCA-UBA-CONICET. Marcelo T. de Alvear 2270. 1122AAJ. Buenos Aires, Argentina. ininca@fmed.uba.ar.

The frequency of coronary intimal hyperplasia did not depend on the group, i.e.: cyanotic CHD group (66%) and non-cyanotic CHD group (64%). However, the frequency of coronary intimal hyperplasia was higher in patients with surgically repaired CHD than in patients without surgical intervention (80% vs. 47% respectively, p=0.0002).

The degree of positive immunostaining for TGF-β_1 or ERα did not depend on the group. i.e.: cyanotic and non-cyanotic type. On the other hand, examination of the intimal layer showed that TGF-β_1 expression was higher and expression of ERα was smaller in patients with surgically repaired CHD compared with those without surgery.

The relationship between the frequency of intimal hyperplasia and the expression of TGF-β_1 and ERα in arteries from 98 pediatric patients with congenital heart defects indicated that: 1) intimal hyperplasia was a common finding in the coronary tree of these patients, 2) both TGF-β_1 and ERα seemed to play a major role in this phenomenon and 3) surgical correction of CHD was associated with further coronary vascular remodeling.

Introduction

Congenital heart disease (CHD) patients represent a risk group for premature atherosclerotic coronary artery disease [1]. Certain congenital heart defects, or the process of their repair, may lead to an increased risk for adult cardiovascular disease compared with the general population on the basis of two major mechanisms: abnormal coronary origin and obstructive lesions of the left ventricle and aorta [1,2]. Congenital anomalies of coronary origin have been reported to portend a high incidence of coronary atheromas, likely due to abnormal blood flow patterns [1]. On the other hand, patients with cyanotic CHD have been reported to present a low incidence of coronary atherosclerosis due to hypocholesterolemia, up regulation of nitric oxide, hyperbilirubinemia and low platelet count [3].

Years ago fatty streaks were described as the earliest manifestation of atherosclerosis [4]. However, the proliferation of intimal smooth muscle cells (SMCs), which causes intimal thickening prior to any visible lipid deposition, was proposed to be the initial lesion [5-8].

Coronary intimal hyperplasia/thickening consists primarily of proliferation of SMCs, which are α-actin positive, surrounded by a proteoglycan-rich matrix but rarely have macrophages [9-11].

The increasing trend to consider coronary intimal thickening as a possible preatherosclerotic lesion [9-11] is based on several findings. First, some papers show that atherosclerotic lesions arise almost exclusively from intimal thickenings in the coronary arteries of hypercholesterolemic swines [12]. Also, a correlation was established between the distribution of intimal hyperplasia in children and the localization of characteristic atherosclerotic lesions observed in adult humans (i.e. first segment of the left anterior descending coronary artery) [13,14]. Additionally the majority of erosions occur over areas of intimal thickening, with minimal or no presence of a lipid core [9]. We previously found that early coronary artery lesions may range from focal areas with mild myointimal thickening in prenatal life to early soft plaques in infants, with c-fos gene activation in the SMCs of the media of coronary arteries, which may also present as intermingled lesions with components of both categories, more frequently observed with increasing age [11-15].

Of note, in 1976 Becu et al. described varying degrees of coronary lumen occlusions consisting of prominent intimal proliferation of (SMCs), media muscle disarray and fragmentation and/or disappearance of the internal elastic lamina in patients aged 6 days to 9 years subjected to pulmonary valvotomy for 'isolated' pulmonary valve stenosis [16].

The transforming growth factor beta 1 (TGF-β_1) and the estrogen receptor alpha (ERα) might be involved in the intimal hyperplasia formation [17].

TGF-β_1 is a secreted multifunctional factor that modulates proliferation of many cell types, including vascular cells, and regulates their interaction with the extracellular matrix. Its signaling plays pivotal roles in SMC differentiation during vascular development and is involved in the development of many cardiovascular diseases [18,19].

Smooth muscle cells are capable of reversibly modulating their phenotype during postnatal development and can de-differentiate into proliferative matrix synthetic cells in response to vascular injury [17-20]. Transforming growth factor-β_1 regulates both SMC differentiation during embryonic development and postnatal phenotypic switching [21]. In this connection, it was observed that over-expression of TGF-β_1 in normal arteries resulted in substantial extracellular matrix production accompanied by intimal and medial hyperplasia [22].

On the other hand, estrogens play an important role in cardiovascular protection. Estrogens stimulate endothelial cell proliferation in the vasculature [23], while inhibiting vascular smooth muscle cell (VSMC) proliferation [24] and migration [25], i.e.: two key steps involved in intimal hyperplasia [10,15]. Estrogens induce a variety of effects through interaction with three estrogen receptors (ER): receptor-α (ERα), receptor-β (ERβ), and transmembrane G protein coupled estrogen receptor (gpER) [26]. Estrogen receptor alpha appears to be largely responsible for the protective effects of estrogens against atherosclerotic vascular disease [27-29] and mediates the inhibition of the vascular injury response by estrogen [30]. It is noteworthy that ER expression has been previously observed in the arterial wall of both men and women [31,32] suggesting a possible role for ER in vascular function aside from its typical function in fertility.

The possibility of reviewing the original microscopic slides belonging to Becu's pioneer paper [16] encouraged us to evaluate the frequency of coronary intimal hyperplasia in CHD in order to assess a connection with the observed accelerated atherosclerosis in patients presenting: 1) abnormal coronary origin 2) surgical repair 3) obstruction of the left ventricle and aorta, 4) cyanotic and non-cyanotic heart disease, and to get insight into the possible role of TGF-β_1 and ERα in the genesis of these lesions as well.

Presence of intimal thickening in arteries was studied in 350 coronary artery samples belonging to 98 patients (range 15 days-9 years, mean age 2.4 years) of the CHD group and 10 controls.

Intimal proliferation was defined as muscle-elastic thickening characterized by: a) proliferation of SMCs; b) scarce monocytes, and rare lymphocytes, embedded by amorphous deposits within the internal elastic membrane; c) endothelium above the lesion morphologically intact, with smooth surface and devoid of thrombi [11,15]. Differential diagnosis with intimal ridges responsible of vessel bifurcation was made with the aid of serial axial sections and longitudinal sections.

Sixty percent (61%) of the CHD cases and all control patients presented at least one coronary vessel with intimal hyperplasia. Hyperplasia was highest in the left main coronary artery (LMCA) followed by the right coronary artery (RCA), the left anterior descending coronary artery (LAD) and posterior descending coronary artery (PDCA), and the circumflex artery (CX).

Most patients presented complex cases with combined CHD. As an example, a 15 days old patient, 2.62 kg weight, 29 cm height, with a heart of 25 g, showing pericarditis, perimembranous ventricular septal defect, right aortic arch and polycystic kidney. In the histological study, the LMCA presented coronary intimal hyperplasia with two components: the first in contact with the arterial lumen resembling a soft plaque with scarce nuclei surrounded by loose connective tissue, and a second component in contact with the media layer characterized by smooth muscle cell proliferation and dense connective tissue (Figure 1).

Therefore, the combination of multiple structural anomalies in one same patient made it difficult to link the occurrence of intimal hyperplasia to one specific congenital heart disease.

In 81 out of 98 autopsies a correct assessment of the coronary origin was made, in the remaining 17 cases there was discrepancy among observers given the reduced size of the hearts. Nine out of 81 patients were found to have anomalous coronary origin. Among these patients with anomalous coronary artery origin eight presented at least one vessel with intimal hyperplasia.

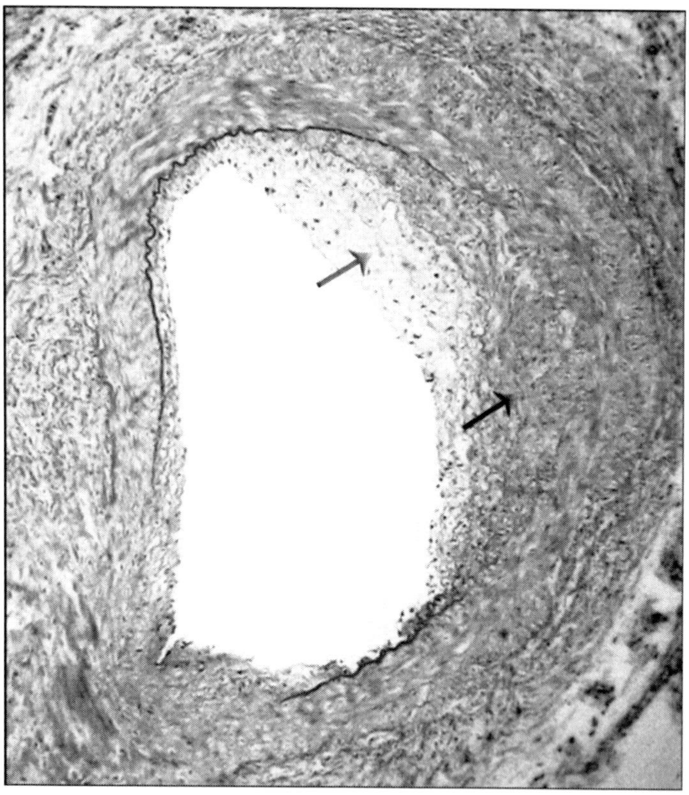

Figure 1. Soft plaque in a CHD patient. Left coronary trunk from a 15 days old female patient presenting an interventricular communication type I, pericarditis and polycystic kidney. A plaque with two components can be seen; the first is in contact with the lumen and resembles a soft, hypocelular plaque, with few nuclei belonging to mononuclear cells surrounding the loose connective tissue (gray arrow). The second, in contact with the media layer, is characterized by SMC proliferation and dense connective tissue (black arrow). It should also be noted the interruption and duplication of the limiting membrane, due to a severe media layer distortion and SMC proliferation. (H-E stain, X40). Reprinted from Ref. [42].

Intimal Hyperplasia in Patients with Cyanotic and Non-Cyanotic CHD

Fifty-four percent of the CHD cases were of the cyanotic type. Difference between presence of coronary intimal hyperplasia in patients with cyanotic CHD (66.1%) and non-cyanotic CHD (64.3%) did not achieve statistical significance (Fisher's exact test, p=0.735).

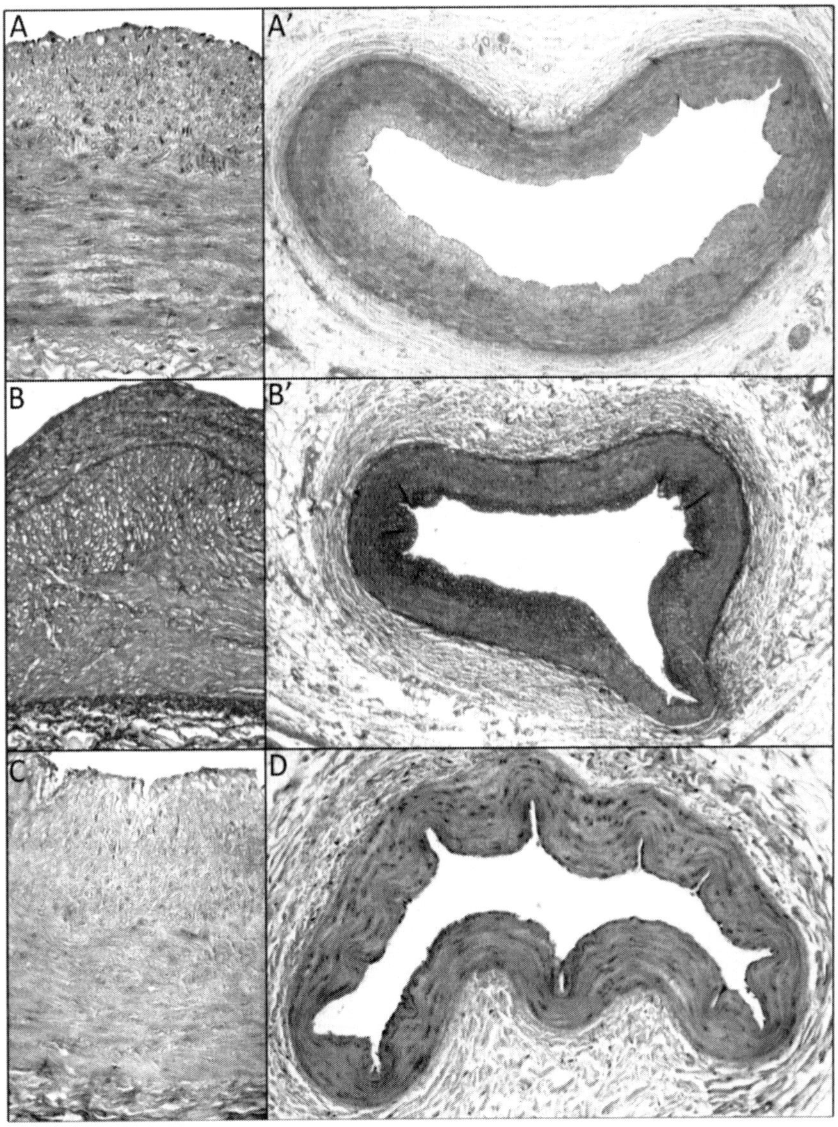

Figure 2. Diffuse intimal thickening in an artery of a CHD patient. Surgically corrected tetralogy of Fallot in a male patient that shows diffuse intimal hyperplasia in the right coronary artery (A), left anterior descending coronary artery (B), left main coronary artery (C), with a normal circumflex artery (D). (A and C: H-E stain, B: Victoria Blue stain, A to C: X25 and A' to C': X10. Reprinted from Ref. [42].

These findings would imply that cyanosis should have no role in influencing CHD propensity to develop atherosclerosis. Yet, the available information suggests that the incidence of atherosclerosis is low in cyanotic CHD [3]. However, it must be noticed that coronary angiography, as used by Fyfe et al. [3], is not well suited for visualizing non-raised lesions which do not significantly reduce visible vessel lumen, and therefore the actual frequency of coronary disease may be underestimated. Furthermore, these patients present hypocholesterolemia, up-regulation of nitric oxide, hyperbilirubinemia and low platelet count, all factors that may contribute to reduce the formation of atherosclerotic plaque.

Intimal Hyperplasia in CHD Patients with Surgical Intervention

Thirty-two percent of the cases of CHD with surgical repair were also analyzed. Eighty percent of these patients died within one month of surgery because of complex CHD, hemodynamic impairment and difficult surgeries (Figure 2).

Surgically repaired CHD presented a higher number of coronary intimal hyperplasia than the group without surgical intervention. Given that some patients may present only one affected vessel while others may have several, two criteria were used for comparison: 1) Percentage of coronary arteries with intimal hyperplasia and 2) Percentage of patients with at least one coronary artery with intimal hyperplasia.

Eighty percent of surgically repaired CHD patients presented at least one coronary artery with intimal hyperplasia in contrast with 47% observed in the non-surgical group (two-tailed Fisher's exact test, $p=0.0002$). In addition, 68% of coronary arteries of the surgically repaired group presented intimal hyperplasia in more than one artery compared with 25% in the CHD group without intervention (Fisher's test, $p<0.0001$). Age and sex were discarded as possible confounding variables.

In view that most patients died within a month of the surgical intervention because of the severity of the CHD it is difficult to determine whether the observed lesions were permanent or transient.

Intimal Hyperplasia in CHD Patients with Obstruction of Left Ventricle or Aorta

The group included aortic coarctation (31%), subaortic stenosis (8%) and aortic valvular stenosis (61%) with left ventricular hypertrophy. All the patients presented coronary intimal hyperplasia compromising at least one vessel. The rest of the congenital cardiopathies presented this condition in 61% of the cases. The difference between both groups was significant (two-tailed Fisher's test, $p=0.0039$). Special mention deserves the case of a 10 years' old male patient presenting subaortic stenosis, left ventricular hypertrophy and moderate mitral insufficiency. The coronary tree showed intimal hyperplasia in each main vessel, with the exception of the CX. The LMCA presented a diffuse and incomplete intimal thickening that occluded 55.4% of the arterial lumen (Figure 3).

The fact that all patients with congenital subaortic stenosis, coarctation of the aorta and left ventricular hypertrophy, presented coronary intimal hyperplasia may lend support to epidemiologic studies revealing that this group has a higher risk for developing coronary atherosclerosis [1]. Coarctation of the aorta is linked to systemic hypertension [33] and left ventricular hypertrophy is an independent risk factor for cardiovascular disease morbility and mortality in adults [2,34]. The association between intimal hyperplasia in these patients, and the high risk of accelerated atherosclerosis described in epidemiological studies [1] are consistent with the hypothesis that intimal hyperplasia can be observed as the first atherogenic event [10,11,35].

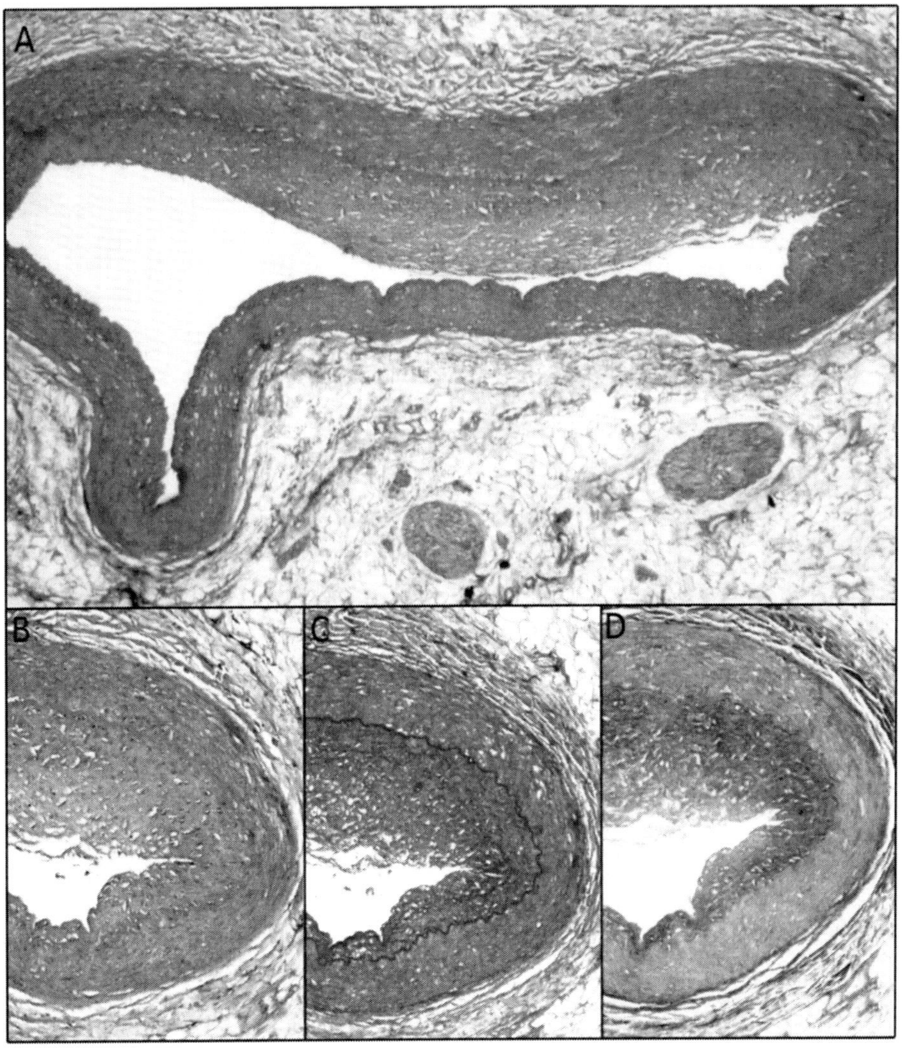

Figure 3. Focal intimal thickening in an artery of a CHD patient. LAD of a 10 year old patient with Ebstein's Anomaly and a surgically corrected ventricular septal defect. Focal intimal hyperplasia can be observed on this vessel. The elastic internal membrane remains intact (Type I). The thickened intima occludes 55.4% of the arterial lumen. Images B, C, and D represent the right quadrant from image A: A-HE X3.5. B: H-E X10. C: Victoria Blue stain X10. D: Masson trichrome X10. Reprinted from Ref. [42].

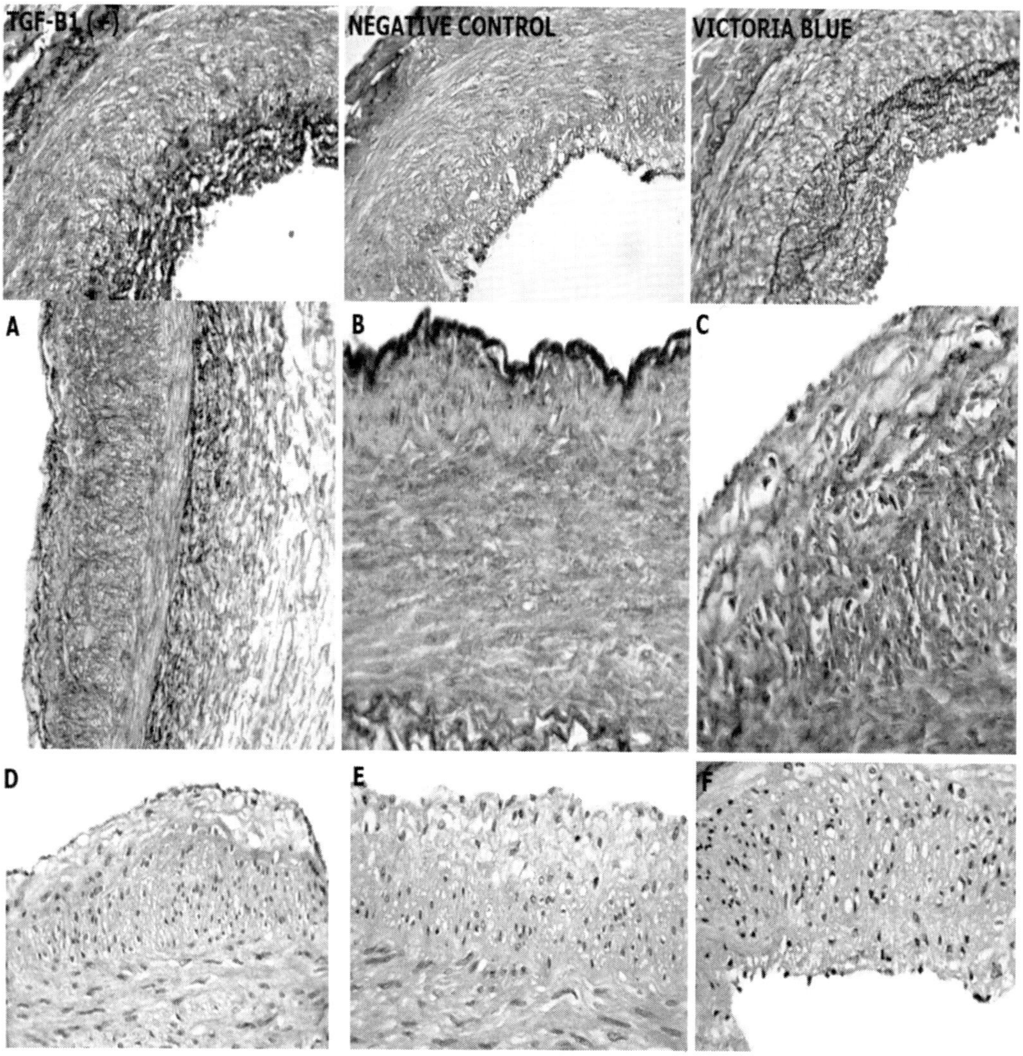

Figure 4. Immunohistochemical staining for TGF-β_1. Different patterns are shown. On the top row we show immunostaining for TGF-β_1, its negative control stained with H-E to corroborate the absence of nonspecific stain and Victoria Blue stain for elastic fibers (x40) performed on the proximal segment of the right coronary artery of a patient with transposition of the great vessels. In the middle row, different patterns of TGF-β_1 can be observed. A: Left coronary trunk from a 4 days old male patient, 48 cm high, 3185 g weight. The autopsy revealed a 30 g heart with a truncus arteriosus and interatrial communication. X10. B: Right coronary artery from a 2 month female patient, 50 cm high, 2200 g weight, who presented coarctation of the aorta and biventricular hypertrophy. X25. C: Left coronary trunk from a patient with truncus arteriosus. In bottom, proximal segment from the right coronary artery is shown. In the bottom row the absence of TGF-β_1 expression can be observed in the population with no CHD, D- Right coronary artery from a 5 year old male patient who died from intracranial hypertension. E- Right coronary artery from a 9 year old male patient who died from meningitis. F- Right coronary artery from a 7 year old male patient who died from acute hydrocephalus. Reprinted from Ref. [42].

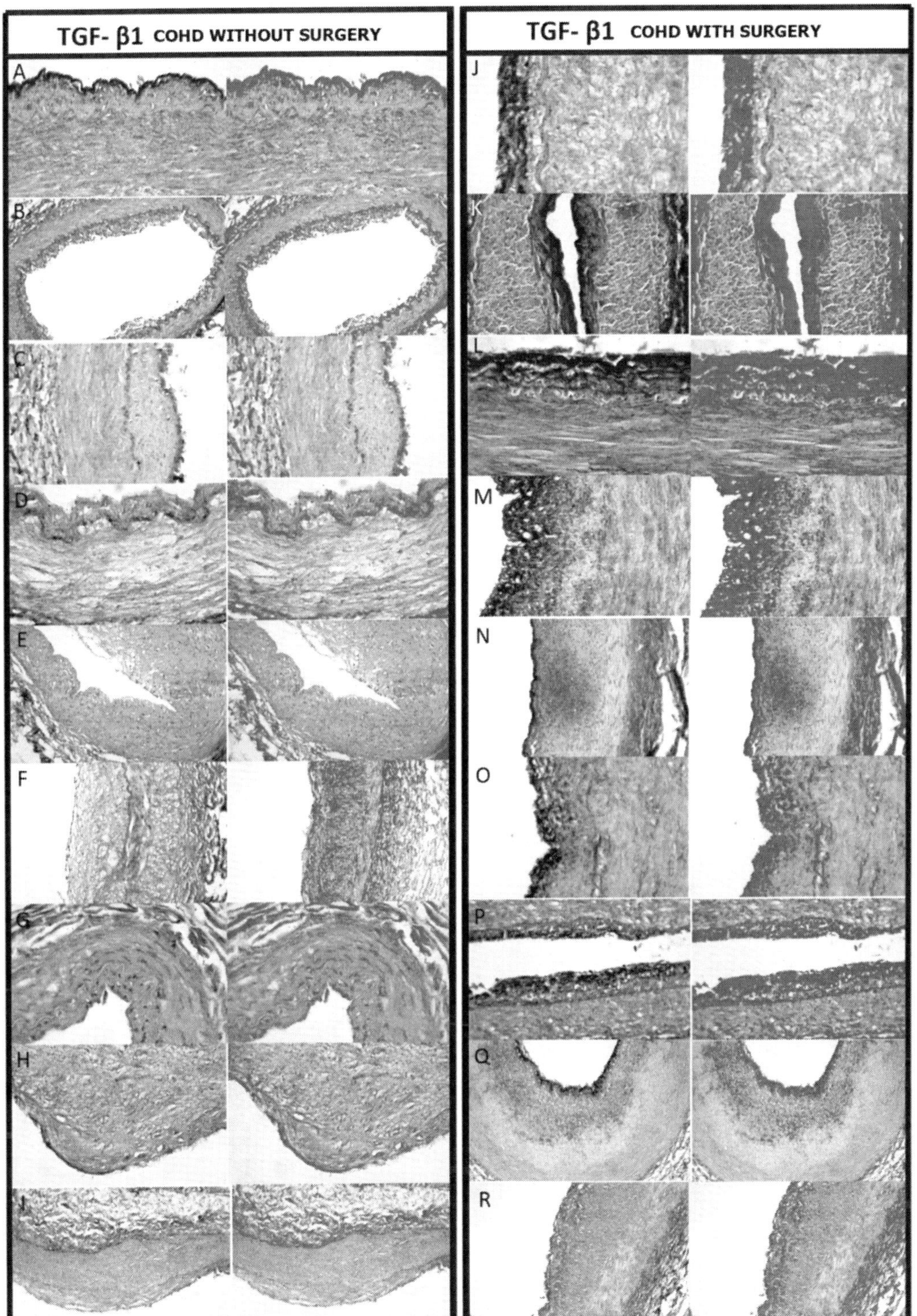

Figure 5. Immunostaining for TGF-β_1 in surgical and non surgical-repaired patients. A to I: non-surgical repaired CHD patients. J to R: Surgically intervened CHD patients. The Image J® analysis is shown in red. Reprinted from Ref. [42].

Immunohistochemistry for TGF-β_1

The expression of TGF-β_1 was analyzed in samples of CHD patients (Figure 4). There were no differences between cyanotic and non-cyanotic CHD patients (% of reactive area was 37.2 ± 12.2 and 25.9 ± 4.9 respectively). Moreover, TGF-β_1 expression was almost undetected in any of the 10 cases of pediatric population (aged ≤9) presenting arterial coronary intimal hyperplasia/ thickening but who died from causes other than CHD (Figure 4).

On the contrary, when immunostaining for TGF-β_1 was analyzed in patients with or without surgical repair, a striking difference was observed between them (mean intimal area positive for TGF-β_1: 50.43% vs. 15.91% respectively; two-tailed Mann-Whitney U-test, $p=0.0005$) (Figure 5).

The non-parametric comparison of repaired CHD, non-repaired CHD and pediatric population without CHD revealed that the difference was significant (Kruskal-Wallis test, $p<0.0001$) (Figure 6).

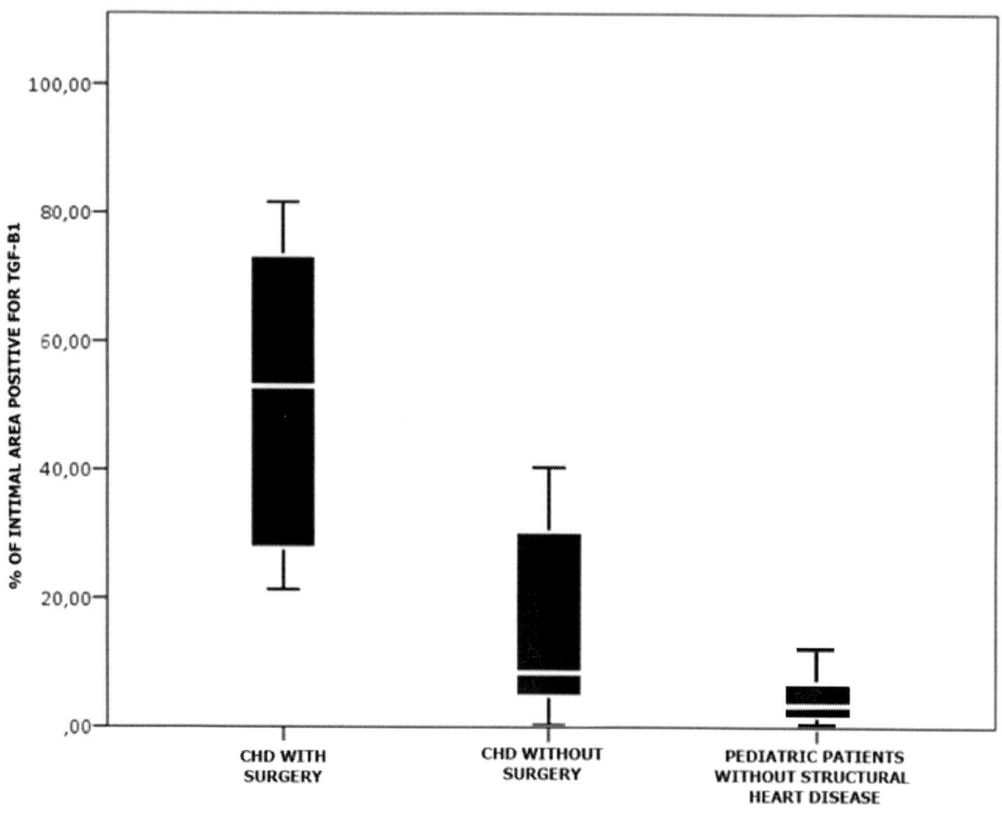

Figure 6. Quantification of immunostaining for TGF-β_1 in surgical and non surgical-repaired patients. Difference in the percentage of intimal area positive for TGF-β_1 between the surgical CHD group, the non-surgical CHD group and the pediatric population with no CHD. Bars indicate maximum and minimum values. Reprinted from Ref. [42].

The presence of intimal hyperplasia and TGF-β_1 expression was more evident in LMCA and RCA compared with the remaining coronary arteries though the differences were not significant.

The relative degree of intimal hyperplasia (intima/media ratio) and the percentage of intimal area stained with TGF-β_1 were not correlated (Spearman's rank correlation coefficient= -0.2955, $IC_{95\%}$ (-0.61 to 0.11, p=0.134).

As stated above, TGF-β_1 has been identified as an underlying factor in reparative process after injury in various organs [36] and the over-production of this growth factor has been implicated as one causative agent in tissue repair processes characterized by increased production of extracellular matrix and fibrosis [37].

The reasons why patients with CHD subjected to surgical repair present TGF-β_1 levels significantly higher are not completely clear. It may be speculated that cardiac surgery is a cause of vascular injury that leads to activation of this pathway. Thus, a “stressor” during the surgical procedure induces the production of TGF-β_1, which in turn leads to intimal hyperplasia. A stressor could be endothelial hypoxia-ischemia. This occurs during arterial clamping [38], external compression of the vessels, extracorporeal circulation or during cardiac preservation before transplant. Hypoxia leads to an increase of TGF-β_1 in human pulmonary artery [39] and human dermal fibroblast [40]. It has also been postulated that hypoxia could stimulate TGF-β_1 through changes in redox state [36]. On the other hand, the patients that were submitted to surgery were the most hemodynamically impaired. Because of this, hypoperfusion and thus low shear stress would likely contribute to inflammation more than in the non surgical patients. This would also contribute to the increase in intimal hyperplasia.

It is not surprising that intimal hyperplasia was found in our control population. We have reported that pediatric patients develop intimal hyperplasia in the absence of substantial TGF-β_1 expression [7,14]. However, the control group was constituted by children who died of non-cardiac disease. Our data seem to indicate that the mechanisms behind intimal hyperplasia are multiple: TGF-β_1 is remarkably increased in children with CHD, and even more so in those who are hemodynamically unstable and/or were subjected to surgery, and hence it may contribute to development of intimal hyperplasia in those subjects; on the other hand, other factors, different than TGF-β_1 may operate in children who died from causes different from CHD.

Intimal hyperplasia may regress by apoptosis, may stay asymptomatic or it may retain lipids and evolve into atherosclerotic lesions [11]. However, the pathophysiology of surgical patients seems to be different due to TGF-β_1 activation. A study on coronary arteries of rats that over-expressed TGF-β_1 proved that this growth factor stimulates intimal hyperplasia rich in extracellular matrix with reversibility of coronary intimal hyperplasia by apoptosis after 8 weeks [41].

Therefore, it seems that clinical implications of intimal hyperplasia in surgical patients due mainly to TGF-β_1 over-expression depend on the reversibility of these lesions once the adverse stimulus disappears. This is not the case of intimal hyperplasia found in the pediatric population, as they do not appear to be related to activation of the TGF-β_1 cascade [11,42].

On the other hand, we found no association between the degree of intimal hyperplasia and TGF-β_1 expression. However, a high incidence of mild intimal hyperplasia was observed on surgical patients with intense TGF-β1 expression, while severe intimal hyperplasia lesions in non-surgical patients and in patients with no CHD were negative for TGF-β_1.

A direct relationship between intimal hyperplasia and TGF-β_1 is difficult to investigate in these patients because the signal transduction of TGF-β_1 is very complex and it interacts with multiple agents. For instance vascular SMC growth can be stimulated or inhibited by TGF-β_1 *in vitro*, depending on cell density, cell age, co-culture factors, and the concentration of TGF-β_1 [43-45]. The identification of a second marker together with the TGF-β_1 may represent a step forward in the elucidation of these discrepancies.

Likewise, it would be necessary an acute temporal study indicating the injury time, TGF-β_1 expression and intimal hyperplasia development, difficult to obtain in human beings.

The intimal hyperplasia has also an important role in restenosis after coronary stent placement, in pulmonary hypertension and in coronary artery lesions after cardiac transplant [46,47]. Yutani et al. reported positivity for TGF-β_1 in the intimal layer of 80% of restenosed coronary arteries [48]. Furthermore, TGF-β_1 administration previous to carotid balloon angioplasty resulted in more extensive intimal hyperplasia after the procedure [49].

The hypoxic theory also might explain the increase of TGF-β1 and posterior coronary intimal hyperplasia after stent implant or balloon angioplasty as both interventions are associated with arterial wall hypoxia and neo-vessels formation in the adventitial layer [50].

Immunohistochemistry for ERα

Overall, ERα expression was evident in all layers of SMCs of arteries (media, endothelium, and intima) and it was quantified as a percentage of the ERα-positive area, considering the whole artery, media or intimal layers. No significant differences between male and female patients were found in the areas studied (Figure 7).

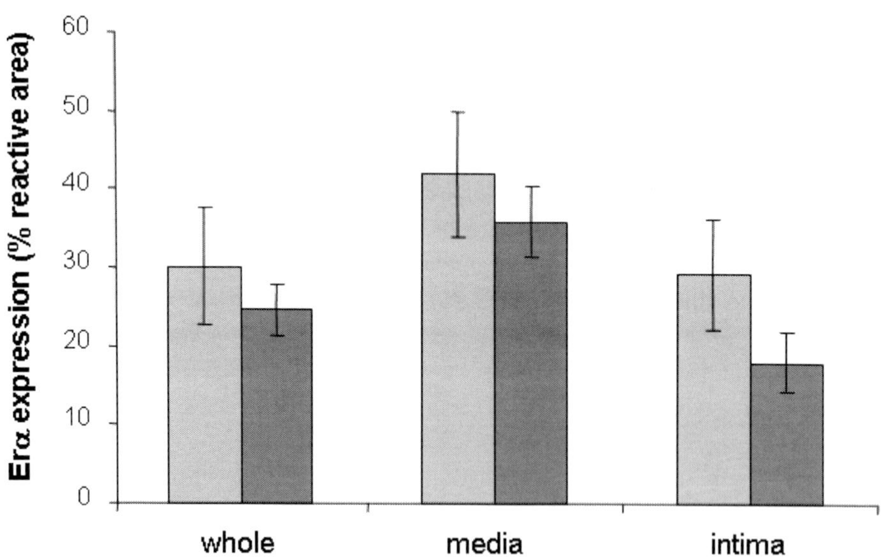

Figure 7. ERα expression in CHD patients according to sex. Plot of ERα reactive area (percentage) considering the whole artery, media or intimal layer of arteries from male and female CDH patients (light-grey bands: female CHD patients, dark-grey bands: male CHD patients). Values are expressed as the mean ± SEM. No significant differences were observed between the groups (non parametric Mann-Whitney U test).

ERα, ERβ and gpER expression was observed previously in the arterial wall of both men and women [31,32]. Consistent with our results, other authors have reported no sex differences in ERα expression as well [51].

Additionally, ERα expression was comparable in cyanotic and noncyanotic CHD patients (Figure 8). Then, the ERα expression obtained in the arteries of controls and CHD patients was evaluated. No significant differences were observed between controls and non-surgically-treated patients.

Since surgery was previously found to impact the incidence of intimal hyperplasia, differences in ERα expression within CHD patients were evaluated according to whether patients had undergone surgical repair or not. A higher staining of ERα was evident in intimal thickenings from non-surgically repaired CHD patients compared with a lower expression observed in surgically treated ones (Figure 9A and B). When ERα expression was quantified considering the whole artery, a significant decrease ($p<0.05$) was evident in surgically repaired CHD patients (Figure 9C), which was almost entirely due to a striking decrease (61.6%) in the intimal layer of the coronary artery of surgically repaired CHD patients, whereas expression in the media was unchanged. This also indicated that the decrease observed was not a consequence of nonspecific degradation of the sample.

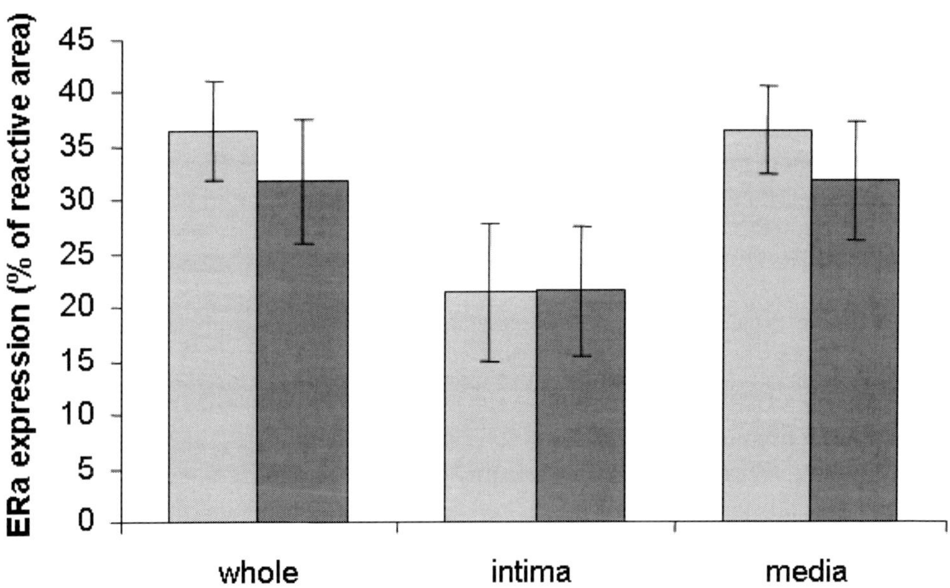

Figure 8. ERα expression in cyanotic and non-cyanotic CHD patients. Plot of ERα reactive area (percentage) considering the whole artery, media or intimal layer of arteries from cyanotic and non cyanotic CDH patients (light-grey bands: cyanotic CHD patients, dark-grey bands: non-cyanotic CHD patients). Values are expressed as the mean ± SEM. No significant differences were observed between the groups (non parametric Mann-Whitney U test). Analysis of ERα expression in control patients and CHD patients with or without surgical repair is shown in Panel C (white bands: control patients, light-grey bands: non-surgically repaired CHD patients, dark-grey bands: surgically repaired CHD patients). Values are expressed as the mean ± SEM. * $p<0.05$, ** $p<0.01$ (non parametric Mann-Whitney U test)

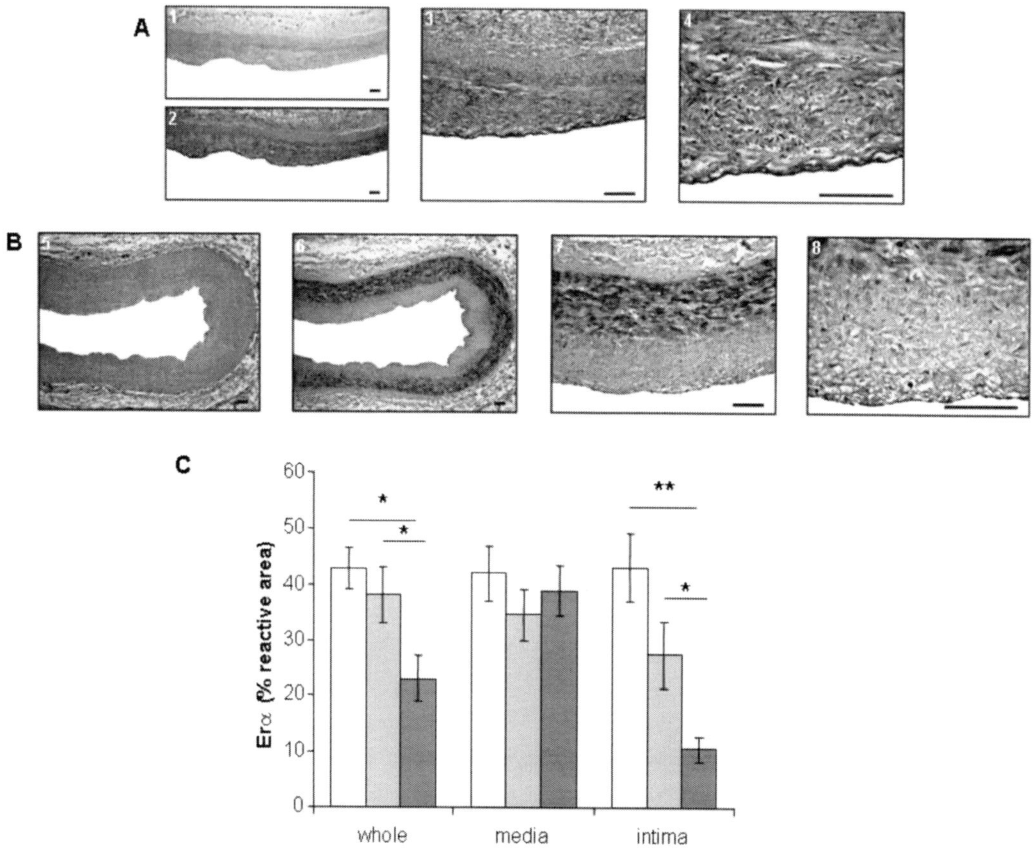

Figure 9. Expression of ERα in CHD patients with and without reparatory surgery. Arteries from CHD pediatric patients were used for immunological determination of ERα. Representative arteries of patients with (Panel B) or without reparatory surgery (Panel A) are shown. Immunohistochemistry was performed in the absence (Pictures 1 and 5) or presence of anti-ERα antibody and observed at 3.5X (Pictures 1, 2, 5 and 6), 10X (Pictures 3 and 7) or 25X (Pictures 4 and 8). Bars indicate 20 μm.

The relationship between CHD and intimal thickenings may involve different mechanisms, whether direct or indirect, acquired or iatrogenic, and depending, in part, on the type of defect and surgical intervention. For this reason, it is difficult to find an immediate explanation for the reduction in ERα expression. As stated above, as possible mechanisms, it should be emphasized that hypoxia induces hypoxia-inducible factor (HIF-1α), which is able to repress the transcription of the ERα gene in human breast cancer cells [52]. Both TGF-β1 and HIF-1α lead to increased proteasome-dependent degradation of ERα in cancer cell lines [53,54]. Provided such mechanisms also operate in SMCs, they might explain the reduction in ERα expression in the intimal layer of these CHD patients.

A decrease in ER was previously regarded as a risk factor for the development of atherosclerosis. Losordo et al. showed that ER expression was reduced in atherosclerotic arteries compared with normal coronary arteries of premenopausal women [55].

On the other hand, restenosis studies have shown that the local delivery of 17β-estradiol inhibits neointimal proliferation without affecting endothelial repair and function [56].

ERα participation in SMC hyperplasia has also been observed. First, ERα is involved in the process of restenosis [57]. Likewise, the length of the nucleotide repeat regulatory region of the ERα gene has been associated with severity of coronary artery disease in men [58]. The authors have suggested that carriers of the long-repeat variant have a lower expression of the ERα gene and that this may reduce the benefits derived from the cardiovascular protective effects of the ER [58]. Accordingly, recent studies [12] also show an important role of gpER in regulating coronary artery SMC growth and promoting redifferentiation and a contractile phenotype in VSMC [59].

Ultimately, this large autopsy study reports on several potentially important findings: 1) Intimal hyperplasia is a frequent finding in the coronary tree of young patients with congenital heart disease (CHD), 2) TGF-β_1 and ERα seem to play a major role in this phenomenon and 3) Surgical correction of CHD is associated with further coronary vascular remodeling.

The high incidence of intimal hyperplasia in patients with surgically repaired CHD is likely related to an increase in TGF-β_1 expression and to a decrease in ERα expression in the intimal layer. Accordingly the increase in TGF-β_1 expression and the decrease in ERα expression might represent risk factors for the development of pre-atherosclerotic lesions in coronary arteries in CHD patients.

Conclusion

The high incidence of intimal hyperplasia in patients with surgically repaired CHD was correlated with an increment in TGF-β_1 expression and a decrease in ERα expression. Augmented expression of TGF-β_1 and a decrease in ERα expression may contribute to the development of atherosclerotic coronary artery disease in CHD patients.

Acknowledgments

The authors are grateful to the National Scientific and Technical Research Council (CONICET) for funding the studies mentioned in this chapter.

References

[1] Kavey, R; Allada, V; Daniels, SR; Hayman, LL; McCrindle, BW; Newburger, JW; Parekh, RS; Steinberger, J. Cardiovascular risk reduction in high-risk pediatric patients: a scientific statement from the American Heart Association Expert Panel on Population and Prevention Science; the Councils on Cardiovascular Disease in the Young, Epidemiology and Prevention, Nutrition, Physical Activity and Metabolism, High Blood Pressure Research, Cardiovascular Nursing, and the Kidney in Heart Disease; and the Interdisciplinary Working Group on Quality of Care and Outcomes Research: endorsed by the American Academy of Pediatrics. *Circulation* 2006, 114, 2710-38.

[2] Levy, D; Garrison, RJ; Savage, DD; Kannel, WB; Castelli, WP. Prognostic implications of echocardiographically determined left ventricular mass in the Framingham Heart Study. *N Engl J Med* 1990, 322, 1561-6.

[3] Fyfe, A; Perloff, JK; Niwa, K; Child, JS; Miner, PD. Cyanotic congenital heart disease and coronary artery atherogenesis. *Am J Cardiol* 2005, 96, 283-90.

[4] Stary, HC; Blankenhorn, DH; Chandler, AB; Glagov, S; Insull, W Jr.; Richardson, M; Rosenfeld, ME; Schaffer, SA; Schwartz, CJ; Wagner, WD; et al. A definition of the intima of human arteries and of its atherosclerosis-prone regions. A report from the Committee on Vascular Lesions of the Council on Arteriosclerosis, American Heart Association. *Arterioscler Thromb* 1992, 12, 120-34.

[5] Stehbens, WE. The pathogenesis of arterial aneurysms and associated lesions. *Cardiovasc Res* 1997, 34, 431-4.

[6] Ikari, Y; McManus, BM; Kenyon, J; Schwartz, SM. Neonatal intima formation in the human coronary artery. *Arterioscler Thromb Vasc Biol* 1999, 19, 2036-40.

[7] Davies, H. Atherogenesis and the coronary arteries of childhood. *Int J Cardiol* 1990, 28, 283-91.

[8] Pesonen, E. Preliminary and early stages of atherosclerosis in childhood. Zentralbl *Allg Pathol* 1989, 135, 545-8.

[9] Virmani, R; Kolodgie, FD; Burke, AP; Farb, A; Schwartz, SM. Lessons from sudden coronary death: a comprehensive morphological classification scheme for atherosclerotic lesions. *Arterioscler Thromb Vasc Biol* 2000, 20, 1262-75.

[10] Nakashima, Y; Wight, TN; Sueishi, K. Early atherosclerosis in humans: role of diffuse intimal thickening and extracellular matrix proteoglycans. *Cardiovasc Res* 2008, 79, 14-23.

[11] Milei, J; Grana, DR; Navari, C; Azzato, F; Guerri-Guttenberg, RA; Ambrosio, G. Coronary intimal thickening in newborn babies and <or=1-year-old infants. *Angiology* 2010, 61, 350-6.

[12] Kim, DN; Schmee, J; Lee, KT; Thomas, WA. Atherosclerotic lesions in the coronary arteries of hyperlipidemic swine. Part 1. Cell increases, divisions, losses and cells of origin in first 90 days on diet. *Atherosclerosis* 1987, 64, 231-42.

[13] Velican, D; Velican, C. Atherosclerotic involvement of the coronary arteries of adolescents and young adults. *Atherosclerosis* 1980, 36, 449-60.

[14] Schwartz, SM; de Blois, D; O'Brien, ER. The intima. Soil for atherosclerosis and restenosis. *Circ Res* 1995, 77, 445-65.

[15] Milei, J; Ottaviano, G; Lavezzi, AM; Grana, DR; Stella, I; Matturri, L. Perinatal and infant early atherosclerotic coronary lesions. *Can J Cardiol 2008*, 24, 137-41.

[16] Becu, L; Somerville, J; Gallo, A. 'Isolated' pulmonary valve stenosis as part of more widespread cardiovascular disease. *Br Heart J* 1976, 38, 472-82.

[17] Mosse, PR; Campbell, GR; Campbell, JH. Smooth muscle phenotypic expression in human carotid arteries. II. Atherosclerosis-free diffuse intimal thickenings compared with the media. *Arteriosclerosis* 1986, 6, 664-9.

[18] Deng, HB; Jiang, CQ; Tomlinson, B; Liu, B; Lin, JM; Wong, KS; Cheung, BM; Lam, TH; Thomas, GN. A polymorphism in transforming growth factor-beta1 is associated with carotid plaques and increased carotid intima-media thickness in older Chinese men, the Guangzhou Biobank Cohort Study-Cardiovascular Disease Subcohort. *Atherosclerosis* 2011, 214, 391-6.

[19] Saltis, J; Agrotis, A; Bobik, A. Regulation and interactions of transforming growth factor-beta with cardiovascular cells: implications for development and disease. *Clin Exp Pharmacol Physiol* 1996, 23, 193-200.

[20] Owens, GK; Kumar, MS; Wamhoff, BR. Molecular regulation of vascular smooth muscle cell differentiation in development and disease. *Physiol Rev* 2004, 84, 767-801.

[21] Mack, CP. Signaling mechanisms that regulate smooth muscle cell differentiation. *Arterioscler Thromb Vasc Biol* 2011, 31, 1495-505.

[22] Nabel, EG; Shum, L; Pompili, VJ; Yang, ZY; San, H; Shu, HB; Liptay, S; Gold, L; Gordon, D; Derynck, R; et al. Direct transfer of transforming growth factor beta 1 gene into arteries stimulates fibrocellular hyperplasia. *Proc Natl Acad Sci USA* 1993, 90, 10759-63.

[23] Lavigne, MC; Ramwell, PW; Clarke, R. Inhibition of estrogen receptor function promotes porcine coronary artery smooth muscle cell proliferation. *Steroids* 1999, 64, 472-80.

[24] Sousa, JE; Costa, MA; Sousa, AG; Abizaid, AC; Seixas, AC; Abizaid, AS; Feres, F; Mattos, LA; Falotico, R; Jaeger, J; Popma, JJ; Serruys, PW. Two-year angiographic and intravascular ultrasound follow-up after implantation of sirolimus-eluting stents in human coronary arteries. *Circulation* 2003, 107, 381-3.

[25] Grube, E; Silber, S; Hauptmann, KE; Mueller, R; Buellesfeld L; Gerckens. U; Russell. ME. TAXUS I: six- and twelve-month results from a randomized; double-blind trial on a slow-release paclitaxel-eluting stent for de novo coronary lesions. *Circulation* 2003, 107, 38-42.

[26] Meyer. MR; Haas. E; Prossnitz. ER; Barton. M. Non-genomic regulation of vascular cell function and growth by estrogen. *Mol Cell Endocrinol* 2009, 308, 9-16.

[27] Hodgin. JB; Krege. JH; Reddick. RL; Korach. KS; Smithies. O; Maeda. N. Estrogen receptor alpha is a major mediator of 17beta-estradiol's atheroprotective effects on lesion size in Apoe$^{-/-}$ mice. *J Clin Invest* 2001, 107, 333-40.

[28] Sudhir, K; Chou, TM; Chatterjee, K; Smith, EP; Williams, TC; Kane, JP; Malloy, MJ; Korach, KS; Rubanyi, GM. Premature coronary artery disease associated with a disruptive mutation in the estrogen receptor gene in a man. *Circulation* 1997, 96, 3774-7.

[29] Rubanyi, GM; Kauser, K; Johns, A. Role of estrogen receptors in the vascular system. *Vascul Pharmacol* 2002, 38, 81-8.

[30] Otsuki, M; Dahlman-Wright, K; Gustafsson, JA. Cardiovascular roles of estrogen receptors: insights gained from knockout models. *Nucl Recept Signal* 2003, 1, e003..

[31] Meyer, MR; Haas, E; Barton, M. Gender differences of cardiovascular disease: new perspectives for estrogen receptor signaling. *Hypertension* 2006, 47, 1019-26.

[32] Haas, E; Meyer, MR; Schurr, U; Bhattacharya, I; Minotti, R; Nguyen, HH; Heigl, A; Lachat, M; Genoni, M; Barton, M. Differential effects of 17beta-estradiol on function and expression of estrogen receptor alpha, estrogen receptor beta, and GPR30 in arteries and veins of patients with atherosclerosis. *Hypertension* 2007, 49, 1358-63.

[33] Costa, M. A Simon, DI. Molecular basis of restenosis and drug-eluting stents. *Circulation* 2005, 111, 2257-73.

[34] Verdecchia, P; Porcellati, C; Reboldi, G; Gattobigio, R; Borgioni, C; Pearson, TA; Ambrosio, G. Left ventricular hypertrophy as an independent predictor of acute cerebrovascular events in essential hypertension. *Circulation* 2001, 104, 2039-44.

[35] Nakashima, Y; Fujii, H; Sumiyoshi, S; Wight, TN; Sueishi, K. Early human atherosclerosis: accumulation of lipid and proteoglycans in intimal thickenings followed by macrophage infiltration. *Arterioscler Thromb Vasc Biol* 2007, 27, 1159-65.

[36] Sporn, MB; Roberts, AB. Transforming growth factor-beta: recent progress and new challenges. *J Cell Biol* 1992, 119, 1017-21.

[37] Border, W. A.; Ruoslahti E. Transforming growth factor-beta in disease: the dark side of tissue repair. *J Clin Invest* 1992, 90, 1-7.

[38] Milei, J; Forcada, P; Fraga, CG; Grana, DR; Iannelli, G; Chiariello, M; Tritto, I; Ambrosio, G. Relationship between oxidative stress, lipid peroxidation, and ultrastructural damage in patients with coronary artery disease undergoing cardioplegic arrest/reperfusion. *Cardiovasc Res* 2007, 73, 710-9.

[39] Ismail, S; Sturrock, A; Wu, P; Cahill, B; Norman, K; Huecksteadt, T; Sanders, K; Kennedy, T; Hoidal, J. NOX4 mediates hypoxia-induced proliferation of human pulmonary artery smooth muscle cells: the role of autocrine production of transforming growth factor-β_1 and insulin-like growth factor binding protein-3. *Am J Physiol Lung Cell Mol Physiol* 2009, 296, L489-99.

[40] Falanga, V; Qian, SW; Danielpour, D; Katz, MH; Roberts, AB; Sporn, MB. Hypoxia upregulates the synthesis of TGF-β_1 by human dermal fibroblasts. *J Invest Dermatol* 1991, 97, 634-7.

[41] Schulick, AH; Taylor, AJ; Zuo, W; Qiu, CB; Dong, G; Woodward, RN; Agah, R; Roberts, AB; Virmani, R; Dichek, DA. Overexpression of transforming growth factor beta1 in arterial endothelium causes hyperplasia, apoptosis, and cartilaginous metaplasia. *Proc Natl Acad Sci USA* 1998, 95, 6983-8..

[42] Guerri-Guttenberg, RA; Castilla, R; Francos, GC; Müller, A; Ambrosio, G; Milei, J. Transforming growth factor β_1 and coronary intimal hyperplasia in pediatric patients with congenital heart disease. *Can J Cardiol* 2013, 29, 849-57.

[43] Barnard, JA; Lyons, RM; Moses, HL. The cell biology of transforming growth factor beta. *Biochim Biophys Acta* 1990; 1032, 79-87.

[44] Owens, GK; Geisterfer, AA; Yang, YW; Komoriya, A. Transforming growth factor-beta-induced growth inhibition and cellular hypertrophy in cultured vascular smooth muscle cells. *J Cell Biol* 1988; 107, 771-80.

[45] Majack, R. A. Beta-type transforming growth factor specifies organizational behavior in vascular smooth muscle cell cultures. *J Cell Biol* 1987, 105, 465-71.

[46] Ramzy, D; Rao, V; Brahm, J; Miriuka, S; Delgado, D; Ross, HJ. Cardiac allograft vasculopathy: a review. *Can J Surg* 2005, 48, 319-27.

[47] Newby, AC; Zaltsman, AB. Molecular mechanisms in intimal hyperplasia. *J Pathol* 2000, 190, 300-9.

[48] Khan, R; Agrotis, A; Bobik, A. Understanding the role of transforming growth factor-$beta_1$ in intimal thickening after vascular injury. *Cardiovasc Res* 2007, 74, 223-34.

[49] Kanzaki, T; Tamura, K; Takahashi, K; Saito, Y; Akikusa, B; Oohashi, H; Kasayuki, N; Ueda, M; Morisaki, N. In vivo effect of TGF-β_1. Enhanced intimal thickening by administration of TGF-β_1 in rabbit arteries injured with a balloon catheter. *Arterioscler Thromb Vasc Biol* 1995, 15, 1951-7.

[50] Cheema, AN; Hong, T; Nili, N; Segev, A; Moffat, JG; Lipson, KE; Howlett, AR; Holdsworth, DW; Cole, MJ; Qiang, B; Kolodgie, F; Virmani, R; Stewart, DJ; Strauss,

BH. Adventitial microvessel formation after coronary stenting and the effects of SU11218, a tyrosine kinase inhibitor. *J Am Coll Cardiol* 2006, 47, 1067-75.

[51] Finking, G; Krauss, N; Romer S; Eckert, S; Lenz, C; Kamenz, J; Menke, A; Brehme, U; Hombach, V; Hanke, H. 17beta-estradiol, gender independently, reduces atheroma development but not neointimal proliferation after balloon injury in the rabbit aorta. *Atherosclerosis* 2001, 154, 39-49.

[52] Ryu, K; Park, C; Lee, Y. Hypoxia-inducible factor 1 alpha represses the transcription of the estrogen receptor alpha gene in human breast cancer cells. *Biochem Biophys Res Commun* 2011, 407, 831-6.

[53] Petrel, TA; Brueggemeier, RW. Increased proteasome-dependent degradation of estrogen receptor-alpha by TGF-β_1 in breast cancer cell lines. *J Cell Biochem* 2003, 88, 181-90.

[54] Cooper, C; Liu, GY; Niu, YL; Santos, S; Murphy, LC; Watson, PH. Intermittent hypoxia induces proteasome-dependent down-regulation of estrogen receptor alpha in human breast carcinoma. *Clin Cancer Res* 2004, 10, 8720-7.

[55] Losordo, DW; Kearney, M; Kim, EA; Jekanowski, J; Isner, JM. Variable expression of the estrogen receptor in normal and atherosclerotic coronary arteries of premenopausal women. *Circulation* 1994, 89, 1501-10.

[56] Abizaid, A; Albertal, M; Costa, MA; Abizaid, AS; Staico, R; Feres, F; Mattos, LA; Sousa, AG; Moses, J; Kipshidize, N; Roubin, GS; Mehran, R; New, G; Leon, MB; Sousa, JE. First human experience with the 17-beta-estradiol-eluting stent: the Estrogen And Stents To Eliminate Restenosis (EASTER) trial. *J Am Coll Cardiol* 2004, 43, 1118-21.

[57] Ferrero, V; Ribichini, F; Matullo, G; Guarrera, S; Carturan, S; Vado, A; Vassanelli, C; Piazza, A; Uslenghi, E; Wijns, W. Estrogen receptor-alpha polymorphisms and angiographic outcome after coronary artery stenting. *Arterioscler Thromb Vasc Biol* 2003, 23, 2223-8.

[58] Kunnas, TA; Laippala, P; Penttila, A; Lehtimaki, T; Karhunen, PJ. Association of polymorphism of human alpha oestrogen receptor gene with coronary artery disease in men: a necropsy study. *Brit Med J* 2000, 321, 273-4.

[59] Li, F; Yu, X; Szynkarski, CK; Meng, C; Zhou, B; Barhoumi, R; White, RE; Heaps, CL; Stallone, JN; Han, G. Activation of GPER Induces Differentiation and Inhibition of coronary artery smooth muscle cell proliferation. *PLoS One* 2013, 8, e 64771.

In: Congenital Heart Diseases
Editor: Raúl Cayré and José Milei

ISBN: 978-1-61122-003-2

Chapter 3

New Diagnostic Techniques in Congenital Heart Disease

Ana Maria de Dios[1*], Judith Ackerman[2], Fernanda Biancolini[2] and Julio Biancolini[3]
Department of Pediatric Cardiology Hospital Pedro Elizalde
Buenos Aires Argentina
[1]Chief of Department
[2]Staff Member
[3]Fellow

Abstract

New diagnostic techniques can help to understand the myocardial function in congenital heart disease. Echocardiography is a reliable, noninvasive tool to evaluate heart structure and contractile function of the left and right ventricle in children and adults. 2D color Doppler imaging of the myocardium enables rapid qualitative assessment of wall dynamics, providing a good spatial resolution to differentiate between velocity profiles of subendocardial and subepicardial layers, and allows simultaneous analysis of various myocardial regions. Tissue Doppler velocity imaging (TDI) offers a different approach, as it does not rely on geometric assumptions. Possibly, the best option for the evaluation ventricular function is the combination of different methods: TAPSE, TDI and index of myocardial performance. Two-Dimensional (2D) Speckle-Tracking Echocardiography (STE) is a relatively new, angle independent technique that is used for the evaluation of global and segmental myocardial function. Myocardial strain values regional ventricular deformation. Myocardial strain rate (SR) is a time derivative of strain and has shown to correlate linearly with left ventricle (LV) peak elastance, which is a load-independent global measure of ventricular systolic function.

Conclusion: New echo technology can identify early left and right ventricular dysfunction. This may allow earlier intervention and help to avoid irreversible damage to the myocardium in congenital heart disease.

[*] E-mail: ana.dedios@gmail.com.

Introduction

Echocardiography is a reliable, noninvasive tool used for the evaluation of heart structure and function in children and adults. Many important clinical decisions are routinely based on the absolute sizes of cardiac structures. [1] Evaluation is highly dependent on the quality of the measurements but also on the quality of the reference values with which these measurements are compared.

The American Society of Echocardiography Pediatric and Congenital Heart Disease Council recently published recommendations for quantification methods during the performance of pediatric echocardiography. [2, 3].

Unbiased reference values require appropriate ''normal'' subjects, standardized reproducible measurements, and appropriate sample sizes. [3] In children, reference values are also highly dependent on accurate adjustment for body size.

Conventional indices of regional and global ventricular function, defined by endocardial excursion, are considered to be mostly load-dependent and based on geometric assumptions.

Tricuspid and Mitral Annular Plane Systolic Excursion

The measurement of the tricuspid and mitral annular plane systolic excursion (TAPSE and MAPSE), estimates right ventricle (RV) and LV systolic function by measuring the level of systolic excursion of the lateral tricuspid and mitral valve annulus toward the apex in the four-chamber view. [4, 5].

These methods represent the movement of the heart from the base to the apex. A significant correlation was demonstrated between the TAPSE and ejection fraction (EF), as assessed by radionuclide angiography and MRI-derived volumes.

Normal values increase with age during childhood until finally adult values. In adult patients TAPSE or MAPSE > 1.8 cm suggests biventricular normal systolic function. This approach is reproducible and has proven to be a strong predictor of prognosis in "heart failure" when the TAPSE or MAPSE is less than 1.5 cm in the adult patient, suggesting a certain degree of systolic dysfunction in the right or left ventricle.

Tissue Doppler Imaging

Tissue Doppler imaging (TDI) is another echocardiographic technique that directly measures myocardial velocities (range from 0 to 20 cm/s). TDI-measured myocardial velocities, as an index of regional ventricular function, [6] do not rely on geometric assumptions but rather are inherently one-dimensional, angle-dependent, and relatively load-dependent. Doppler gain settings also must be increased to adequately visualize TDI waveforms.

Tissue Doppler Imaging techniques: Pulsed and color TDI have been used for the assessment of myocardial function; however, both techniques have advantages and disadvantages. [7] With color TDI of the myocardium, we can superimpose wall motion velocity on the two dimension (2D) echocardiographic imaging by velocity color-coding. Pulsed Doppler techniques obtain high quality Doppler signals, measure, mean and instantaneous local acceleration, and obtain quantitative wall motion information. Nevertheless, it requires manual mapping, and it is difficult to distinguish subendocardial and subepicardial myocardial velocities.

2D color Doppler imaging of the myocardium enables rapid qualitative assessment of wall dynamics, provides a good spatial resolution to differentiate between velocity profiles of subendocardial and subepicardial layers, and allows simultaneous analysis of various myocardial regions. However, it is limited by temporal resolution.

In contrast, M mode color-coded tissue imaging: is characterized by a high spatial and temporal resolution, although sampling is only performed along a single line.

Velocities are typically are measured at the myocardium on the longitudinal axis in the four chambers or two-chamber view to minimize the effect of cardiac translation.

To study each point, the sample is placed at the level of interest and is recorded during apnea to minimize errors. We can visualize three waveforms during the cardiac cycle (Figure 1): the peak systolic wave (S' wave), early diastolic wave (E' wave), and end diastolic wave produced by atrial contraction (A' wave).

Other recommended measurements are isovolumic contraction time (IVCT) and isovolumic relaxation time (IVRT). (Figure 1).

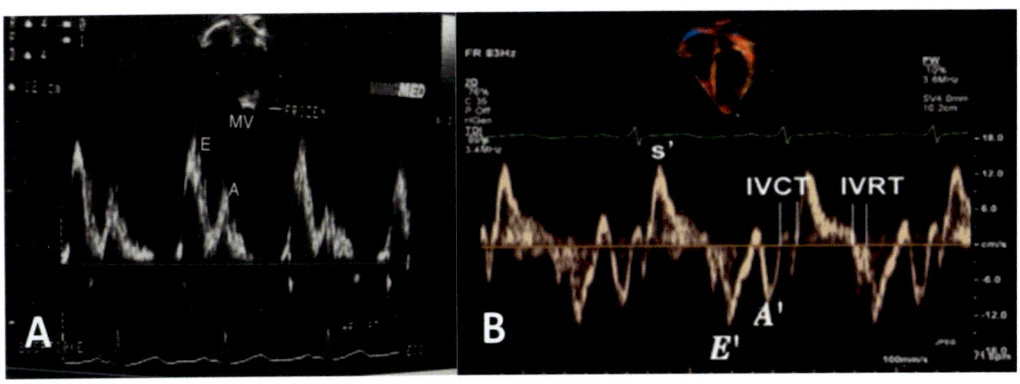

A: Pulsed Eco Doppler (Pw): Lateral mitral annular E wave peak velocity during early ventricular diastole.

B: Tissue Doppler (TDI) tracing. S': peak velocity during ventricular systole; E': peak velocity during early ventricular diastole; A': Peak velocity during atrial contraction; IVCT: isovolumic contraction time; IVRT: isovolumic relaxation time.

Figure 1. Cardiac Cycle, compare: A) Pulsed Doppler. B) Tissue Doppler (TDI).

It is possible to calculate the Pw E/E' ratio (Pw E obtained by pulse Doppler, and E' obtained by TDI), to estimate pressure in the left atrium.

The pulsed Doppler early mitral inflow peak velocity E divided by TDI early diastolic mitral annular velocity (E') correlates well with pulmonary wedge pressure (PCWP).

In the assessment of diastolic function, velocities typically are measured at the annuli or myocardium in the longitudinal axis to minimize the effect of cardiac translation.

From either the apical four chamber or two chamber acoustic windows, the region of interest is placed at the level of the mitral annulus on the septal, lateral, anterior, or posterior aspect. Recordings are obtained during apnea.

By TDI the measured at the longitudinal axis in the four chambers view, the velocities are higher in the base and decrease towards the apex. Systolic and diastolic velocities increase with heart growth.

In short axis views the myocardial velocities are higher at the posterior wall than at the anteroseptal wall (average value 6.3±1.7 cm/s versus 9.3±3 cm/s). [5, 8]

Other recommended measurements are: the isovolumic acceleration slope (IVA): this is the presystolic velocity slope and it is expressed in m/s2.

IVA as assessed by Tissue Doppler Imaging (TDI) has been proposed as a measure of left ventricular (LV) contractility. IVA is believed to be less dependent on preload. This measurement is also the less age-dependent value and is less grown-dependent than myocardial velocities. (Figure2).

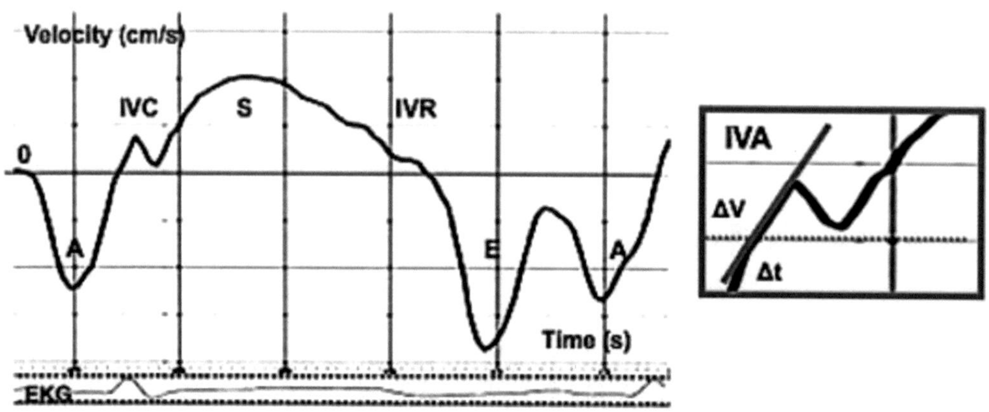

IVA: express Δ velocities / Δ time. IVA is less growth dependent than myocardial velocities.

Figure 2. This image shows the representation of IVA slope.

IVA can be used as an index to evaluate the contractile function of the left ventricle. It was introduced as a measure unaffected by physiological changes, including changes in preload. [8-10].

Normal values for age, heart rate and body surface area (BSA) are standardized.

Table 1, shows normal values for longitudinal Doppler tissue imaging (TDI): systolic wave (S'), early diastolic wave (E'), and late diastolic wave (A') in the left ventricle at mitral valve annulus (MV) base level, and mid level in pediatric patients. [11]. The table also shows the relation between shortening fraction (FA%), Tei index, and TDI systolic tissues Doppler (S') wave, Early (E') and Late (A') wave in m/s and isovolumic acceleration slope (IVA) in m/s2; with body surface at base and mid LV (statistical significance was express with $p<0.05$). We can also see here that the Tei index, FA%, and IVA m/s2 values were not influenced by body surface, while S' and E' waves increased with it.

Table 1. Normal values for longitudinal Doppler tissue imaging (TDI): systolic wave (S'), early diastolic wave (E'), and late diastolic wave (A') in the left ventricle at mitral valve annulus (MV) base level, and mid level in pediatric patients

Body surface	X 0.33		X: 074		X: 1.14		X: 1.85		p
	X	DS	X	DS	X	DS	X	DS	
FA%	37,34	3,17	37,59	8,86	39,6	6,54	35,4	4,34	ns
ITei	0,47	0.01	0,59	0,13	0,35	0,16	0,43	0,11	ns
Base LV:									
S'	0,08	0	0,09	0,04	0,11	0,02	0,13	0,03	0,00
E'	0,09	0,08	0,17	0,04	0,18	0,04	0,18	0,01	0,00
A'	0,1	0,04	0,07	0,01	0,08	0,03	0,04	0,04	0,00
IVAm/s2	1,98	0,25	1,77	0,46	1,66	0,54	1,74	1,29	ns
Mid LV									
S'	0,09	0,04	0,1	0,04	0,09	0,02	0,15	0,01	ns
E'	0,1	0,08	0,17	0,03	0,17	0,03	0,21	0,02	0,00
A'	0,08	0,04	0,19	0,33	0,07	0,04	0,06	0	ns
IVA m/s2	2	1,2	2,41	0,52	2,1	0,67	2,3	0.01	ns

Referens: FA: shortening fraction, ITei: Tei index. Base LV TDI: systolic tissues Doppler velocity in m/s (S') and diastolic wave: Early (E') and Late (A') wave in m/s, isovolumic acceleration slope (IVA) in m/s2. The statistical significance (P) was express with $p<0.05$, ns: no signifative.

The S´ wave and the E' wave correlate negatively with heart rate (HR), decrease with tachycardia and increase in bradycardia; correlate positively with age, increase with age and body surface, and have a strong correlation at the mitral, septal and tricuspid annulus. The A' wave has a strong positive correlation with HR and a strong negative correlation with body surface and age at the tricuspid valve site only. [12] In conclusion, TDI measures changes with aging and is influenced by anthropometry, heart rate and left ventricular growth in pediatric population. [13, 14].

Such dependency of TDI-measured myocardial velocities may limit its utility as an independent index when comparing ventricular function across differing age and loading conditions in the pediatric population. [15, 16].

In adults, TDI is a recommended component of routine echocardiography and is particularly useful in the assessment of diastolic function of the left ventricle.

Myocardial mitral annular or base segmental in systolic and early diastolic velocities have been shown to predict mortality or cardiovascular events. In particular, those with reduced S´ or E´ values of <3 cm/s have a very poor prognosis. [17, 18].

In contrast, color and pulsed-wave TDI velocities are less accepted in pediatrics, perhaps due to their strong age dependence in children [19].

Myocardial velocities increase during normal childhood heart development, starting from fetal life, and these changes vary by cardiac segment. TDI velocity maturation opens an interesting window into the normal development of myocardial mechanics in childhood, but makes it difficult to interpret data in an individual child. Moreover, there is a wider range of normal values for any given pediatric age than in adults. In the individual child, a given measurement may not be very informative if the baseline is unknown. In the clinical situation, serial measurements in the same patient may in part overcome this problem. Nevertheless, TDI has been useful in the monitoring of systolic heart function in children with cardiomyopathy or after heart transplantation. Following orthotopic cardiac transplant in childhood, patients have diminished right heart TDI velocities for reasons that are incompletely understood. [20, 21] This begins at the time of transplant and may show some improvement during recovery, but not normalization. [22].

In children with volume overload of the right ventricle due to atrial septal defects, tricuspid ring velocities are slightly higher than normal during childhood. [23]

Right ventricular systolic function: Assessment of right heart function with TDI velocities has been used widely, with a considerable body of clinical studies documenting its utility in adults and children. Peak S' velocity near the tricuspid ring is useful in the assessment of right ventricular longitudinal wall motion. The most widely studied heart defect is tetralogy of Fallot (TOF). [24, 25].

The number of studies using TDI to assess right heart function in children with congenital heart disease or pulmonary hypertension is steading increasing. TDI has been used in the assessment of RV diastolic function. [26]

In Tetralogy of Fallot (TOF), tricuspid ring velocities are reduced (in presence of severe overload caused by severe pulmonary regurgitation). Studies have shown a correlation between QRS complex duration on electrocardiogram and tricuspid ring velocities. In addition, on exercise stress testing, patients with TOF showed less contractile reserve than healthy controls. [27, 28].

A similar pattern with diminished tricuspid ring S velocities is also seen in patients with systemic right ventricle after atrial switch operation for transposition of the great arteries [29].

TDI studies have revealed diastolic dysfunction in obese children and in cancer survivors with preclinical anthracycline cardiomyopathy.

Another potential strength of TDI velocities is the study of myocardial dyssynchrony where color TDI is well-suited for rapid pediatric heart rates, even on fetal echocardiogram.

Some studies have used peak S´ velocity in attempt to quantify global systolic function in single-ventricle hearts. [30, 31] Conventional assessment of function in univentricular hearts is problematic due to the unusual configuration of these hearts. Tissue Doppler velocity imaging offers a different approach that does not rely on geometric assumptions. It represents a paradigm shift away from the familiar approach to quantify cardiac function by assessing cardiac output. [32] TDI studies give information about the properties of the heart muscle rather than the pump function. However, TDI measurements should be interpreted with caution in the single-ventricle setting as wall-motion abnormalities and abnormal loading conditions may preclude a straightforward interpretation of the S velocity measurements. At the same time, for individual patients, serial measurements may still be informative in the individual patient.

Tissue Doppler echocardiography has been used in the assessment of RV diastolic function. [33]

The E/E' ratio, is a strong indicator of increased filling pressure in hypertrophic cardiomyopathies. A RV E/E' ratio >6 suggests a mean pulmonary pressure >10 mm Hg. [34, 35].

E/E'annular mitral ratio: The early diastolic velocity of the longitudinal motion of the mitral annulus (E') reflects the rate of myocardial relaxation. [36] The velocity of the mitral annulus can be recorded by TDI, and this has become an essential part of evaluating diastolic function by echocardiography. [37, 38] In normal subjects, E' increases as transmitral gradient increases with exertion or increased preload, whereas in patients with impaired myocardial relaxation E' is reduced at baseline and does not increase as much as in normal subjects with increased preload. Lateral annulus early diastolic velocity is usually higher than septal annulus E'. The E' increases with increasing transmitral gradient in healthy individuals, so that E/E' is similar at rest and with exercise (usually < 8). A decreased in E' is one of the earliest markers for diastolic dysfunction and is present in all stages of diastolic dysfunction. Because E' annular mitral velocity remains reduced and mitral E velocity increases with higher filling pressure, the ratio between transmitral E and E' tisular (E/E') correlates well with LV filling pressure or pulmonary capillary wedge pressure.

If the PCWP is ≥20 mmHg: E/E'annular is ≥15.

If the PCWP is normal: E/E' annular is <8.

Because PCWP has been shown to be a prognostic indicator in patients with heart failure (HF), it is reasonable to expect E/E' to be a similarly powerful prognosticator in various cardiac diseases. Indeed, both E/E'≥15 and B-type natriuretic peptide ≥250 pg./ml have carried independent prognostic value in patients with heart failure (HF). The independent predictive value of E/E'≥15 for cardiac mortality or HF hospitalization has been confirmed in patients with LV dysfunction. [39, 40]

Strengths and Weaknesses of TDI: The major strength of TDI is that it is readily available and allows objective quantitative evaluation of local myocardial dynamics. Over the past decade, this ability triggered extensive research in a variety of disease states that affect myocardial function, either globally or regionally, as reflected by the large body of literature involving this methodology. It is well established that peak tissue velocities are sufficiently reproducible, which is crucial for serial evaluations. Also, spectral pulsed TDI has the advantage of online measurements of velocities and time intervals with excellent temporal resolution. The major weakness of TDI is its angle dependency, as any Doppler-based methodology can by definition only measure velocities along the ultrasound beam, while velocity components perpendicular to the beam remain undetected. The best option may be to measure the ventricular function is the combination with different methods: TAPSE, TDI and index of myocardial performance.

The Doppler Index of Myocardial Performance (MPI) or TEI Index

MPI is another non-geometric index of global ventricular function [41]. It is expressed as a ratio obtained by adding the isovolumic contraction time (IVCT) and isovolumic relaxation time (IVRT) and then dividing the result by the ejection time (ET): MPI = (IVCT + IVRT)/ET.

The normal value for the Tei index is: <0.45 (0.39 ± 0.05). [41] But there are some limitations: atrial fibrillation, atrioventricular (AV) block, valvulopathies, and restrictive myocardiopathy. There is an excellent correlation between ejection fraction (EF) and TAPSE, DTI and MPI. [42, 43]

Increased TEI values correlate with increased ventricular dysfunction. It has been established that MPI or TEI index is established that it is actually unaffected by heart rate, loading conditions or the presence and the severity of regurgitation. An MPI of >0.4 has 100% sensitivity and negative predictive value in identifying abnormal EF.

When EF is between 30-50%, MPI is near 0.6 (0.59±0.1), but when severe dysfunction is present with EF less than 30%, this value is near 1 (1.06±0.24). [42]

The combination of TDI with MPI is the best predictor and discriminator of EF<50% by Simpson's method.

Independent and Additive Prognostic Value of right ventricular systolic function and pulmonary artery pressure in patients with chronic heart failure are: right ventricular fraction ejection (RVFE) by each 5 unit decrement; NYHA function class (III-IV versus II); left ventricular end systolic diameter (LVESDI) per each 5 mm increment; and mean pressure arterial pulmonary (PAP) per each 5 mmHg increment. [43]

Other methods used in evaluation of left ventricle function:

- The relationship between rate corrected mean velocity of circumferential fiber shortening and systolic wall stress has been shown to be independent of heart rate, preload, and afterload.
- The rate of pressure development (dp/dt max) is also used as an index of contractility. As demonstrated by numerous studies, dp/dt max is significantly affected by loading conditions and cannot be used as a reliable index of contractility. [44]

Tissue Track (TT)

TT is another technique derived from color TDI and represents longitudinal displacement of atrioventricular annulus in mm.

This parameter decreases in dilated myocardiopathy but is affected late when severe dysfunction is established. This is also seen in surgically corrected tetralogy of Fallot with significant overload due to chronic pulmonary regurgitation.

Two-Dimensional (2D) Speckle-Tracking Echocardiography (STE)

STE is a relatively new, largely angle-independent technique used for the evaluation of myocardial function. The speckles seen in gray scale B-mode images are the result of constructive and destructive interference of ultrasound backscattered from structures smaller than the ultrasound wavelength. With this technology, random noise is filtered out, while keeping small temporally stable and unique myocardial features, referred to as speckles.

Blocks or kernels of speckles can be tracked from frame to frame (simultaneously in multiple regions within an image plane) using block matching and provide local displacement information, from which parameters of myocardial function such as velocity, strain, and strain rate (SR) can be derived. [45].

Strain - Strain Rate

During the past several years, strain and strain rate (SR) imaging have emerged as a quantitative technique to accurately estimate myocardial function and contractility. [46] Strain is a dimensionless parameter representing deformation of an object, relative to its original shape. Strain is expressed as the percent (or fractional) change from the original dimension:

$$S=\Delta L/L0 = L\text{-}L0/L0 \quad (1)$$

(1) Where S is longitudinal strain, ΔL is absolute change in length (L), and L0 is the baseline length.

SR is the local rate of deformation or strain per unit time, which equals velocity difference per length unit:

$$SR=S/\Delta t= (\Delta L/L0)/\Delta t= (\Delta L/\Delta t)/L0= \Delta V/L0 \quad (2)$$

(2) Where ΔV is the velocity gradient in the segment studied.

From the above equations it can be seen that strain and SR measurements can be obtained from data acquired by Doppler tissue imaging. SR is calculated from the instantaneous spatial velocity gradient in a small myocardial segment. Integrating these SR values allows calculation of strain.

Myocardial strain is a dimensionless measure of regional ventricular deformation. Myocardial strain rate (SR), a time derivative of strain, has been shown to correlate linearly with LV peak elastance, which is a load-independent global measure of ventricular systolic function. [47, 48] Reference values for longitudinal systolic strain and SR are necessary in evaluating pathologic alteration in LV function. The septal and lateral longitudinal systolic strain defined are relatively independent of maturational changes and changing hemodynamic parameters of resting heart rate (in physiologic range) through the first 18 years of life. [49].

Longitudinal Strain (septal -18.30% ± 6.67% and lateral -20.68% ± 8.08%) did not change significantly with maturation and declining heart rate from birth to 18 years. This may partly be attributed to the fact that LV geometry (represented by the LV length-diameter ratio) remains constant from infancy to adulthood, leading to normalized torsion [50], which is considered a major mechanism for the deformation of the myocardium. [51, 52].

Peak strain can be measured as peak systolic strain (positive or negative), peak strain at end-systole (at time of aortic valve closure), or peak strain regardless of timing (in systole or early diastole). The time point to be used to measure peak strain in the assessment of systolic function depends on the specific question one wishes to answer. [53, 54].

Assessment of 2D strain by STE can be applied to both ventricles and atria. However, because of the thin wall of the atria and right ventricle, signal quality may be suboptimal. In contrast, all LV segments can be analyzed successfully in most patients. Feasibility is best for longitudinal and circumferential strain and is more challenging for radial strain. Because LV rotation increases toward the apex, it is important to standardize the apical short-axis view. In contrast to TDI, analysis of these velocity vectors allows the quantification of strain and SR in any direction within the imaging plane. Depending on spatial resolution, selective analysis of epicardial, midwall, and endocardial function may be possible as well.

In conclusion, from a color Doppler TDI we can obtain Strain, SR and TT waves at each point of interest. (Figure 3)

Function parameters derived from one region of interest (yellow dot) within the same color Doppler data set: (A) velocity; (B) displacement; (C) SR; and (D) strain. Electrocardiogram. Opening and closing artifacts allow the exact definition of the cardiac time intervals. Note that in this case, the baseline is arbitrarily set to the curve value (red arrows) at the automatically recognized beginning of the QRS complex (red open bracket).

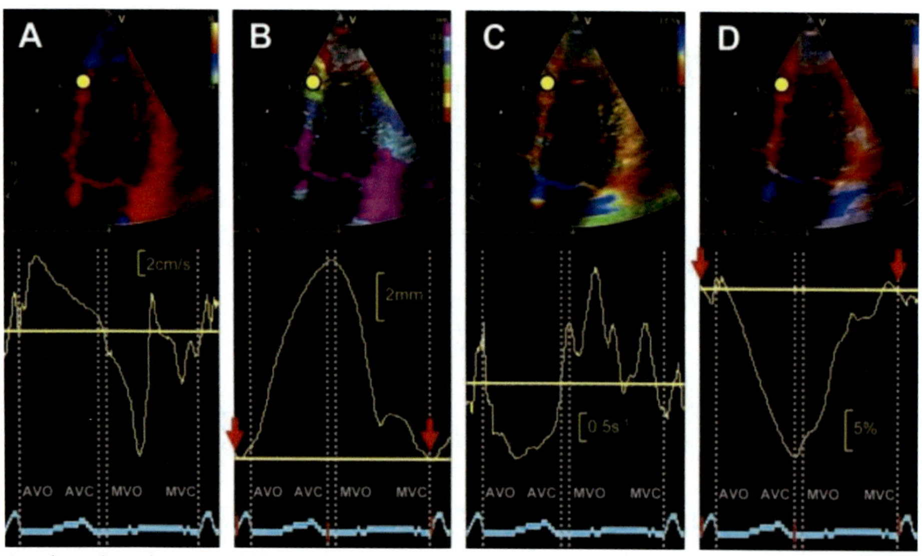

AVC, Aortic valve closure; *AVO,* aortic valve opening; *MVC,* mitral valve closure; *MVO,* mitral valve opening.

Figure 3. Different techniques derived from color TDI: (Top). With Color-coded displays (below), and corresponding time curves. (Bottom).

(A) TDI (m/s), (B) Tissue Track (mm), (C) Strain rate (1/s), (D) Strain (%).

Strengths and Weaknesses of 2D STE:

Both TDI and STE measure motion against a fixed external point in space (i.e., the transducer). However, STE has the advantage of being able to measure this motion in any direction within the image plane, whereas TDI is limited to the velocity component toward or away from the probe. This property of STE allows measurement of circumferential and radial components irrespective of the direction of the beam. Note, however, that STE is not completely angle independent, because ultrasound images normally have better resolution along the ultrasound beam direction compared with the perpendicular direction. Therefore, in principle, speckle tracking works better for measurements of motion and deformation along the ultrasound beam direction than in other directions. Similar to other 2D imaging techniques, STE relies on good image quality as well as the assumption that morphologic details can be tracked from one frame to the next (i.e., that they can be identified in consecutive frames), which may not be true when out of plane motion occurs. Because speckle tracking relies on sufficiently high temporal resolution, TDI may prove advantageous when evaluating patients with higher heart rates (i.e., during stress echocardiography) or if short-lived events need to be tracked (isovolumic phases, diastole, etc.). Validation studies on 2-dimensional speckle tracking echocardiography (2DSE) suggest that the method is reliable and angle-independent. [55, 56].

Longitudinal and Circumferential Mechanics: During preejection, reshaping of LV geometry causes simultaneous shortening and stretch of the early and the late activated regions, respectively. Thus, shortening of subendocardial fibers is accompanied by simultaneous subepicardial fiber stretching. Segmental stretch may also be seen in the late activated regions of the subendocardium, particularly near the base posterolateral region, which is the last area of the ventricle to activate. The onset of longitudinal and circumferential shortening therefore shows substantial transmural and apex-to-base heterogeneity. Subendocardial and subepicardial layers shorten concurrently during ejection. The magnitude of circumferential strains during ejection exceeds that of longitudinal strains. Furthermore, longitudinal and circumferential shortening strains during ejection show a small apex-to-base gradient, such that successive shortening strains are higher at apical and mid segments compared with the LV base. Acute ischemia produces, within a few minutes, a local reduction in myocardial contractility. In studies looking at strain and SR during coronary angioplasty, typical changes could be found that were shown to have high sensitivity and specificity for the diagnosis of ischemia. During acute ischemic insult, there is a decrease in peak systolic strain (longitudinal and radial) and a decrease in peak systolic SR. In addition, segmental relaxation is impaired, resulting in loss of the early diastolic thinning and lengthening. These are replaced by local early diastolic thickening and shortening, known as post- systolic strain. [53, 54] Several studies have shown that the combination of reduced peak systolic strain with significant increase in post- systolic strain is a highly sensitive marker for acute ischemia.

Automatic Function Imaging (AFI) or Bidimensional Myocardial Deformation

This technique derives from speckle tracking. It is also known as non-Doppler 2D Strain imaging and is a new echocardiographic technique that allows the measurement of myocardial strain and strain rate. It analyzes motion by tracking speckles in the ultrasonic image in two dimensions and requires only one cardiac cycle to be acquired. Further processing and interpretation can be done after image data acquisition.

Because AFI is not based on tissue Doppler measurements, it is angle independent. 2D strain images are quickly achieved. This technique may prove to be of significant clinical value, enabling rapid and accurate assessment of global and segmental myocardial function.

The end-systolic frame is first defined in the apical long-axis (3-chamber) view, where the aortic valve is directly visible. Aortic valve closure time is marked. The software then measures the R wave to aortic valve closure time. Subsequently, the same R wave to aortic valve closure time distance is used as a reference on the other loops. The time distance is also checked against the mitral valve opening, which is easily seen in any apical plane. This allows accurate timing of systole, diastole, and aortic valve closure on all views. [57]

Within the end-systolic frames, an estimation of the LV myocardium is traced in a click-to-point approach. Subsequently, the software automatically defines an epicardial and mid myocardial line and processes all frames of the loop. Endocardial border is identified by edge detection, based on black-and-white transition recognition on a single frame. The myocardium is defined by empiric estimation of myocardial thickness and can then be further corrected by the operator. Motion is evaluated by tracking speckles (natural acoustic markers) in the ultrasonic image in two dimensions. By tracking the entire LV myocardium, the new border is determined without the need for repeated border location by edge detection. On all apical views, end-diastolic volume, end-systolic volume and EF are calculated based on the modified Simpson's rule. Motion and velocities are then analyzed by calculating frame-to-frame changes. The final result showing is a continuous cineloop, tracking the acoustic markers and superimposing color points on the gray scale image. A visual control for the individual tracking quality is directly performed thereafter.

Tracking quality is based on several criteria:

- each speckle is followed for several consecutive frames forward and backward. Return to baseline coordinates is considered evidence for adequate tracking.
- adjacent speckles (that are in close proximity within the tissue) are assumed to have similar velocities. If a significant difference in tissue velocities is detected, the software rejects the tracking.
- the software evaluates the drift compensation that is required.

The strain at the beginning and the end of a cardiac cycle should be the same. The larger the required drift compensation, the lower the tracking quality scores. The automatically obtained tracking process may be accepted or rejected by the reader.

The myocardium in each of the 3 standard apical planes is automatically divided into 6 segments, and the analyzed values within the middle points for all resulting 18 segments are shown as traces in specific diagrams. These diagrams can display different parameters (strain, SR, displacement, velocities), which are all derived from the instantaneous angle-independent speckle velocities. [58] The resulting signal is a continuous tracking cineloop. (Figure 4).

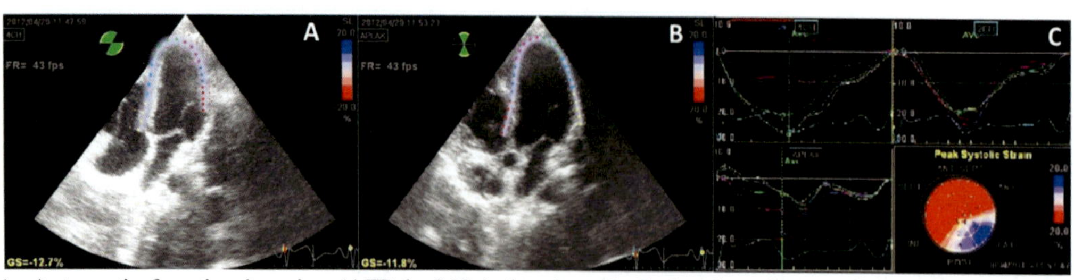

A: Automatic function imaging (AFI) in LV 4 chamber; B: 5 chamber views and C: strain waves and bull eye.

Figure 4. Shows the myocardial deformation in left ventricle with new technics.

The greatest advantages of AFI are that it analyzes wall motion in real time and allows an automatic assessment of ventricular function. It simultaneously obtains the curved anatomical M mode and it´s scale deformation. (Figure 5)

It also shows deformation waves in time of each region and a dotted average wave.

Bidimensional myocardial deformation gives information about systolic and diastolic function in three dimensions: longitudinal, radial and circumferential; and it can be measured both regional or globally. [59]

During ventricular systole, longitudinal fibers shorten towards the apex while radial fibers thicken. Circumferential fibers converge towards the center, decreasing its axis. [60]

Longitudinal deformation images are acquired from apical views.

Longitudinal deformation is larger in apical than in base segments. Radial and circumferential deformation images should be achieved in transversal minor axis views. The incidence of major events is significantly higher in patients with biventricular dysfunction rather than in isolated left ventricular dysfunction (45% versus 11%, $p < 0.0001$). [61, 62]

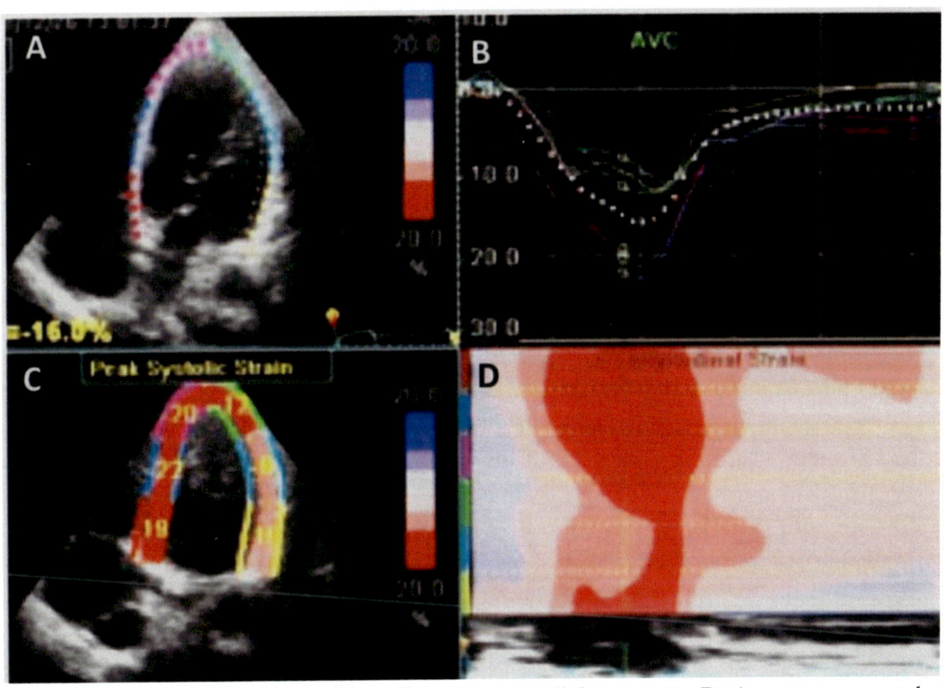

A: Tracked apical loop with color-coding of the 6-myocardial segments. B: Average segmental strain graphically displaced. Each color line corresponds to the same color-coded myocardial segment. C: Color display of peak systolic strain. Color scale shown on the right corner. D: M mode representation of peak systolic strain. Myocardial segments are color-coded, strain color scale same as in C.

Figure 5. The Left ventricular dysfunction in a patient with surgically repaired ventricular septal defect (VSD). In Apical 4-chamber "quad" view.

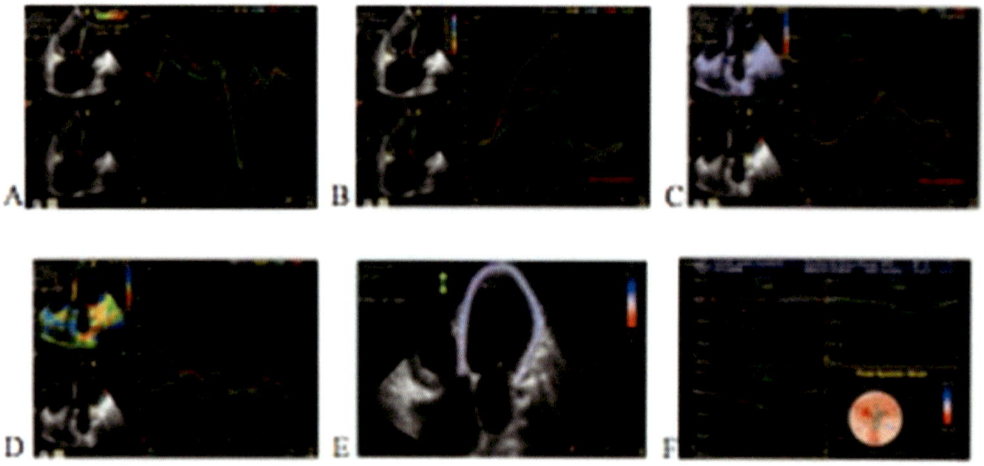

A-TSI: shows apical dyssynchrony. B- Tissue Track: normal. C- The Strain is opponent at base, mid and apical level in LV. D- The Strain rate is opponent at the three levels. E- 2D myocardial deformation in LV. F- The Bull eye shows the LV dysfunction.

Figure 6. Severe LV dysfunction in a surgically repaired VSD:

Peak strain is assessed in 16 LV segments at aortic valve closure (peak systolic strain). Peak systolic strain from each segment is average to global longitudinal strain (GLS) from a 16-segment LV model.

It is possible to obtain all of the following functions derived from a TDI color loop: TSI (time synchronic image), Tissue track (longitudinal movement), Strain (myocardial deformation), Strain rate (myocardial deformation in time). Speckle tracking permits the analysis of bidimensional myocardial deformation, as is shown in the example of a surgically repaired VSD with severe biventricular dysfunction. (Figure 6).

Electromechanical dyssynchrony is an important consequence of and contributor to ventricular dysfunction. [63, 64] Echocardiography can be useful to assess the mechanisms underlying mechanical dyssynchrony, to evaluate the impact of mechanical dyssynchrony on ventricular function, and to try to predict the therapeutic response to cardiac resynchronization therapy (CRT).

Regional bidimensional myocardial deformation represents the regional ejection fraction (EF), while end systolic global deformation represents left ventricular EF. There is a significant correlation between apical view 4-chamber peak systolic global longitudinal strain and Magnetic Resonance Imaging left ventricular EF (in the pathologic adult population). [65].

The most important benefit of STE in the pediatric age range is the angle independence and lack of geometric assumptions. [66] Mechanical dyssynchrony has been demonstrated in several pediatric acquired and congenital cardiac conditions, but experience is still limited. Understanding mechanisms of electromechanical dyssynchrony by echocardiography seems promising, at least in left bundle branch block (LBBB), but may be limited in children due to the uncommon occurrence of LBBB in this population. [67].

LV Torsion

LV torsion is due to the contraction of subepicardial oblique fibers towards the apex with a counterclockwise rotation. In contrast, subendocardial fibers rotate clockwise.

By convention, counterclockwise rotation is displayed as positive when viewed from the apex. In the normal heart, there is a wringing motion with an early counterclockwise and then more dominant clockwise rotation at the base, and counterclockwise rotation at the apex during systole. [68] This motion results in a net gradient between the base–apex and it is referred to as net LV twist and is expressed in degrees (°). [69]

LV torsion seems to have an important role in normal systolic function and the diastolic "detorsion" allows a normal LV filling by a suction mechanism. Diminished LV "detorsion" with less diastolic suction contributes to diastolic dysfunction in sick hearts.

Tetralogy of Fallot (TOF)

The Right Ventricle (RV) responds with spherical dilatation to volume over load and with hypertrophy to pressure over load. [70] The knowledge of RV remodeling is important for understanding its response and discovering the mechanisms of ventricular dysfunction.

TOF patients develop not only dilatation of the RV but also, to a lesser degree, of the LV and with lower EF in both cases; there is also rectification of the interventricular septum, suggesting interdependency of both ventricles.

In these patients RV has an increased end diastolic area at the expense of the free wall. (Figure 7) Muscle fibers distribution generates a mid ventricular muscular waist that only allows ventricular dilatation in the base and apical area. [70] The interventricular septum occupies less space and the apex of the heart becomes rounded.

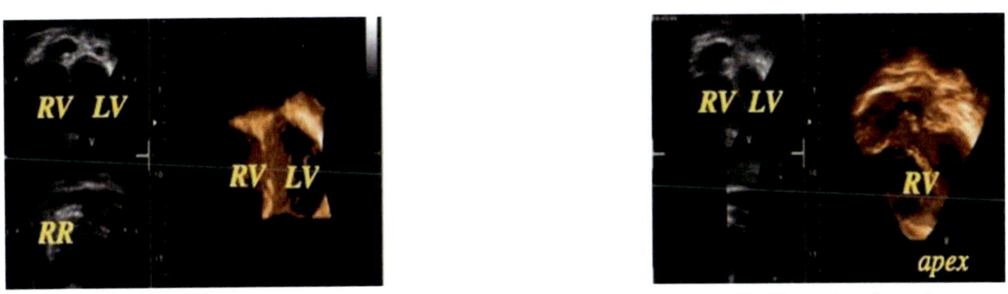

A: Transversal view B: Four chamber view.

The interventricular septum occupies less space. The apex of the heart becomes rounded.

Figure 7. 3D echo: TOF with right ventricle dilatation in short axis view and four-chamber view.

63 patients with severe pulmonary regurgitation after surgical correction of tetralogy of Fallot were studied in our hospital by echocardiographic assessment of the right and left ventricular systolic function in response to volume overload. [71, 72].

The median (X) age of the group was: 14±4y, surgical correction was done at X: 2.7±1y. The patients were divided into 3 groups depending on end diastolic volume overload of the right ventricle secondary to pulmonary regurgitation: 1) RV less than100ml/m2; 2) RV 100-120 ml/m2; and 3) RV more than120ml/m2

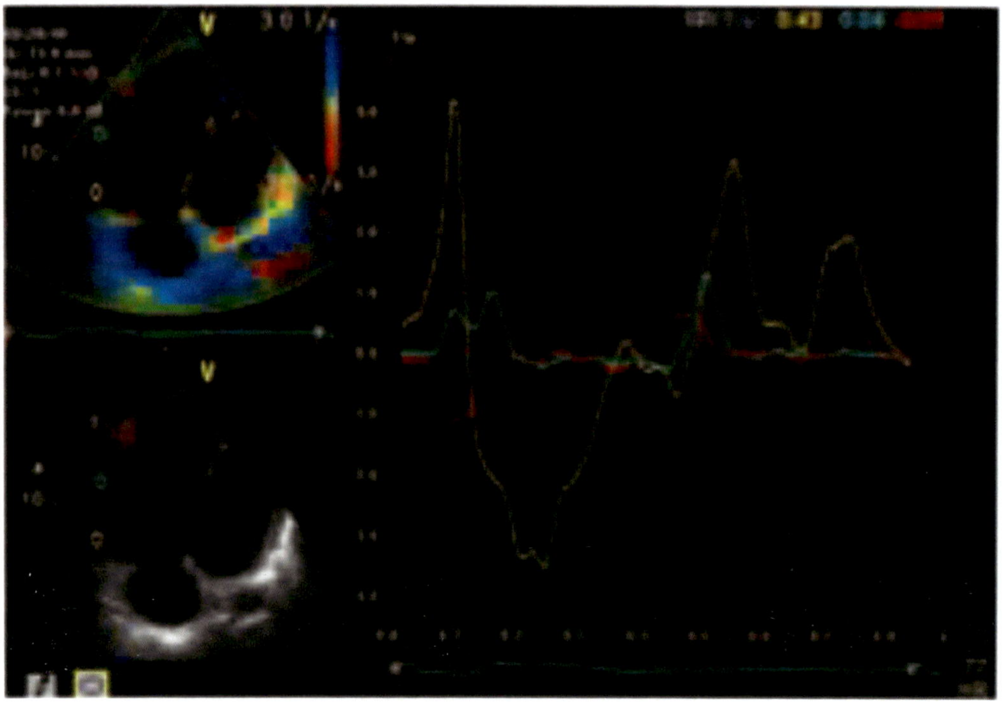

A: TDI: the sample in mid RV showing decreased systolic and diastolic peak velocities waves.
B: decreased mid RV strain and strain rate, and normal waves in base RV.

Figure 8. First group: *mild RV volume overload* secondary to pulmonary regurgitation.

Echocardiographic evaluation of myocardial function was assessed using new techniques: two-dimensional speckle tracking, longitudinal strain and strain rate of the right and left ventricle. The X follow-up was: 11.8±6y.

The first group (RV less than 100ml/m2) with mild RV volume overload secondary to pulmonary regurgitation showed decreased mid RV tissue Doppler systolic velocity (S'), diastolic E' wave and isovolumic acceleration time, with minimal RV two-dimensional speckle tracking dysfunction and altered mid RV Strain and Strain Rate. Annular TDI was not affected, with normal Strain and Strain Rate waves at base RV. (Figure 8).

The second group with moderate overload (RV 100-120 ml/m2): evidenced both right and left dysfunction. RV TDI showed decreased systolic and diastolic peak waves at base and mid RV, including diastolic E/A inversion. It also demonstrated more positive strain values and SR opponent waves in base and mid RV; with opponent base strain and strain rate waves in the left ventricle. Figure 9.

The third group with severe overload (RV more than120ml/m2): showed the same tissue Doppler affection in RV and LV, including E/A ratio inversion in the right ventricle.

A decreased E' wave is one of the earliest markers of diastolic dysfunction and is present in all stages of diastolic dysfunction. Base and mid right ventricle strain turned more positive with opponent strain rate waves. Base and mid left ventricle strain rate turned opponent to normal display. (Figure10).

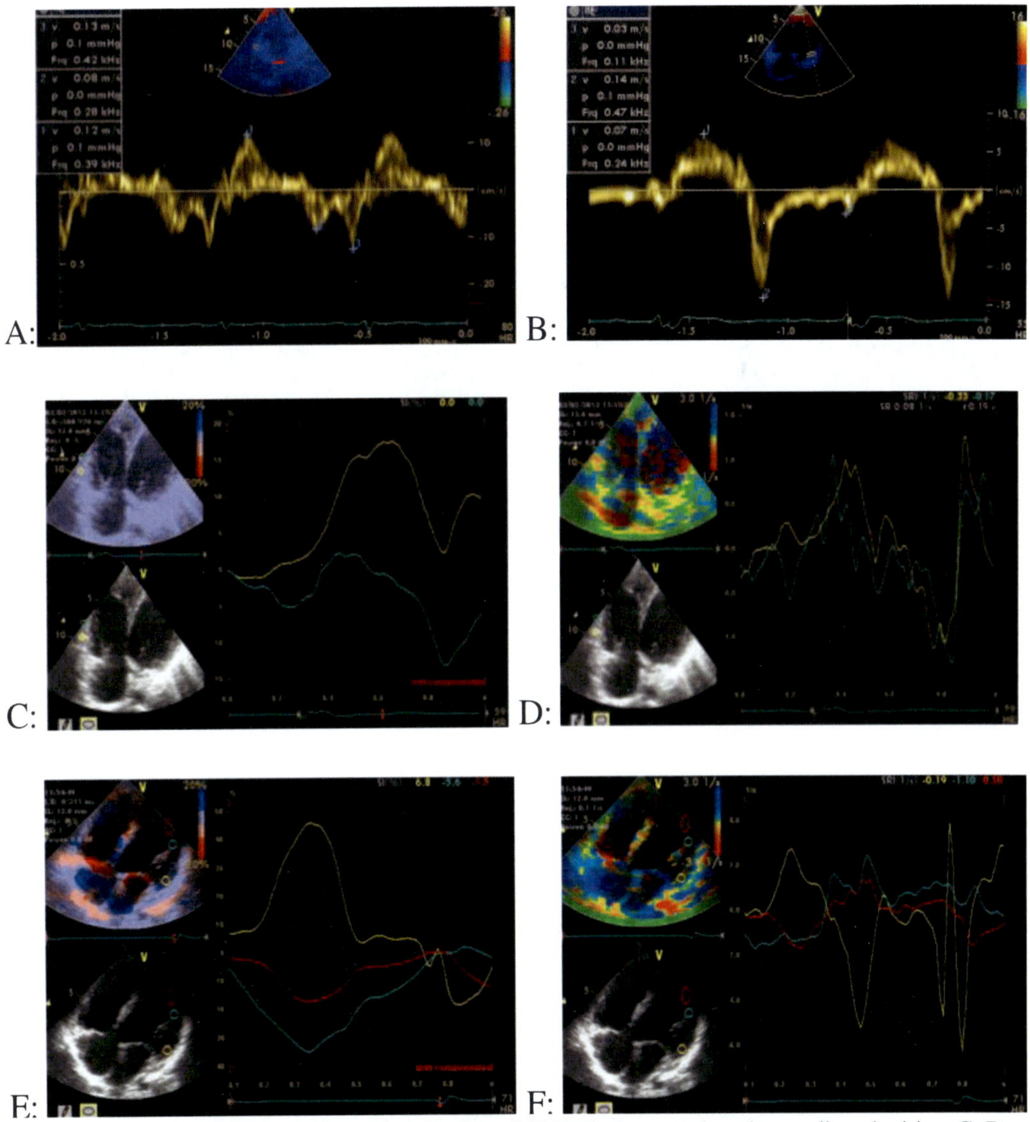

A: Base RV TDI: diastolic E/A inversion. B: Base LV TDI: decreased peak systolic velocities. C: Base and mid RV strain opponent. D: Base and mid RV Strain rate. E: Base LV: Strain, positive waves. F: Strain Rate, opponent base waves.

Figure 9. In presence of moderate to severe overload: base RV and LV function is affected.

2D speckle tracking echocardiography showed longitudinal and circumferential strain measurements, evidencing the severity of the pulmonary regurgitation overload. In the first group with RV <100 ml/m2, two-dimensional speckle tracking showed only a slight alteration in right ventricle function (average -17%), with normal values in the left ventricle or minimal repercussion.

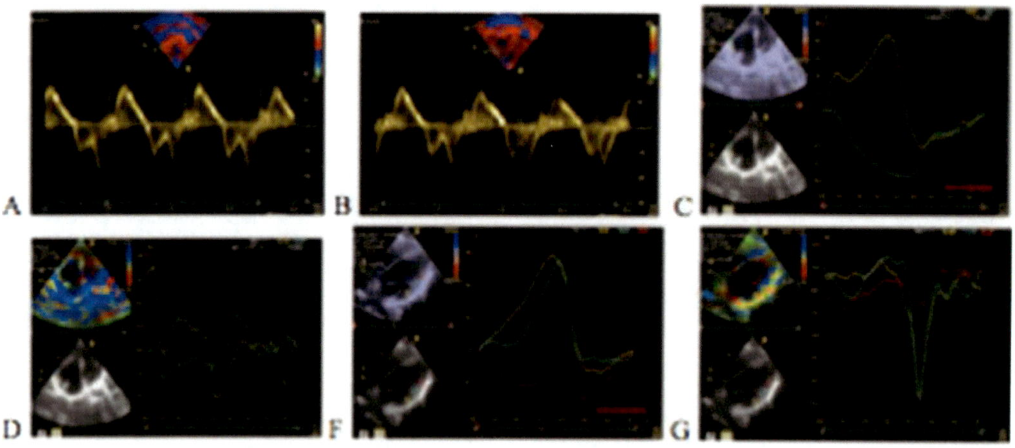

A: sample at base RV TDI shows inversion of E'/A' ratio. B: the sample at mid RV, shows TDI with inversion E'/A' ratio. C: sample at Base RV shows opponent strain. D: sample at Base RV shows opponent strain rate. F: samples at base and mid LV, shows opponent strain. G: samples at base and mid LV, shows opponent strain rate.

Figure 10. In presence of severe overload: base RV and LV function is affected.

However, when the overload increased, the dysfunction was seen first in the RV; 2D speckle tracking then showed left ventricular dysfunction as well, with strain and strain rate anormal in base and mid LV. Figure 10.

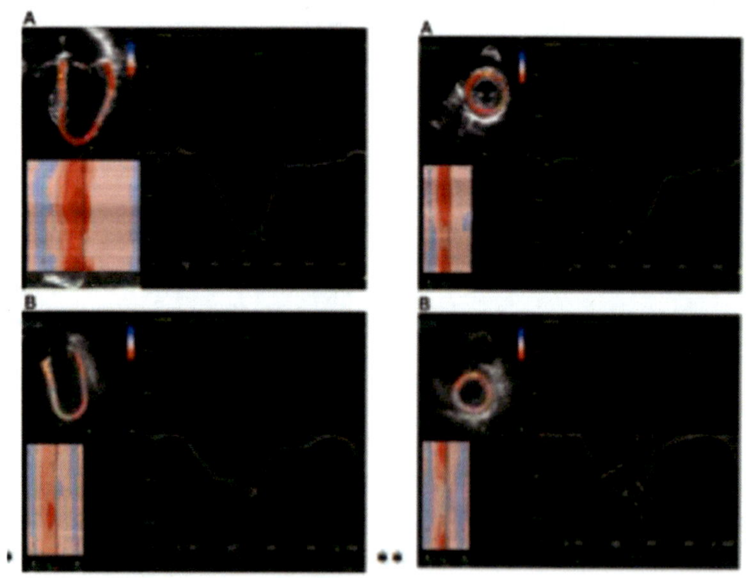

*Longitudinal: **Circumferential:

2D speckle tracking echocardiography: (A) On the right side, longitudinal view and on the left, circumferential view in a normal child. (B) After repair of TOF: on the right, LV longitudinal strain; on the left, circumferential view of peak strain and time to peak strain in various segments. The dotted white line in both represents the global average of the segmental strain.

Figure 11. LV longitudinal and circumferential strain measured by 2D speckle tracking echocardiography.

In this example, LV longitudinal and circumferential Strain are measured by 2D speckle tracking. The peak strain and time to peak strain in different segments are shown.

The white arrows indicate the peak strain in multiple segments.

Note the lower circumferential strain in patients with TOF in the posterior and inferior segments as compare with the healthy patients.

This was a common finding. The dotted white line represents the global circumferential strain (the average of the segmental strains). [73].

When the overload was severe (RV more than 120 ml/m2), the left ventricle showed significant repercussion. (Figure 12)

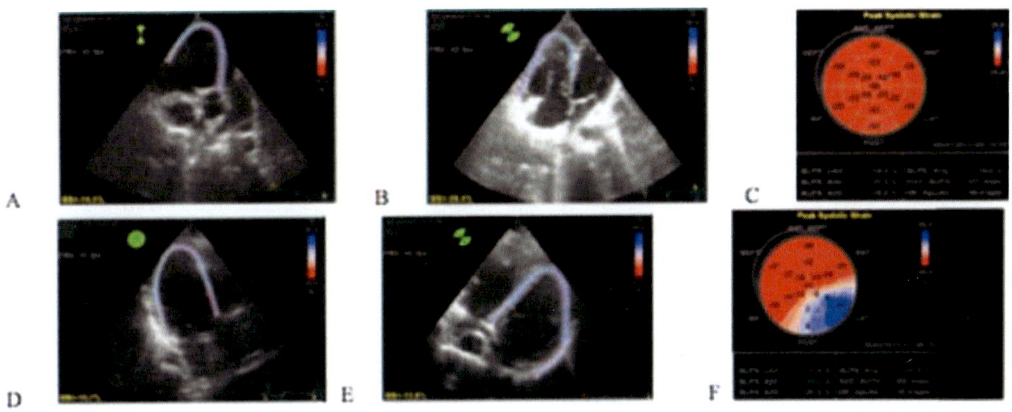

In moderate overload: the dysfunction started in the RV outlet (A) with moderate alteration of the RV 2D speckle tracking in four-chamber view. (B) While the left ventricle showed little repercussion in the bull's eye (C).

In severe overload: the right (D) and the left ventricle (E) showed severe repercussion in the 2D speckle tracking as shown in the bull eye shows (F).

Figure 12. 2D speckle tracking echocardiograph: in a patients with moderate (A, B, C) and severe (D, E, F) overload secondary to pulmonary regurgitation.

The same observation of the direct relationship between the RV and the LV ejection fraction affection due to the right overload was evidenced in 2D speckle tracking echocardiography. When the overload was severe in the RV, the dysfunction in the left ventricle was severe as well.

RV end-systolic volume index <90 mL/m^2 and QRS duration <140 ms are associated with optimal postoperative outcome (normal RV size and function), and RV ejection fraction <45% and QRS duration ≥160 ms are associated with suboptimal postoperative outcome (RV dilatation and dysfunction). The regional myocardial deformation may be altered and can be prospectively evaluated from echocardiography-derived speckle-tracking analysis to measure myocardial strain and provide direct information about the contractile performance of the right ventricle. [64].

RV basal wall peak diastolic velocity tended to be lower for the patients with restrictive physiology, likely reflecting impaired relaxation of the noncompliant right ventricle. Likewise, their peak RV basal and mid wall diastolic strain rates were higher than those with nonrestrictive physiology, with values similar to those recently reported by Friedberg et al., [65] and decreased in comparison with controls.

These regional trends may be related to chronic volume overload of the right ventricle from pulmonary regurgitation (PR), which is greater for those with restrictive physiology (46% vs 28%, P = .002). [66].

RV end diastolic volume (EDV) indexed to body surface area, RV EDV ≥160 ml/m2 (Z score >5) and RV end-systolic volume (ESV) indexed to body surface area, RV ESV ≥70 ml/m2, predicted poor RV remodeling and recovery of RV function after pulmonary valve replacement (PVR). Likewise, LV ESV less than 65 ml/m2, RV EF less than 45% and aneurism in outlet RV are predictors of poor outcomes.

- RV ESV is a strong independent predictor of decreased RV EF (OR= 5.3 for each 10 ml/m2 increase)
- RV dysfunction is a strong independent predictor of a worse functional score (OR for a score ≥4= 4.33 for each decrease 10%).
- Other independent predictors of a worse score are: age at TOF repair (>3 years), decreased LV EDV; repaired TOF or similar physiology with moderate or severe pulmonary regurgitation (PR) with regurgitation fraction of ≥25% by MRI and ≥2 of the following criteria: RV EDV ≥160 ml/m2 (Z score >5), RV ESV ≥70 ml/m2, LV EDV ≤65 ml/m2, RV EF ≤45%; and RV outflow aneurysm. Clinical criteria included: exercise intolerance, heart failure, symptoms, syncope, and sustained ventricular tachycardia. Additional hemodynamic burden: ≥ moderate tricuspid regurgitation, residual VSD, and severe aortic regurgitation. QRS duration, RV end-systolic volume, or RV ejection fraction are useful criteria in determining the need for PVR. The elimination of sources of RV volume overload does not always permit total recovery of the left and right ventricular function. Elimination of PR was associated with a marked reduction in RV EDV and RV ESV, unchanged RV EF and increased LV EDV, and unchanged exercise parameters but significant improvements in symptoms and functional status. RV remodeling after PVR was not associated with a measurable benefit 6 months after surgery [73]. In our experience, RV remodeling occurs within the first 2 to 4 years after PVR.

  After Pulmonary Valve Replacement (PVR), some patients recover RV function but persist with LV dysfunction. (Figure 13).

  New echo technology can identify early LV repercussion. Early PVR may be the new criteria in the prevention of irreversible LV damage when dysfunction is detected through the use of this technology.

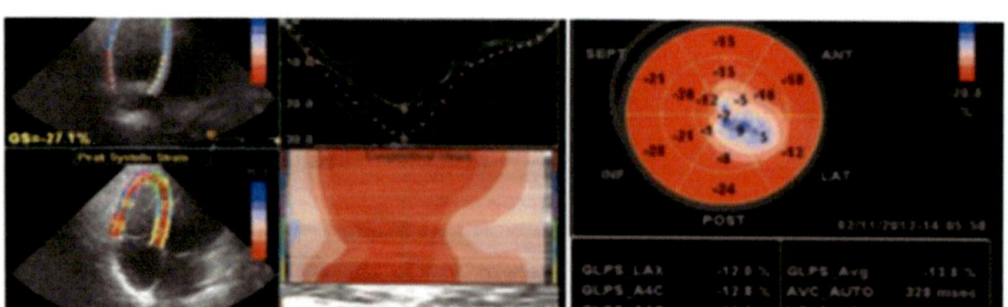

RV normal LV abnormal.

Figure 13. Post PVR: normalized RV 2D speckle tracking, still LV dysfunction.

References

[1] Lipshultz SE, Miller TL. Establishing norms for echocardiographic measurements of cardiovascular structures and function in children. *J. Appl. Physiol.* 2005; 99: 386-88.

[2] Lopez L, Colan SD, Frommelt PC et al., Recommendations for quantification methods during the performance of a pediatric echocardiogram: a report from the Pediatric Measurements Writing Group of the American Society of Echocardiography Pediatric and Congenital Heart Disease Council. *J. Am. Soc. Echocardiogr.* 2010; 23: 465-95.

[3] Mawad W, Drolet C, Dahdah N et al., A review and critique of the statistical methods used to generate reference values in pediatric echocardiography. *J. Am. Soc. Echocardiogr.* 2013; 26: 29-37.

[4] Ghio S, Recusani F, Klersy C et al., Prognostic usefulness of the tricuspid annular plane systolic excursion in patients with congestive heart failure secondary to idiopathic or ischemic dilated cardiomyopathy. *Am. J. Cardiol.* 2000; 85: 837-42.

[5] Leary PJ, Kurtz CE, Hough CL et al., Three-dimensional analysis of right ventricular shape and function in pulmonary hypertension. Pulmonary Circulation (online). April 2012; 2: 34-40. Available at http://www.pulmonarycirculation.org/article DOI: 10.4103/2045-8932.94828 5.

[6] Lopez-Candales A, Rajagopalan N, Saxena N et al., Right ventricular systolic function is not the sole determinant of tricuspid annular motion. *Am. J. Cardiol.* 2006; 98: 973-77.

[7] Desai MY, Klein AL. Assessment of diastolic function by echocardiography. In: Otto CM, ed. The practice of clinical echocardiography. 3rd. Edition. Philadelphia, PA: Saunders Elsevier, 2007: 237-261.

[8] Gorcsan J III, Strum DP, Mandarino WA, Gulati VK, Pinsky MR. Quantitative assessment of alterations in regional left ventricular contractility with color-coded tissue Doppler echocardiography. *Circulation* 1997;95: 2423-33.

[9] Dalsgaard M, Snyder EM, Kjaergaard J et al., Isovolumic acceleration measured by tissue Doppler echocardiography is preload independent in healthy subjects. *Echocardiography* 2007: 24: 572-79. DOI:10.1111/j.1540-8175.2007.00454.x.

[10] Vogel M, Cheung MM, Li J, et al: Non invasive assessment of left ventricular force-frequency relationship using tissue Doppler-derived isovolumic acceleration. Validation in an animal model. *Circulation* 2003; 107(12): 1647–52.

[11] Levantini F, Gonzalez G, Vaccari M, et al., Doppler Tisular Normal en edad pediátrica. *Rev. Arg. de Cardiol.* 2010. Vol. 78. Sup 2: 101.

[12] Roberson DA, Cui W, Chen Z, Madronero LF, Cuneo BF. Annular and septal Doppler tissue imaging in children: Normal *z-score*. Tables and effects of age, heart rate, and body surface area. *J. Am. Soc. Echocardiogr.* 2007; 20: 1276-84.

[13] Pauliks L. Tissue Doppler myocardial velocity imaging in infants and children- a window into developmental changes of myocardial mechanics. *Echocardiography* 2013; 30: 439-46.

[14] Eidem BW, McMahon CJ, Cohen RR et al., Impact of cardiac growth on Doppler tissue imaging velocities: a study in healthy children. *J. Am. Soc. Echocardiogr.* 2004; 17: 212-21.

[15] Hees PS, Fleg JL, Dong SJ, Shapiro EP. MRI and echocardiographic assessment of the diastolic dysfunction of normal aging: altered LV pressure decline or load? *Am. J. Physiol. – Heart Circ. Physiol.* 2004; 286: H782-88 DOI: 10.1152/ajpheart. 01092.2002

[16] Cannesson M, Jacques D, Pinsky MR, Gorcsan J III. Effects of modulation of left ventricular contractile state and loading conditions on tissue Doppler myocardial performance index. *Am. J. Physiol. – Heart Circ. Physiol.* 2006; 290: H1952-59. DOI: 10.1152/ajpheart.01090.2005.

[17] Hsiao SH, Huang WC, Sy CL, Lin SK, Lee TY, Liu CP. Doppler tissue imaging and color M-mode flow propagation velocity: are they really preload independent? *J. Am. Soc. Echocardiogr.* 2005; 18: 1277-84.

[18] Yu CM, Sanderson JE, Marwick TH, Oh JK. Tissue Doppler imaging. A new prognosticator for cardiovascular diseases. *J. Am. Coll. Cardiol.* 2007; 49: 1903–14.

[19] Pauliks LB, Undar A, Clark JB, Myers JL. Segmental differences of impaired diastolic relaxation following cardiopulmonary bypass surgery in children: a tissue Doppler study. *Artif. Organs* 2009; 33: 904-08.

[20] Pauliks LB, Pietra BA, DeGroff CG et al., Non-invasive detection of acute allograft rejection in children by tissue Doppler imaging: myocardial velocities and myocardial acceleration during isovolumic contraction. *J. Heart Lung Transplant* 2005; 24 (7 Suppl): S239–48.

[21] Fyfe DA, Ketchum D, Lewis R et al., Tissue Doppler imaging detects severely abnormal myocardial velocities that identify children with pre-terminal cardiac graft failure after heart transplantation. J Heart Lung Transplant 2006; 25: 510–17.

[22] Lunze FI, Colan SD, Gauvreau K et al., Cardiac allograft function during the first year after transplantation in rejection-free children and young adults. *Circ. Cardiovasc. Imaging* 2012; 5: 756–64.

[23] Pauliks LB, Chan KC, Chang D et al., Regional myocardial velocities and isovolumic contraction acceleration before and after device closure of atrial septal defects: a color tissue Doppler study. *Am. Heart J.* 2005: 150: 294-301.

[24] Vogel M, Sponring J, Cullen S, Deanfield JE, Redington AN. Regional wall motion and abnormalities of electrical depolarization and repolarization in patients after surgical repair of tetralogy of Fallot. *Circulation* 2001; 103: 1669–73.

[25] Roche SL, Grosse-Wortmann L, Redington AN et al., Exercise induces biventricular mechanical dyssynchrony in children with repaired tetralogy of Fallot. *Heart* 2010; 96: 2010–15.

[26] Shiina Y, Funabashi N, Lee K et al., Right atrium contractility and right ventricular diastolic function assessed by pulsed tissue Doppler imaging can predict brain natriuretic peptide in adults with acquired pulmonary hypertension. *Int. J. Cardiol.* 2009; 135: 53–59.

[27] Harada K, Toyono M, Yamamoto F: Assessment of right ventricular function during exercise with quantitative Doppler tissue imaging in children late after repair of tetralogy of Fallot. *J. Am. Soc. Echocardiogr.* 2004; 17: 863–869.

[28] Brili S, Stamatopoulos I, Barbetseas J et al., Usefulness of dobutamine stress echocardiography with tissue Doppler imaging for the evaluation and follow-up of patients with repaired tetralogy of Fallot. *J. Am. Soc. Echocardiogr.* 2008; 21: 1093–98.

[29] Rentzsch A, Abd El Rahman MY, Hui W et al., Assessment of myocardial function of the systemic right ventricle in patients with D-transposition of the great arteries after atrial switch operation by tissue Doppler echocardiography. *Z Kardiol* 2005; 94: 524-31.

[30] Khoo NS, Smallhorn JF, Kaneko S, Myers K, Kutty S, Tham EB. Novel insights into RV adaptation and function in hypoplastic left heart syndrome between the first 2 stages of surgical palliation. *J. Am. Coll. Cardiol. Img* 2011; 4: 128–37. doi:10.1016/j.jcmg.2010.09.022.

[31] Rhodes J, Margossian R, Sleeper LA et al., Non-geometric echocardiographic indices of ventricular function in patients with a Fontan circulation. *J. Am. Soc. Echocardiogr.* 2011; 24: 1213–19.

[32] Lindqvist P, Waldenström A, Henein M, Mörner S, Kazzam E. Regional and global right ventricular function in healthy individuals aged 20–90 years: A pulsed Doppler tissue imaging study Umeå General Population Heart Study. *Echocardiography* 2005; 22: 305–14.

[33] Nageh MF, Kopelen HA, Zoghbi WA, Quinones MA, Nagueh SF. Estimation of mean right atrial pressure using tissue Doppler imaging. *Am. J. Cardiol.* 1999; 84:1448–1451

[34] Nagueh SF, Sun H, Kopelen HA, Middleton KJ, Khoury DS. Hemodynamic determinants of the mitral annulus diastolic velocities by tissue Doppler. *J. Am. Coll. Cardiol.* 2001; 37(1): 278-285.

[35] Sohn DW, Chai IH, Lee DJ et al., Assessment of mitral annulus velocity by Doppler tissue imaging in the evaluation of left ventricular diastolic function. *J. Am. Coll. Cardiol.* 1997; 30: 474–80.

[36] Ommen SR, Nishimura RA, Appleton CP, et al., Clinical utility of Doppler echocardiography and tissue Doppler imaging in the estimation of left ventricular filling pressures: a comparative simultaneous Doppler-catheterization study. *Circulation* 2000; 102: 1788–94.

[37] Yamamoto T, Oki T, Yamada H, et al., Prognostic value of the atrial systolic mitral annular motion velocity in patients with left ventricular systolic dysfunction. *J. Am. Soc. Echocardiogr.* 2003; 16: 333–9.

[38] Eidem BW, Tei C, O'Leary PW, Cetta F, Seward JB. Nongeometric quantitative assessment of right and left ventricular function: myocardial performance index in normal children and patients with Ebstein anomaly. *J. Am. Soc. Echocardiogr.* 1998; 11: 849–56.

[39] Hsiao SH, Yang SH, Wang WC, Lee CY, Lin SK, Liu CP. Usefulness of regional myocardial performance index to diagnose pulmonary embolism in patients with echocardiographic signs of pulmonary hypertension. *Am. J. Cardiol.* 2006; 98: 1652–55.

[40] Goldstein JA. Pathophysiology and management of right heart ischemia. *J. Am. Coll. Cardiol.* 2002; 40:841-853.

[41] Tei C, Dujardin KS, Hodge DO et al., Doppler echocardiographic index for assessment of global right ventricular function. *J. Am. Soc. Echocardiogr.* 1996; 9: 838-47.

[42] Miller D, Farah MG, Liner A et al., The relation between quantitative right ventricular ejection fraction and indices of tricuspid annular motion and myocardial performance. *J. Am. Soc. Echocardiogr.* 2004; 17: 443-47.

[43] Ghio S, Gavazzi A, Campana C et al., Independent and additive prognostic value of right ventricular systolic function and pulmonary artery pressure in patients with chronic heart failure. *J. Am. Coll. Cardiol.* 2001; 37: 183-88.

[44] Hoffmann R, Lethen H, Marwick T et al., Analysis of interinstitutional observer agreement in interpretation of dobutamine stress echocardiograms. *J. Am. Coll. Cardiol.* 1996; 27: 330-36.

[45] Kvitting JPE, Wigström L, Strotmann JM, Sutherland GR. How accurate is visual assessment of synchronicity in myocardial motion? An in vitro study with computer-simulated regional delay in myocardial motion: clinical implications for rest and stress Echocardiography studies. *J. Am. Soc. Echocardiogr.* 1999; 12: 698-05.

[46] Greenberg NL, Firstenberg MS, Castro PL, Main M, Travaglini A, Oda- bashian JA, et al., Doppler-derived myocardial systolic strain rate is a strong index of left ventricular contractility. *Circulation* 2002; 105: 99-105.

[47] Gorcsan J III, Deswal A, Mankad S et al., Quantification of the myocardial response to low-dose dobutamine using tissue Doppler echocardiographic measures of velocity and velocity gradient. *Am. J. Cardiol.* 1998; 81: 615-23.

[48] Lorch SM, Ludomirsky A Singh GK. Maturational and growth-related changes in left ventricular longitudinal strain and strain rate measured by two-dimensional speckle tracking echocardiography in healthy pediatric population. *J. Am. Soc. Echocardiogr.* 2008; 21: 1207-15.

[49] Ingels NB Jr, Hansen DE, Daughters GT 2nd, Stinson EB, Alderman EL, Miller DC. Relation between longitudinal, circumferential, and oblique shortening and torsional deformation in the left ventricle of the trans- planted human heart. *Circ. Res.* 1989; 64: 915-27.

[50] Liu W, Ashford MW, Chen J, Watkins MP, Williams TA, Wickline SA et al., MR tagging demonstrates quantitative differences in regional ventricular wall motion in mice, rats, and men. *Am. J. Physiol. Heart Circ. Physiol.* 2006; 291: H2515-21.

[51] Korinek J, Wang J, Sengupta PP et al., Two-dimensional strain-a Doppler-independent ultrasound method for quantitation of regional deformation: validation in vitro and in vivo. *J. Am. Soc. Echocardiogr.* 2005; 18: 1247-53.

[52] Kukulski T, Jamal F, D'hooge J, Bijnens B, De Scheerder I, Shuterland GR. Acute changes in systolic and diastolic events during clinical coronary angioplasty: A comparison of regional velocity, strain rate, and strain measurement. *J. Am. Soc. Echocardiogr.* 2002; 15: 1-12.

[53] Voigt JU, Lindenmeier G, Exner B et al., Incidence and characteristics of segmental postsystolic longitudinal shortening in normal, acutely ischemic and scarred myocardium. *J. Am. Soc. Echocardiogr.* 2003; 16: 415-23.

[54] Leitman M, Lysyansky P, Sidenko S, et al., Two-dimensional strain—a novel software for real-time quantitative echocardiographic assessment of myocardial function. *J. Am. Soc. Echocardiogr.* 2004; 17: 1021-9.

[55] Toyoda T, Baba H, Akasaka T et al., Assessment of regional myocardial strain by a novel automated tracking system from digital image files. *J. Am. Soc. Echocardiogr.* 2004; 17: 1234-38.

[56] Perk G, Tunick PA, Kronzon I. Non-Doppler two-dimensional strain imaging by echocardiography –from technical considerations to clinical applications. *J. Am. Soc. Echocardiogr.* 2007; 20: 234-43.

[57] La Vecchia L, Paccanaro M, Bonnano C, Varotto L, Ometto R, Vincenzi M. Left ventricular versus biventricular dysfunction in idiopathic dilated cardiomyopathy. *Am. J. Cardiol.* 1999; 83:120-22.

[58] Fernandes FP, Manlhiot C, Roche SL et al., Impaired left ventricular myocardial mechanics and their relation to pulmonary regurgitation, right ventricular enlargement and exercise capacity in asymptomatic children after repair of tetralogy of Fallot. *J. Am. Soc. Echocardiogr.* 2012; 25: 494-03.

[59] Sjoli B, Orn S, Grenne B, Ihlen H, Edvardsen T, Brunvand H. Diagnostic capability and reproducibility of strain by Doppler and by speckle tracking in patients with acute myocardial infarction. *J. Am. Coll. Cardiol. Img.* 2009; 2: 24–33. doi: 10.1016/j.jcmg.2008.10.007.

[60] Gjesdal O, Hopp E, Vartdal T et al., Global longitudinal strain measured by two-dimensional speckle tracking echocardiography is closely related to myocardial infarct size in chronic ischemic heart disease. *Clin. Sci. Lond.* 2007; 113: 287–96.

[61] Pirat B, McCulloch ML, Zoghbi WA. Evaluation of global and regional right ventricular systolic function in patients with pulmonary hypertension using a novel speckle tracking method. *Am. J. Cardiol.* 2006; 98: 699-04.

[62] Amundsen BH, Crosby J, Steen PA, Torp H, Slørdahl SA, Støylen A. Regional myocardial long-axis strain and strain rate measured by different tissue Doppler and speckle tracking echocardiography methods: a comparison with tagged magnetic resonance imaging. *Eur. J. Echocardiogr* 2009; 10: 229-37.

[63] Friedberg MK, Fernandes FP, Roche SL et al., Impaired right and left ventricular diastolic myocardial mechanics and filling in asymptomatic children and adolescents after repair of tetralogy of Fallot. *Eur. Heart J. Cardiovasc. Imaging* 2012; 13: 905-13.

[64] Samyn MM, Kwon EN, Gorentz JS et al., Restrictive versus nonrestrictive physiology following repair of tetralogy of Fallot: is there a difference?. *J. Am. Soc. Echocardiogr.* 2013; 26: 746-55.

[65] Brown J, Jenkins C, Marwick TH: Use of myocardial strain to assess global left ventricular function: a comparison with cardiac magnetic resonance and 3-dimensional echocardiography. *Am. Heart J.* 2009; 157: 102.e1-e5. doi: 10.1016/j.ahj.2008.08.032.

[66] Forsey J, Friedberg MK, Mertens L. Speckle Tracking Echocardiography in Pediatric and Congenital Heart Disease. *Echocardiography* 2013; 30: 447-59.

[67] Friedberg MK, Mertens L. Echocardiographic assessment of ventricular synchrony in congenital and acquired heart disease in children. *Echocardiography* 2013 Apr; 30 (4): 460-71.

[68] Takahashi K, Al Naami G, Thompson R, Inage A, Mackie AS, Smallhorn JF. Normal rotational, torsion and untwisting data in children, adolescents and young adults. *J. Am. Soc. Echocardiogr.*. 2010; 23: 286–93.

[69] Sengupta PP, Tajik AJ, Chandrasekaran K, Khandheria BK. Twist mechanics of the left ventricle: principles and application. *J. Am. Coll. Cardiol. Img* 2008; 1: 366–76.

[70] Sheehan FH, Ge Shuping, Vick III W., et al., Three-dimensional shape analysis of right ventricular remodeling in repaired tetralogy of Fallot. *Am. J. Cardiol.* 2008; 101: 107–113.

[71] de Dios A., Carugati R., Biancolini MF, Levantini Florencia, et al., Nuevas técnicas ecocardiográficas en el Fallot alejado con insuficiencia pulmonar severa para identificar disfunción ventricular. *Rev. Arg. Cardiol.* Vol. 80 Sup3- Octubre 2012: 58.

[72] Geva T, Sandweiss BM, Gauvreau K, Lock JE, Powell AJ. Factors associated with impaired clinical status in long-term survivors of tetralogy of Fallot repair evaluated by magnetic resonance imaging. *J. Am. Coll. Cardiol.* 2004: 43: 1068-74.

[73] Geva T, Gauvreau K, Powell AJ et al., Randomized trial of pulmonary valve replacement with and without right ventricular remodeling surgery. *Circulation* 2010: 122 (Suppl 1): S201-S208.

In: Congenital Heart Diseases
Editor: Raúl Cayré and José Milei
ISBN: 978-1-61122-003-2

Chapter 4

Use of Coronary Computed Tomography Angiography in the Diagnosis of Coronary Artery Anomalies

Augusto Pablo Bayol*
Instituto de Cardiología "J.F.Cabral",
Department of Radiology, Corrientes, Argentina

Abstract

Coronary artery anomalies are some of the most confusing, neglected topics in cardiology. The occurrence of coronary artery abnormalities is reported to be approximately 0.2% to 5.6 %. These anomalies are usually not symptomatic and have no clinical significance, although in some particular cases can be fatal. Recently Coronary Computed Tomography Angiography, replaces the method of choice, coronary invasive angiography, for detecting coronary anomalies, based on its ability to accurately depict the anatomy of the heart and thorax. A useful classification it is very important to understand the complex topic of coronary artery anomalies (CAAs). There are four types: Anomalies of origination and course, anomalies of intrinsic coronary arterial anatomy, anomalies of coronary termination and anomalous collateral vessels. Each tipe has differents items that are shown in correlative figures in this chapter. The Malignant type, it is also reported as anomalous origination of a coronary artery from the opposite sinus (ACAOS) with intussusception of the ectopic proximal vessel, which is the subgroup of CAAs that has the most potential for clinical repercussions, specifically sudden death in the Young. It is very important the adequate knowledge of these anomalies in order to achieve an appropriate and accurate diagnosis, that can be the key for the good prognosis of this group of patients.

* E-mail: pablobayol@hotmail.com; pablobayol@gmail.com.

Introduction

Coronary artery anomalies (CAAs) are some of the most confusing, neglected topics in cardiology [1]. The occurrence of coronary artery abnormalities in the general population is reported to be approximately 0.2% to 2 % based on the adult population [2, 3]. Angelini and coworkers [1] found a 5.6% incidence in an ad hoc study of 1950 consecutive cineangiograms to rule out coronary artery disease. These anomalies are usually not symptomatic and have no clinical significance. Although the medical community and general public are increasingly aware that coronary anomalies can be fatal [1]. Certain types of coronary artery abnormalities, the ones called malignant or hemodynamically significant [4], were related to sudden death, particularly in young athletes. According to the report of the Sudden Death Committee of the American Heart Association, approximately 19% of sudden death in athletes may be related to these anomalies [5]. Other studies also report that sudden cardiac death due to coronary anomalies, especially those which course between the root of the aorta and the pulmonary artery (range from 19% to 33% in healthy young individuals) [6, 7]. Coronary angiography and autopsy were used to detect coronary artery anomalies, but these procedures have limitations because of their invasiveness. Coronary Computed Tomography Angiography (CTA), replaces the method of choice for detecting coronary anomalies [8]. Because of its ability to accurately depict the anatomy of the heart and thorax, coronary CTA has been deemed appropriate for evaluation of coronary anomalies. In the 2010 guidelines from the American College of Cardiology and American Heart Association (ACC/AHA) for the management of adults with congenital heart disease, the use of coronary CTA is a Class I recommendation for initial screening of congenital coronary anomalies of ectopic origin in centers with expertise in such imaging [9, 10].

Definitions

Any anatomic or morphologic finding found in >1% of the general population is defined as normal. A normal variant describes an alternative, relatively unusual finding that is observed in >1% of the same population [11]. An anomaly is a morphologic feature seen in <1% of the general population [11, 12]. Angelini and col. [12] concluded that a comprehensive and widely agreed-upon scheme to define and classify Coronary Artery Anomalies should initially consider all possible coronary anatomic variations independently from the clinical and hemodynamic repercussions of individual CAAs. Such a scheme should include the normal coronary anatomy (described in terms of quantitative and qualitative criteria), and once the normal features have been excluded, the remaining features should be considered to define abnormality and should be used to generate a classification order. The following criteria are proposed to define each coronary artery:

1. The right coronary artery (RCA) is the vessel that provides blood flow to the right ventricular free wall. It is not essential for the posterior descending branch to originate from the RCA (the most common pattern) or that the ostium of the RCA be located at the right anterior sinus of Valsalva (which is normal).

2. The left anterior descending (LAD) artery is the vessel that provides blood flow to the anterior interventricular septum. It is not essential for the diagonal branch to originate from this vessel (as is normal).
3. The circumflex (LCX) artery is the vessel that provides blood flow to the free wall of the left ventricle, on the obtuse margin of the heart [13].

Incidence

Normal variants of coronary artery anatomy are benign entities with limited clinical significance. In contradistinction, coronary artery anomalies range from benign entities to those associated with a high risk of sudden cardiac death. In the United States, coronary artery anomalies are the second most common cause of sudden death in competitive athletes after hypertrophic cardiomyopathy [13]. Van Camp and coworkers [14] reported that coronary anomalies cause 11.8% of deaths in US high school and college athletes. Moreover, Burke and colleagues [15] reported that, in 14 to 40 year old individuals, coronary anomalies are involved in 12% of sports-related sudden cardiac deaths versus 1.2% of non–sports-related deaths [16]. Recent data suggests that the prevalence of coronary anomalies in patients that underwent coronary CTA in different nations varies from 1.3 % in China [17] to 2.9 % in Italy [18]. The association between Coronary anomalies and Sudden Cardiac Death (SCD), has been demonstrated in retrospective cohort analyses of autopsy reports for SCDs. In a continuous series of 6.3 million 18-year-old recruits who underwent intense military training for 8 weeks, 277 deaths unrelated to trauma were identified. A review of the clinical and necropsy charts showed that, of 64 cardiac deaths, 21 (33%) were related to Anomalous Origination of a Coronary Artery From the Opposite Sinus (ACAOS) of the Left Coronary Artery [6]. In a study of 134 athletes with SCD, hypertrophic cardiomyopathy was the most common cause of death (36%), followed by ACAOS (13%) [4]. In a retrospective study the prevalence of CAAs in patients who underwent Coronary CTA at the Instituto de Cardiología "J.F. Cabral" Corrientes Argentina was 3.2 % (42 of 1300 patients), and 2 (4.7%) correspond of left ACAOS.

Classification

A useful classification it is very important to understand the complex topic of coronary anomalies. The lack of a uniform classification system is due in part to the exhaustive nature of classification schemes required to encompass some of the rarer variants and also to the difficulty of developing a system that is intuitive but still sufficiently inclusive [7]. A basic principle of coronary classification should be that the nature and name of a specific coronary artery are assigned, not according to the site of origin or proximal course, but according to the dependent territory. Angelini´s group proposed a comprehensive classification scheme [12]. There are four types: Anomalies of origination and course, anomalies of intrinsic coronary arterial anatomy, anomalies of coronary termination and anomalous collateral vessels. Each tipe has differents items that are shown in correlative figures in this chapter.

1) Anomalies of Origination and Course

Absent Left Main Trunk (Split Origination of Left Coronary Artery)

The LAD and LCX arteries arise separately with no Left Main Trunk (LMT). Separate ostia of the LAD and LCX artery may occur in a small percentage (0.41%) of individuals with otherwise normal anatomy [19]. (Figure 1) Although multiple ostia represent a technical difficulty for the angiographer, they may also allow alternate collateral sources in patients with proximal coronary artery disease [20].

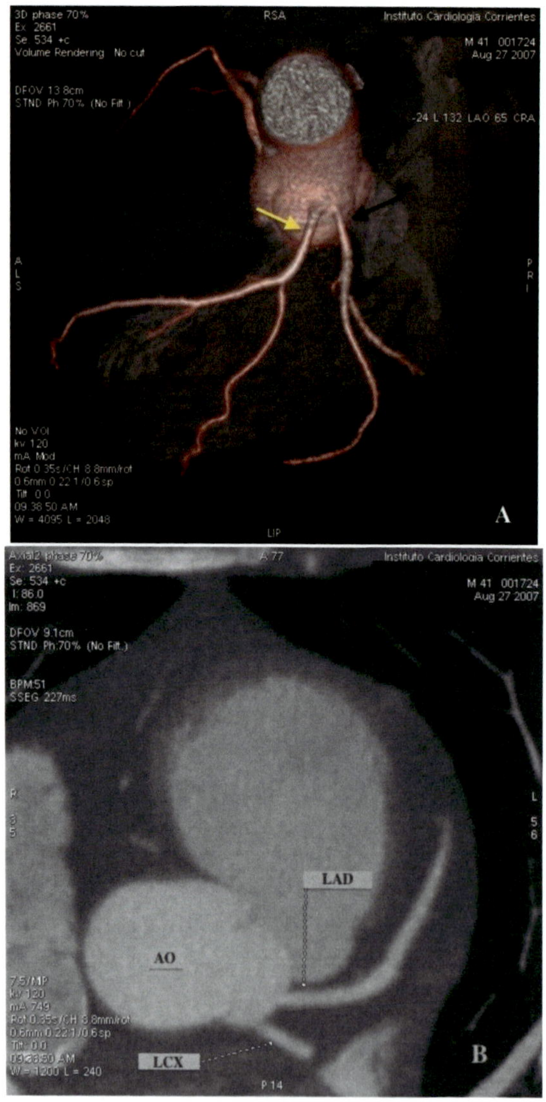

Figure 1. Absent Left Main Trunk (split origination of Left Coronary Artery). Volume Rendered 3-dimensional reconstruction (A) and maximum intensity projection image (B), showing the left anterior descending artery (LAD) (yellow arrow) and left circumflex artery (LCX) (black arrow) arising separately from the left sinus of Valsalva. AO: Aorta.

Anomalous Location of Coronary Ostium within Aortic Root or Near Proper Aortic Sinus of Valsalva

High location: The origin of either the RCA or the LCA at a point above the junctional zone between its sinus and the tubular part of the ascending aorta (Figure 2). 6% of adult hearts were reported to be above the sinotubular junction [21]. This anomaly usually presents no major clinical problems, but it may cause difficulty in cannulating the vessels during coronary arteriography. Selective catheterization of the Right Coronary Artery may be extremely difficult [22]. The location of the coronary ostium could also be low or commissural.

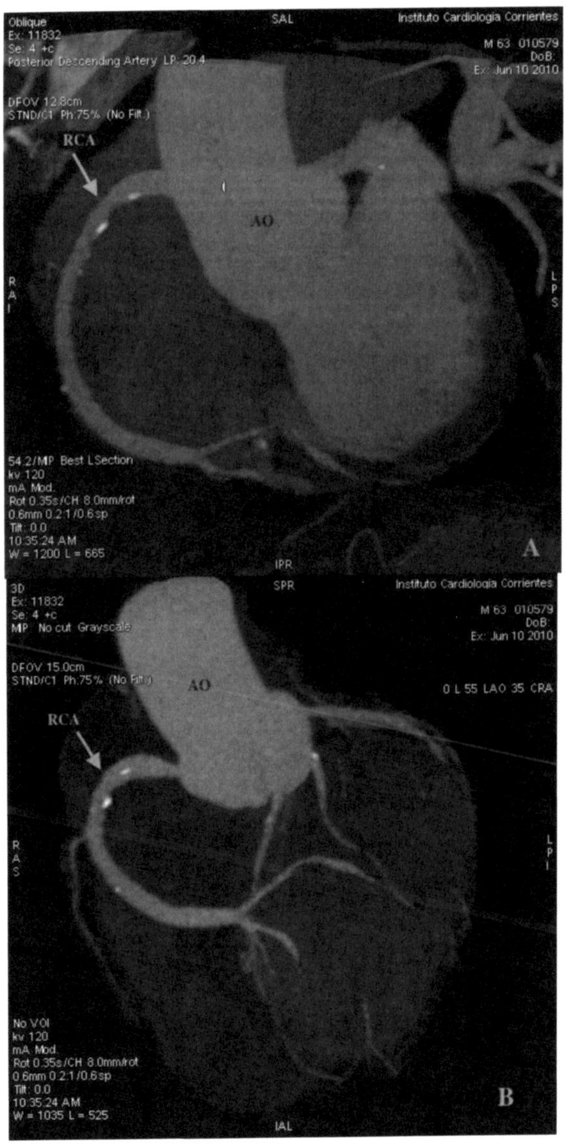

Figure 2. Anomalous location of coronary ostium within aortic root or near proper aortic sinus of Valsalva. (A) Maximum intensity projection displaying origin site of Right Coronary Artery (RCA) above right sinus of Valsalva. (B) Angiographic Reconstruction View. AO: Aorta.

Anomalous Location of Coronary Ostium Outside Normal Coronary Aortic Sinuses

The most common anomaly of this type is the Anomalous origin of the coronary artery from the pulmonary artery (ALCAPA), and is one of the most serious congenital coronary artery anomalies. It has an estimated prevalence of one in 300,000 live births [23]. Most affected patients show symptoms in infancy and early childhood. Approximately 90% of untreated infants die in the 1st year of life, and only a few patients survive to adulthood [24]. In the most common form of this disease, the LCA arises from the pulmonary artery and the RCA arises normally from the aorta (Bland-White-Garland syndrome) (Fig 3) [25]. In infants, it presents as failure to thrive, profuse sweating, dyspnea, pallor, and atypical chest pain on eating or crying. Presentation in adults is extremely rare with symptoms of ischemia, congestive heart failure, mitral regurgitation, and malignant arrhythmias leading to sudden cardiac death [26]. Surgical correction is the elective treatment because uncorrected cases have almost 90% mortality at a mean age of 35 years old [27].

The coronary ostium can also be located in the right or left ventricles, and in the Aorta and or the aorta´s thoracic branches.

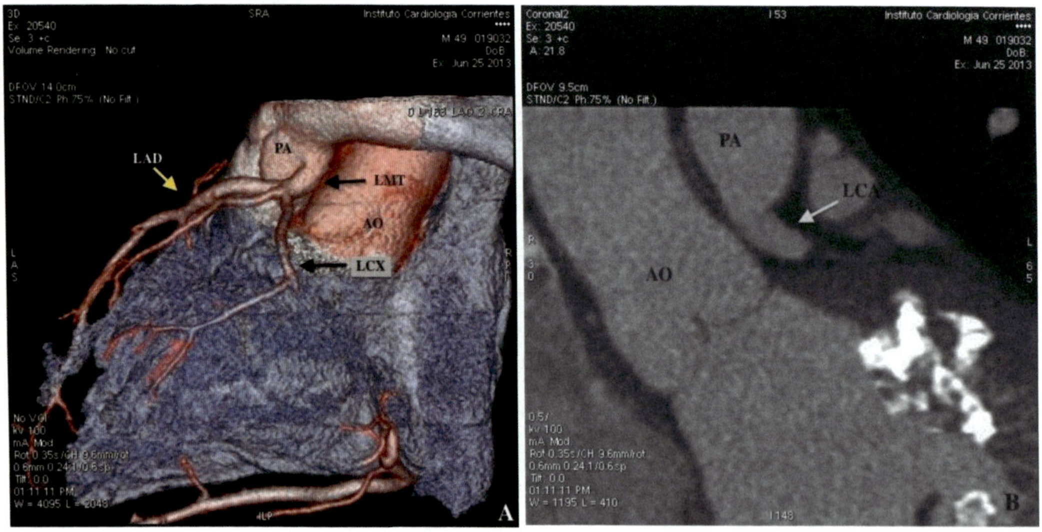

Figure 3. Anomalous origin of the Left Coronary Artery (LCA) arising from posterior facing sinus of the Pulmonary Artery (ALCAPA). (A) Volume Rendered 3 dimensional reconstruction depicting left coronary artery (LCA), Left Main Trunk divided in LAD and LCX, originating from de pulmonary artery (PA). (B) Coronal view showing Left Coronary Artery arising from the pulmonary artery (PA). AO: Aorta, LMT: Left Main Trunk, LAD: Left Anterior Descending Artery, LCX: Left Circumflex Artery.

Anomalous Location of Coronary Ostium at Improper Sinus

The four recognized patterns of an anomalous origin of a coronary artery from the opposite or noncoronary sinus are (a) the RCA arising from the left coronary sinus, (b) the LCA arising from the right coronary sinus, (c) the LCX or LAD artery arising from the right coronary sinus, and (d) the LCA or RCA (or a branch of either artery) arising from the noncoronary sinus. In these anomalies, the coronary ostium may be at the normal level, or the involved artery may have a high or low takeoff [28]. Moreover, a coronary artery arising from the opposite or noncoronary sinus can take any of four common courses, depending on the anatomic relationship of the anomalous vessel to the aorta and the pulmonary trunk: (a) interarterial (i.e., between the aorta and the pulmonary artery), (b) retroaortic, (c) prepulmonic, or (d) septal (subpulmonic) [29]. It is of great clinical importance which course is taken. Although retroaortic, prepulmonic, and septal (subpulmonic) courses seem to be benign, an interarterial course carries a high risk for sudden cardiac death [29, 30].

The LCX artery is the artery that most commonly arises from a separate ostium within the right sinus or as a proximal branch of the RCA (approximately 0.32%–0.67% of the population) [31]. Several reports have shown that this anomalous LCX artery passes behind the aortic root [32-34]; fortunately, this anomaly has not been associated with death.

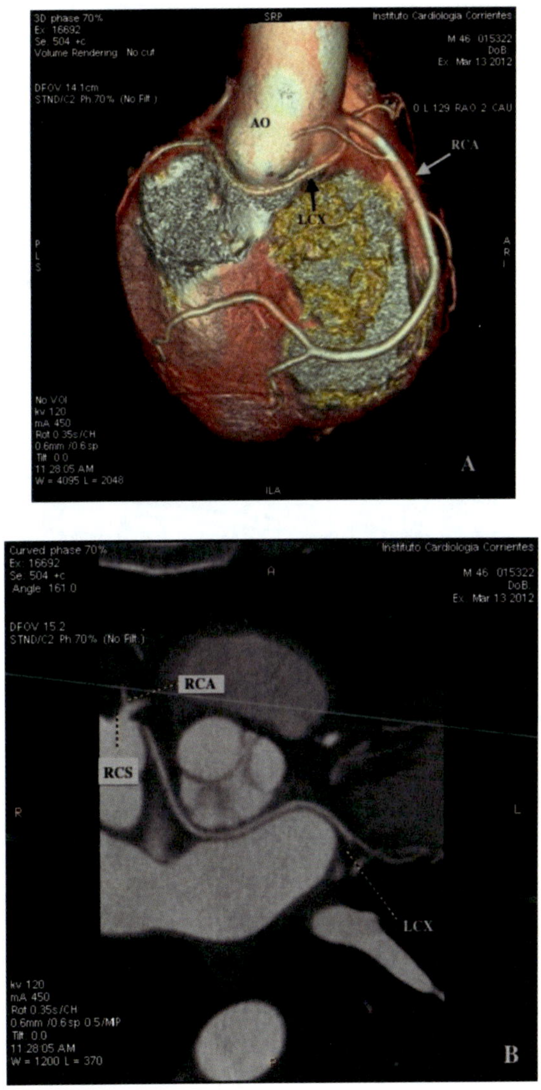

Figure 4. Anomalous location of coronary ostium at improper sinus. Left Circumflex Artery (LCX) that arises from anterior right sinus, with anomalous retroaortic course. (A) Volume rendered 3 dimensional reconstruction. (B) Multiplanar Curve Reconstruction. AO: Aorta, RCA: Right Coronary Artery, RCS: Right Coronary Sinus.

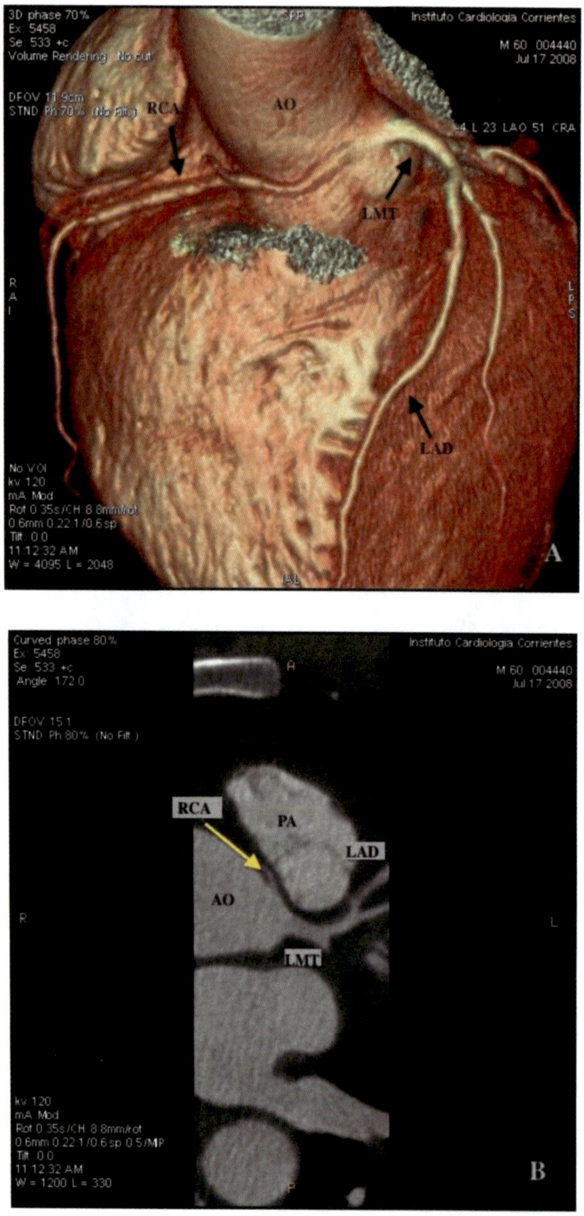

Figure 5. Anomalous location of coronary ostium at improper sinus. Right Coronary Artery (RCA) that arises from left anterior sinus, with anomalous course between aorta and pulmonary artery. (A) Volume rendered 3 Dimensional image. (B) Multiplanar Curve Reconstruction. AO: Aorta, PA: Pulmonary Artery, LMT: Left Main Trunk, LAD: Left Anterior Descending Artery. RCA: Right Coronary Artery.

The RCA arises from the left sinus of Valsalva as a separate vessel or as a branch of a single coronary artery in 0.03%–0.17% of patients who undergo angiography. The most common course of an anomalous RCA arising from the left sinus of Valsalva is interarterial [32] (Figure 5); this variant can be associated with sudden cardiac death in up to 30% of patients [29]. It has been postulated that, when dilation of the aorta occurs during exercise, the anomalous slit-like ostium for the RCA in the left sinus becomes narrower, possibly limiting coronary blood flow and resulting in myocardial infarction [22, 35].

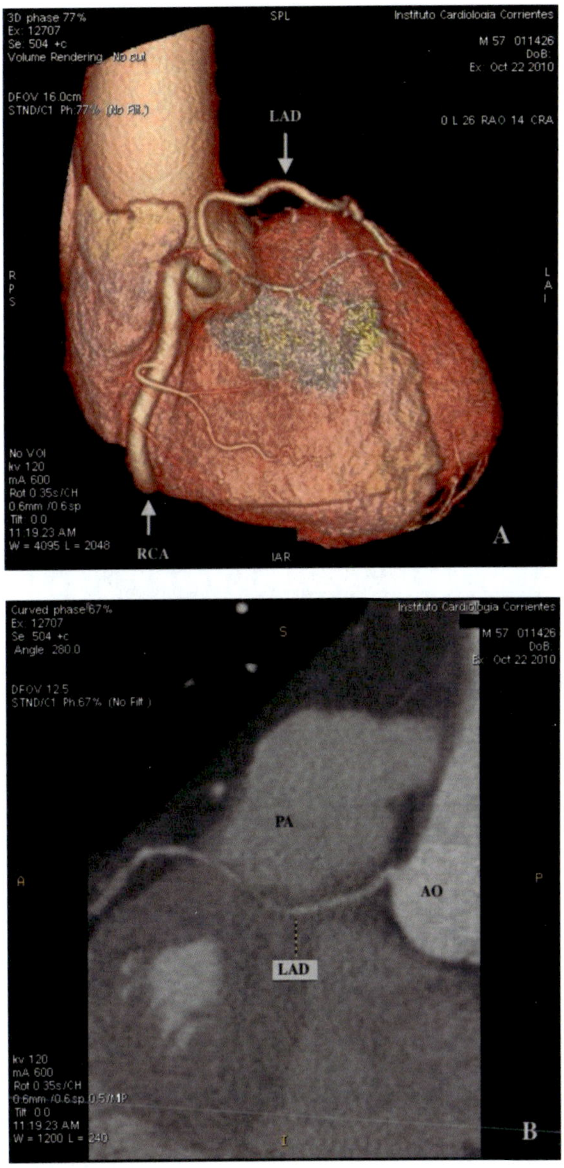

Figure 6. Anomalous location of coronary ostium at improper sinus. Left Anterior Descending (LAD) Artery that arises from right anterior sinus, with anomalous course between aorta and pulmonary artery. This anomaly is also known as Anomalous Coronary Artery From the Opposite Sinus (ACAOS) of the Left Coronary Artery [6]. (A) Volume rendered 3 dimensional reconstruction. (B) Multiplanar Curve Reconstruction. AO: Aorta, RCA: Right Coronary Artery, PA: Pulmonary Artery.

The LCA arises from the right sinus of Valsalva as a separate vessel or as a branch of a single coronary artery in 0.09%–0.11% of patients who undergo angiography. This anomalous LCA may take a retroaortic, prepulmonic, septal (subpulmonic) or interarterial course [31]. An interarterial course (Figure 6), also called the malignant type, may be seen in up to 75% of patients with this anomaly [36], who are at high risk for sudden cardiac death due to the acute angle of the ostium, the stretch of the intramural segment, and the compression between the commissure of the right and left coronary cusps. It is also reported as anomalous origination of a coronary artery from the opposite sinus (ACAOS) [12] (Figure 7) with intussusception of the ectopic proximal vessel, which is the subgroup of CAAs that has the most potential for clinical repercussions, specifically sudden death in the Young.

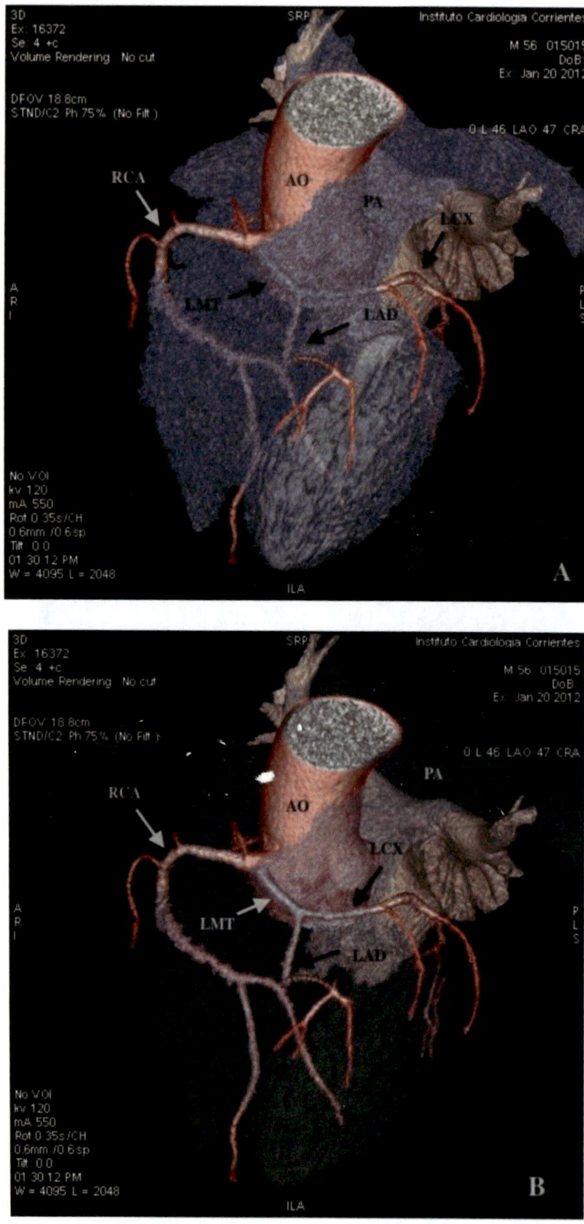

Figure 7. Anomalous location of coronary ostium at improper sinus. Left Anterior Descending (LAD) Artery that arises from right anterior sinus, with anomalous course between aorta and pulmonary artery. This anomaly is also known as Coronary Artery From the Opposite Sinus (ACAOS) of the Left Coronary Artery [6]. (A) Volume rendered 3 dimensional reconstruction, the Left Main Trunk (LMT), LAD and the Left Circumflex Artery (LCX) can be seen behind the Pulmonary Artery (PA) in transparent blue. (B) Volume rendered 3 dimensional reconstruction, the LMT, LAD and LCX) can be seen behind the PA in very transparent blue. AO: Aorta, PA: Pulmonary Artery.

In a continuous series of 6.3 million 18-year-old recruits who underwent intense military training for 8 weeks, the researchers identified 277 deaths unrelated to trauma. A review of the clinical and necropsy charts showed that, of 64 cardiac deaths, 21 (33%) were related to ACAOS of the left coronary artery (left-ACAOS) and that no other CAAs resulted in cardiac death. This was the first large-scale study of CAAs in which the denominator (all candidates at risk) was known, the setting of the clinical events was consistent (extreme physical training), and all the fatal events led to necropsy studies [6].

In comparison, Drory and colleagues [37] studied the incidence of CAAs in a continuous series of 162 patients with sudden unexpected death. The patients were less than 40 years of age and underwent routine autopsy studies in Israel, where an autopsy is obligatory in such cases.

The incidence of CAA related sudden death was 0.6% (1 of 162 cases); taken together with the recent military recruit series [6], this result suggests that extreme exercise plays a powerful role in such deaths. Whereas sudden death is usually associated with extreme exercise in young adults [38], the other manifestations of ACAOS are more frequently seen in older adults and are related to the onset of hypertension. Other authors [39] claimed that sudden death is seen only in young patients, possibly because of progressive hardening of the aortic wall in adults.

2) Anomalies of Intrinsic Coronary Arterial Anatomy

Coronary Ectasia or Aneurysm

Coronary ectasia or aneurysm, (Figure 8) is described as dilation of blood vessel lumen, exceeding the diameter of the adjacent normal segment, or the dilation exceeding the largest diameter of a coronary vessel of a given patient more than 1.5-fold. [40] Others authors [41], proposed a classification of aneurysms, according to the morphological picture and the number of affected arteries. As type 1 they described dilations in all 3 epicardial coronary arteries, type 2 as dilation in 1 blood vessel only with accompanying stenosis in another coronary artery, and type 3 as dilation limited only to 1 artery. Tunick et al., [42] in their work described aneurysms as limited, unusual dilation of the coronary artery with spherical or saccular shape.

Most commonly coronary aneurysms are located in the right coronary artery, and then in decreasing order in the left descending artery, the left circumflex artery, and only exceptionally in the left main coronary artery [43]. Atherosclerosis is the main cause of these anomalies in adults, and Kawasaki disease in children and adolescents [44]. Coronary CTA has been shown to be highly sensitive and specific for coronary artery aneurysms. In a study [45] performed in16 adolescents and young adults with Kawasaki disease. Images were of adequate quality for 96% of the major coronary segments, with 100% sensitivity to detect aneurysms; sensitivity was 87.5% and specificity was 92.5% for significant coronary artery stenosis.

More recently, Chu et al., [46] performed a comparative study and found that Coronary CTA was more sensitive than 2D echocardiography for identifying fusiform and distally located aneurysms.

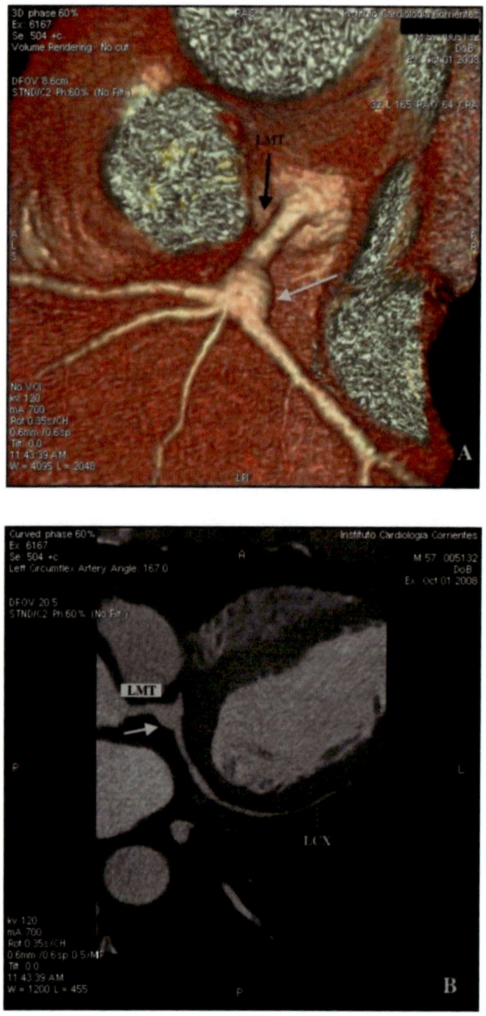

Figure 8. Coronary aneurysm of the left main trunk (LMT). (A) Volume rendered 3 dimensional reconstruction showing aneurysm (white arrow). (B) Multiplanar Curve Reconstruction, showing aneurysm (white arrow) of the LMT. LCX: Left Circumflex Artery.

Intramural Coronary Artery

Intramural coronary artery (muscular bridge), is defined as the presence of an intramyocardial segment of a major coronary artery that normally has an epicardial course [47] (Figure 9). There is some discrepancy between the prevalence of myocardial bridging at angiography (0.5%–2.5%) and that at pathologic analysis (15%–85%) [48]. The cause for this discrepancy is presumed to be the fact that myocardial bridging often occurs without overt symptoms, so that patients are rarely referred for coronary angiography [49]. In some cases, however, myocardial bridging is responsible for angina pectoris, myocardial infarction, life-threatening arrhythmias, or even death [50]. The standard of reference for diagnosing myocardial bridges is coronary angiography, at which a typical "milking" effect and a "step down–step up" phenomenon induced by systolic compression of the tunneled segment may be seen [49]. In contrast, coronary CTA clearly shows the intramyocardial location of the involved coronary arterial segment [48]. The ECG-gated reconstruction window used in standard CTA of the coronary artery is usually positioned within the diastolic phase for maximal vasodilatation and minimal motion artifacts [51]. However, when there is suspicion for myocardial bridging, it is recommended that ECG-gated reconstruction be performed during the systolic phase as well as the diastolic phase. Comparison of the images obtained during the two phases will allow assessment of luminal narrowing during the systolic phase.

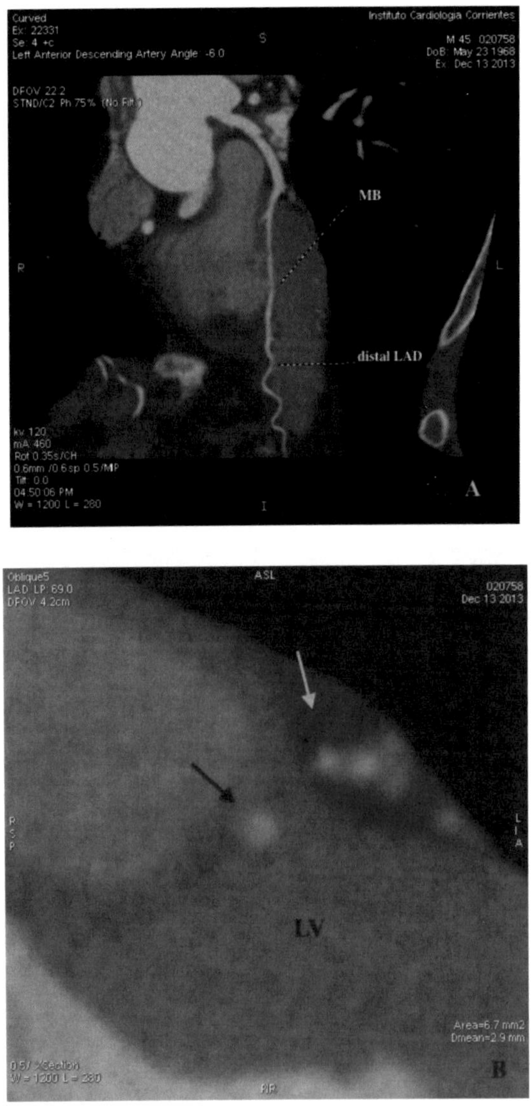

Figure 9. Intramural coronary artery (muscular bridge). (A) Multiplanar curve reconstruction showing left anterior descending artery (LAD) with intramural course. MB: Myocardial Bridge. (B) Orthogonal View of the LAD (black arrow) surrounded by left ventricle myocardium. Left ventricle (LV). Epicardial fat (white arrow).

Coronary Crossing

Although coronary arteries and their branches typically run parallel to one another, published case reports have described anomalous crossing of coronary branches and, less commonly, of the LAD and LCX. This is typically seen as a benign incidental finding on conventional angiography or coronary CTA [52].

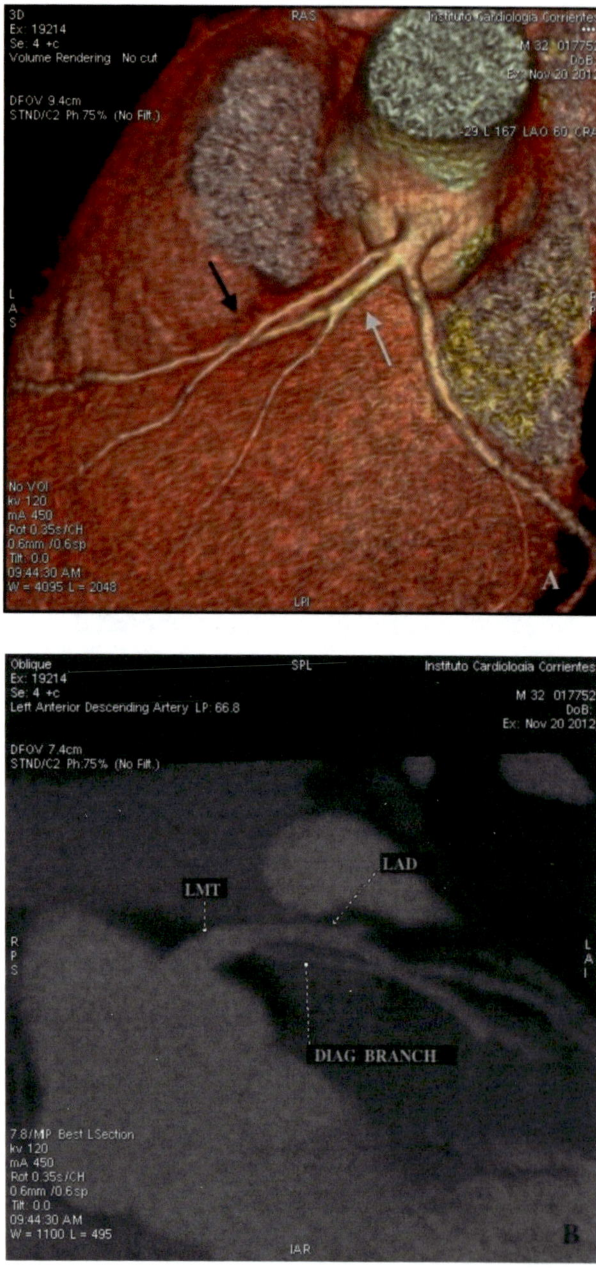

Figure 10. Coronary crossing. (A) Volume rendered 3 Dimensional reconstruction showing a diagonal branch (black arrow) crossing the left anterior descending (LAD) artery (white arrow). (B) Maximum intensity projection. Left Main Trunk (LMT). Left anterior descending artery (LAD). Diagonal branch.

3) Anomalies of Coronary Termination

Coronary Artery Fistula

Coronary artery fistula is a condition in which a communication exists between one or two coronary arteries and either a cardiac chamber, the coronary sinus, the superior vena cava, or the pulmonary artery (Figure 11).

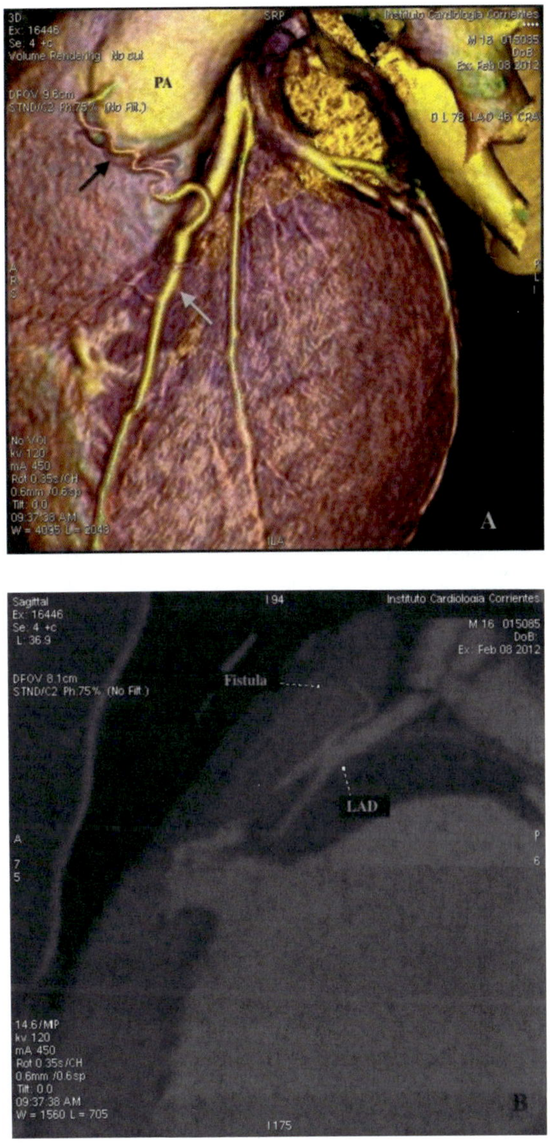

Figure 11. Coronary fistula. (A) Volume rendered 3 dimensional reconstruction showing a coronary fistula (black arrow) between the left descending coronary artery (white arrow) and the pulmonary artery (PA). (B) Maximum intensity projection image showing coronary fistula from left descending coronary artery (LDA) to PA.

This condition is seen in approximately 0.1%–0.2% of all patients who undergo selective coronary angiography [53]. It more commonly involves the RCA (60% of cases) than the LCA (40%) [54]. In less than 5% of cases, fistulas originate from both the LCA and the RCA [55]. In coronary artery fistula, the involved coronary artery is dilated because of increased blood flow and is often tortuous to an extent determined by the shunt volume [56]. In terms of morphologic features, the fistula is variable at its drainage site, with either single or multiple communications or a maze of fine vessels that form a diffuse network, or plexus, with extensive intramural distribution. The drainage site of the fistula has a greater clinical and physiologic importance than does the artery of origin. The most common site of drainage is the right ventricle (45% of cases), followed by the right atrium (25%) and the pulmonary artery (15%) [57].

Diagnosis

For several decades, premorbid diagnosis of coronary artery anomalies was made with angiography. However, it was recently reported that, among patients with anomalous coronary arteries identified consensually with 16 -Multidectector Computed Tomography, conventional angiographic findings alone allowed correct identification of the abnormalities in only 53% of cases [58]. The reason for this discrepancy may be that coronary artery anomalies are very difficult to visualize at angiography, and even if they are visualized, their course may be delineated inaccurately [59].

In addition to coronary angiography, transesophageal echocardiography (TEE) [60, 61] also may clinically detect coronary anomalies, but this method is not totally noninvasive and is too costly for screening large populations. Transthoracic Echocardiography it is commonly used as a routine examination, in a continuous series of 2388 transthoracic echocardiograms [62] obtained in children, 4 anomalies of coronary origination (0.17%) were found; in 1 case, a negative echocardiographic finding was followed by sudden death related to a coronary anomaly newly found at necropsy.

Another available method is the Cardiac Magnetic Resonance Imaging (MRI), which avoids radiation and contrast agents and yields excellent images at expert centers. In determining coronary origination, MRI may surpass conventional angiography, especially in patients with congenital defects. For isolated coronary anomalies, MRI is similarly successful, although series remain small. Its greatest limitation is in determining the distal coronary course [63]. Therefore, this technique is less helpful in evaluating fistulas, coronary origination outside the normal sinuses, and collateral vessels [1].

Recently Coronary CTA emerged as an essential imaging tool for evaluating the coronary arteries, CAAs are easily assessed with this modality, which, compared with conventional angiography, offers superior definition of the ostial origin and proximal path of the anomalous coronary artery. Knowledge of the CT appearances of various coronary artery anomalies and an understanding of the clinical significance of these anomalies are essential for accurate diagnosis [59] of coronary anomalies.

Conclusion

Congenital Coronary Anomalies is a rare but not as uncommon type of coronary pathology. Coronary CTA is a very useful tool in their diagnosis because of its excellent anatomical visualization capability based on volumetric 3 Dimensional reconstruction and its improved temporal and spatial resolution.

It is very important the adequate knowledge of these anomalies in order to achieve an appropriate and accurate diagnosis, that can be the key for the good prognosis of this group of patients.

References

[1] Angelini P, Velasco J A, Flamm S. Coronary Anomalies: Incidence, pathophysiology, and clinical relevance. *Circulation* 2002; 105: 2449-54.

[2] Ghersin E, Litmanovich D, Ofer A, et al., Anomalous origin of right coronary artery: diagnosis and dynamic evaluation with multidetector computed tomography. *J. Comput. Assist. Tomogr* 2004; 28:293-4.

[3] 3.Frescura C, Basso C, Thiene G, et al., Anomalous origin of coronary arteries and risk of sudden death: a study based on an autopsy population of congenital heart disease. *Hum. Pathol.* 1998; 29: 689–95.

[4] Maron BJ, Thompson PD, Puffer JC, et al., Cardiovascular preparticipation screening of competitive athletes. A statement for health professionals from the Sudden Death Committee (clinical cardiology) and Congenital Cardiac Defects Committee (cardiovascular disease in the young), American Heart Association. *Circulation* 1996; 94: 850-6.

[5] Pelliccia A. Congenital coronary artery anomalies in young patients: new perspectives for timely identification. *J. Am. Coll. Cardiol.* 2001; 37: 598-600.

[6] Eckart RE, Scoville SL, Campbell CL, et al., Sudden death in young adults: a 25-year review of autopsies in military recruits. *Ann. Intern. Med.* 2004; 141: 829-34.

[7] Shriki JE, Shinbane JS, Rashid MA, et al., Identifying, characterizing, and classifying congenital anomalies of the coronary arteries. *Radio Graphics* 2012, 32: 453-68.

[8] Park JH, Kwon NH, Kim JH, et al., Prevalence of congenital coronary artery anomalies of korean men detected by coronary computed tomography. *Korean Circ. J.* 2013; 43: 7-12.

[9] Warnes CA, Williams RG, Bashore TM, et al., : ACC/AHA 2008 Guidelines for the Management of Adults with Congenital Heart Disease: a report of the American College of Cardiology/American Heart Association Task Force on Practice Guidelines (writing committee to develop guidelines on the management of adults with congenital heart disease). *Circulation* 2008; 118: e714–e833.

[10] Taylor AJ, Cerqueira M, Hodgson JM, Mark D, Min J, O´Gara P, et al., ACCF/SCCT/ACR/AHA/ASE/ASNC/NASCI/SCAI/SCMR 2010. Appropriate Use Criteria for Cardiac Computed Tomography: A Report of the American College of Cardiology Foundation Appropriate Use Criteria Task Force, the Society of Cardiovascular Computed Tomography, the American College of Radiology, the American Heart Association, the American Society of Echocardiography, the American

Society of Nuclear Cardiology, the North American Society for Cardiovascular Imaging, the Society for Cardiovascular Angiography and Interventions, and the Society for Cardiovascular Magnetic Resonance. *J. Am. Coll. Cardiol.* 2010; 56: 1864-94. Doi:10.1016/j.jacc.2010.07.005.

[11] Angelini P. Normal and anomalous coronary arteries: definitions and classification. *Am. Heart J.* 1989; 117: 418–34.

[12] Angelini P. Coronary artery anomalies: an entity in search of an identity. *Circulation* 2007; 115: 1296–305.

[13] Angelini P, Villason S, Chan AV, Diez JG. Normal and anomalous coronary arteries in humans. In: Angelini P, ed. Coronary artery anomalies: A comprehensive approach. Philadelphia: Lippincott Williams & Wilkins, 1999: 27–150.

[14] Maron BJ, Doerer JJ, Haas TS, Tierney DM, Mueller FO: Sudden deaths in young competitive athletes: analysis of 1866 deaths in the United States, 1980–2006. *Circulation* 2009; 119: 1085–92.

[15] Van Camp SP, Bloor CM, Mueller FO, et al., Nontraumatic sports death in high school and college athletes. *Med. Sci. Sports Exerc.* 1995; 27: 641–47.

[16] Burke AP, Farb A, Virmani R, et al., Sports-related and non-sports-related sudden cardiac death in young adults. *Am. Heart J.* 1991; 121: 568–75.

[17] Zhang LJ, Yang GF, Huang W, Zhou CS, Chen P, Lu GM. Incidence of anomalous origin of coronary artery in 1879 chinese adults on dual source CT angiography. *Neth Heart J.* 2010; 18: 466-70.

[18] Andreini D, Mushtaq S, Pontone G, et al., Additional clinical role of 64-slice multidetector computed tomography in the evaluation of coronary artery variants and anomalies. *Int. J. Cardiol.* 2010; 145: 388-90.

[19] Danias PG, Stuber M, McConnell MV, Manning WJ. The diagnosis of congenital coronary anomalies with magnetic resonance imaging. *Coron Artery Dis.* 2001; 12: 621-26.

[20] Greenberg MA, Fish BG, Spindola-Franco H. Congenital anomalies of coronary artery: classification and significance. *Radiol. Clin. North Am.* 1989; 27: 1127–46.

[21] Vlodaver Z, Neufeld HN, Edwards JE. Pathology of coronary disease. *Semin. Roentgenol.* 1972; 7: 376–94.

[22] Douglas JS, Franch RH, King SB. Coronary artery anomalies. In: King SB, Douglas JS, eds. Coronary arteriography and angioplasty. New York, NY: McGraw Hill, 1985; 33–85.

[23] Dodge-Khatami A, Mavroudis C, Backer CL. Anomalous origin of the left coronary artery from the pulmonary artery: collective review of surgical therapy. *Ann. Thorac. Surg.* 2002; 74: 946–55.

[24] Wesselhoeft H, Fawcett JS, Johnson AL. Anomalous origin of the left coronary artery from the pulmonary trunk: its clinical spectrum, pathology and pathophysiology, based on review of 140 cases with seven further cases. *Circulation* 1968; 38: 403–25.

[25] Bland EF, White PD, Garland J. Congenital anomalies of the coronary arteries: report of an unusual case associated with cardiac hypertrophy. *Am. Heart J.* 1933; 8: 787–801.

[26] Moodie DS, Fyfe D, Gill CC. Anomalous origin of the left coronary artery from the pulmonary artery (Bland-White-Garland syndrome) in adults patients: long-term follow up after surgery. *Am. Heart J.* 1983; 106: 381-88.

[27] Fernandes ED, Kadivar H, Hallman GL. Congenital malformations of the coronary arteries: the Texas Heart Institute experience. *Ann. Thorac. Surg.* 1992; 54: 732-40.
[28] Greenberg MA, Fish BG, Spindola-Franco H. Congenital anomalies of coronary artery: classification and significance. *Radiol. Clin. North Am.* 1989; 27: 1127–46.
[29] Roberts WC, Siegel RJ, Zipes DP. Origin of the right coronary artery from the left sinus of Valsalva and its functional consequences: analysis of 10 necropsy patients. *Am. J. Cardiol.* 1982; 49:863–68.
[30] Cheitlin MD, De Castro CM, McAllister HA. Sudden death as a complication of anomalous left coronary origin from the anterior sinus of Valsalva: a not-so-minor congenital anomaly. *Circulation* 1974; 50: 780–87.
[31] Bunce NH, Lorenz CH, Keegan J, et al., Coronary artery anomalies: assessment with free-breathing three-dimensional coronary MR angiography. *Radiology* 2003; 227: 201–08.
[32] Yamanaka O, Hobbs RE. Coronary artery anomalies in 126,595 patients undergoing coronary angiography. *Cathet Cardiovasc. Diagn* 1990; 21: 28- 40.
[33] Donaldson RM, Raphael M, Radley-Smith R, Yacoub MH, Ross DN. Angiographic identification of primary coronary anomalies causing impaired myocardial perfusion. *Cathet Cardiovasc. Diagn* 1983; 9: 237–49.
[34] Page HL Jr, Engel HJ, Campbell WB, Thomas CS Jr. Anomalous origin of the left circumflex coronary artery: recognition, angiographic demonstration and clinical significance. *Circulation* 1974; 50: 768–73.
[35] Lee J, Choe YH, Kim HJ, Park JE. Magnetic resonance imaging demonstration of anomalous origin of the right coronary artery from the left coronary sinus associated with acute myocardial infarction. *J. Comput. Assist. Tomogr.* 2003; 27: 289–91.
[36] Chaitman BR, Lesperance J, Saltiel J, Bourassa MG. Clinical, angiographic, and hemodynamic findings in patients with anomalous origin of the coronary arteries. *Circulation* 1976; 53: 122–31.
[37] Drory Y, Turetz Y, Hiss Y, Lev B, Fisman EZ, Pines A, Kramer MR. Sudden unexpected death in persons less than 40 years of age. *Am. J. Cardiol.* 1991; 68: 1388–92.
[38] Liberthson RR. Nonatherosclerotic coronary artery disease. In: Eagle KA, ed. The practice of cardiology. Boston: Little Brown and Company, 1989: 614–51.
[39] Cheitlin MD. Coronary anomalies as a cause of sudden death in the athlete. In: Estes NAM, Salem DN, Wang JJP, eds. Sudden Cardiac Death in the Athlete. Armonk NY: Futura Publishing Co, 1998.
[40] Jumbo G, Liu F, Kearney P, et al., Intravascular ultrasound approach to the diagnosis of coronary artery aneurysm. *Am. Heart J.* 1995; 130: 765-81.
[41] Markis JE, Joffe CD, Cohon PF. Clinical significant of coronary arterial ectasia. *Am. J. Cardiol.* 1976: 37: 217-22.
[42] Tunick PA, Slater J, Konzon I, et al., Discrete atherosclerotic coronary artery aneurysms: A study of 20 patients. *J. Am. Coll. Cardiol.* 1990; 15: 279-82.
[43] Daoud A, Pankin D, Tulgan H, et al., Aneurysms of the coronary artery. Report of ten cases and review of literature. *Am. J. Cardiol.* 1963; 11: 228-37.
[44] Gziut AI, Gil RJ. Coronary aneurysms. A review article. *Pol. Arch. Med. Wewn.* 2008; 118: 741-46.

[45] Kanamaru H, Sato Y, Takayam T, et al., Assessment of coronary artery abnormalities by multislice spiral computed tomography in adolescents and young adults with Kawasaki disease. *Am. J. Cardiol.* 2005; 95: 522–25.

[46] Chu WC, Mok GC, Lam WW, Yam MC, Sung RY. Assessment of coronary artery aneurysms in paediatric patients with Kawasaki disease by multidetector row CT angiography: feasibility and comparison with 2D echocardiography. *Pediatr Radiol.* 2006; 36:1148–53.

[47] Geiringer E. The mural coronary. *Am. Heart J.* 1951; 41:359–68.

[48] Amoroso G, Battolla L, Gemignani C, et al., Myocardial bridging on left anterior descending coronary artery evaluated by multidetector computed tomography. *Int. J. Cardiol.* 2004; 95: 335–37.

[49] Mohlenkamp S, Hort W, Ge J, Erbel R. Update on myocardial bridging. *Circulation* 2002; 106: 2616–22.

[50] Tio RA, Van Gelder IC, Boonstra PW, Crijns HJ. Myocardial bridging in a survivor of sudden cardiac near-death: role of intracoronary Doppler flow measurements and angiography during dobutamine stress in the clinical evaluation. *Heart* 1997; 77: 280-82.

[51] Kopp AF, Schroeder S, Kuettner A, et al., Coronary arteries: retrospectively ECG-gated multi–detector row CT angiography with selective optimization of the image reconstruction window. *Radiology* 2001; 221: 683–88.

[52] Pursnani A, Jacobs JE, Saremi F, Coronary CTA assessment of coronary anomalies *Journal of Cardiovascular Computed Tomography* 2012; 6: 48–59.

[53] Said SA, el Gamal MI, van der Werf T. Coronary arteriovenous fistulas: collective review and management of six new cases—changing etiology, presentation, and treatment strategy. *Clin. Cardiol.* 1997; 20: 748–52.

[54] Neufeld HN, Lester RG, Adams P Jr, et al., Congenital communication of a coronary artery with a cardiac chamber or the pulmonary trunk (coronary artery fistula). *Circulation* 1961;24: 171–79.

[55] Reagan K, Boxt LM, Katz J. Introduction to coronary arteriography. *Radiol. Clin. North Am.* 1994; 32: 419–33.

[56] van Geuns RJ, Cademartiri F. Anatomy of the coronary arteries and vein in CT imaging. In: Schoepf UJ, ed. CT of the heart. Totowa, NJ: Humana, 2005: 219–228.

[57] McNamara JJ, Gross RE. Congenital coronary artery fistula. *Surgery* 1969; 65: 59–69.

[58] Shi H, Aschoff AJ, Brambs HJ, Hoffmann MH. Multislice CT imaging of anomalous coronary arteries. *Eur. Radiol.* 2004; 14: 2172–81.

[59] Kim SY, Seo JB, Do KH. Coronary Artery Anomalies: Classification and ECG-gated Multi–Detector Row CT Findings with Angiographic Correlation. *RadioGraphics* 2006; 26: 317–34.

[60] Gaither NS, Rogan KM, Stajduhar K, et al., Anomalous origin and course of coronary arteries in adults: identification and improved imaging utilizing transesophageal echocardiography. *Am. Heart J.* 1991; 122: 69–75.

[61] Giannoccaro PJ, Sochowski RA, Morton BC, et al., Complementary role of transesophageal echocardiography to coronary angiography in the assessment of coronary artery anomalies. *Br. Heart J.* 1993; 70: 70–74.

[62] Davis JA, Cecchin F, Jones TK, et al., Major coronary artery anomalies in a pediatric population: incidence and clinical importance. *J. Am. Coll. Cardiol.* 2001; 37: 593–97.

[63] Taylor AM, Thorne SA, Rubens MB, et al., Coronary artery imaging in grown up congenital heart disease: complementary role of magnetic resonance and x-ray coronary angiography. *Circulation* 2000; 101: 1670–78.

In: Congenital Heart Diseases
Editor: Raúl Cayré and José Milei

ISBN: 978-1-61122-003-2

Chapter 5

Intrauterine Ductus Arteriosus Constriction: An Etiological Overview

Paulo Zielinsky** *and Stefano Busato
Fetal Cardiology Unit, Institute of Cardiology, Porto Alegre, Brazil

Abstract

The ductus arteriosus plays a fundamental role in directing 80–85% of the right ventricular output arising from the superior vena cava, coronary sinus, and a small part from the inferior vena cava to the descending aorta. Its histological structure is predominantly made up by a thick muscular layer, different from the aorta and the pulmonary artery, which increases with gestational age. The fibers have a circumferential orientation, especially at the external layers, facilitating and making effective ductal constriction. These factors may generate lumen alterations, which may cause fetal and neonatal complications, such as heart failure, hydrops, neonatal pulmonary hypertension, and even death. Classically, maternal administration of indomethacin and/or other anti-inflammatory drugs interfere in prostaglandins metabolism, causing ductal constriction. However, many cases of fetal ductal constriction, as well as of persistent neonatal pulmonary artery hypertension, remain without an established etiology, being referred as "idiopathic." In recent years, a growing body of evidence has shown that herbs, fruits, nuts, and a wide diversity of substances commonly used in daily diets have definitive effects upon the metabolic pathway of inflammation, with consequent inhibition of prostaglandins synthesis. This anti-inflammatory action, especially of polyphenols, when ingested during the third trimester of pregnancy, may influence the dynamics of fetal ductus arteriosus flow. The aim of this review is to present these new observations and findings, which may influence dietary orientation during pregnancy.

Keywords: Ductal constriction, Polyphenols, Pulmonary Hypertension, Prostaglandins, Anti-inflammatory substances

* E-mail: paulozie.voy@terra.com.br.

1. Morphology and Physiology of Normal and Abnormal Fetal Ductus Arteriosus

The ductus arteriosus originates from the distal portion of the left sixth aortic arch, which connects the left pulmonary artery to dorsal aorta [1]. Its histological structure is formed by an internal elastic membrane, a tunica media muscular layer and an external adventitial layer. The muscular layer is predominant, which makes the ductal structure different from aorta and pulmonary artery, and increases with gestational age. It has a circumferential orientation, mainly at the external layers, which facilitates and makes ductal constriction effective [2].

The ductus arteriosus is positioned between the pulmonary artery, near the emerging left pulmonary artery, and the aorta, at the zone of the isthmus (Figure 1). At the aortic-pulmonary plan, around 80-85% of the poorly saturated blood (50% oxygen) ejected by the right ventricle into the main pulmonary artery passes through the ductus arteriosus to the descending aorta (around 75 ml/min), and as a result will mix with the blood coming from the left ventricle. Due to the high pulmonary vascular resistance, only 15-20% (near 15 ml/min) are directed to the lungs. Around 40-50% of the descending aorta flow passes through the umbilical arteries and returns to the placenta for hematosis. The remaining blood will nourish the organs and the inferior body half [3].

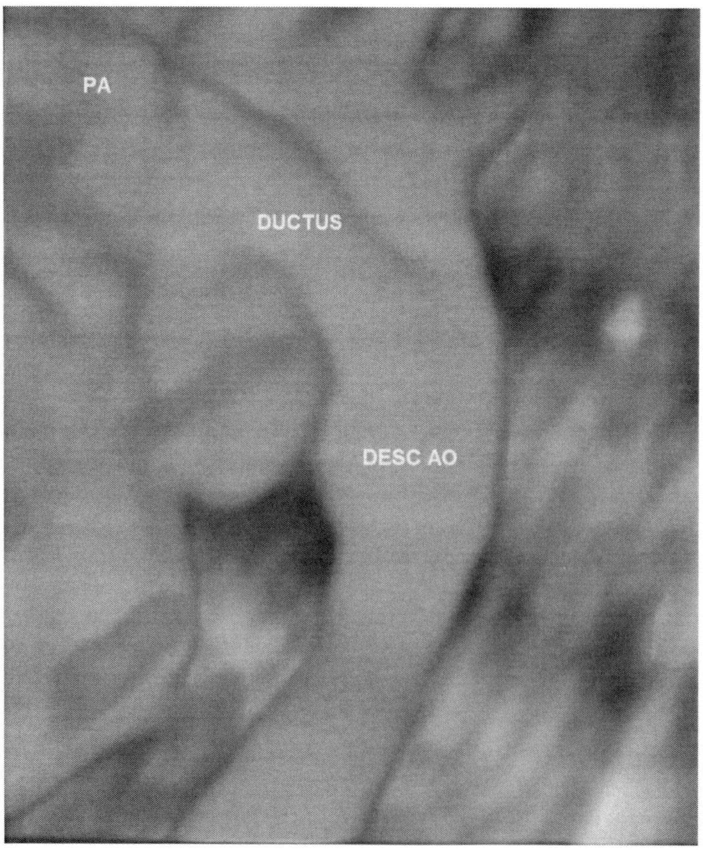

Figure 1. 3D echocardiographic image of the ductus arteriosus in a normal 33 weeks fetus. Notice that the ductus arteriosus inserts in the descending aorta distally to left subclavian artery.

The ductus arteriosus shows a peculiar differentiation program in order to prepare itself for postnatal spontaneous closure [1]. There is a relationship between gestational age and the histological maturation of the ductus [4]. The process of fetal intimal thickening starts at the second trimester of pregnancy and is characteristically a continuous process. This mechanism of intimal thickening seems to be linked to prostacyclin syntase (PGI2 syntase), which has a regulating role on ductal patency [5]. During the ductus arteriosus closing there are higher PGI2 syntase levels in smooth muscle cells at the sites of intimal thickening than in other places. These findings demonstrate the relationship between ductal morphology and the presence of PGI2 syntase [6, 7]. Vascular remodelling also seems to be associated to dedifferentiation of the smooth muscle cells and to apoptosis present in the areas of tunica media and intimal layers [8].

Hemodynamic alterations during the immediate neonatal period occur at the moment of cessation of placentary blood circulation, lung insufflation, pulmonary vasodilation and foramen ovale closure. The sudden increase in systemic vascular resistance and the decrease in pulmonary vascular resistance generate a reverse flow through the ductus arteriosus and an abrupt increase in pulmonary flow. Some minutes after birth, 90% of the blood ejected by the right ventricle is directed to the pulmonary arteries. With the decrease in pulmonary vascular resistance there is an increase in pulmonary blood flow, which culminates with ductal occlusion [9, 10]. The functional closure of ductus arteriosus is initiated by a mechanism induced by the higher blood oxygen concentration [11]. This mechanism, albeit mediated by prostaglandins and endothelins, is intrinsic to smooth muscle cells [12]. It is a potentially reversible phenomenon which occurs 8-72 hours after birth, secondary to muscular constriction. After this event, there is a remodelling of the vascular wall, with neointimal formation caused by proliferation and migration of smooth muscle cells from the tunica media to the subendothelial layers. This seems to be the final event of a process, which initiates at the second trimester of pregnancy, starting with the accumulation of glycosaminoglycans at the subendothelial region [5]. Usually, the ductus arteriosus remains patent for some hours or days in the neonatal period.

Physiological closure of the ductus in the term neonate starts with a phase of functional obliteration secondary to the wall vessel muscular constriction. The closure is gradual and is completed more frequently in 10 to 15 hours after birth[13]. Observations in neonates show that the arterial duct starts to close at the pulmonary arterial end, and then the constriction spreads to the aorta [14]. After completion of ductal occlusion, the arterial ligament is formed [15]. If the ductus arteriosus remains patent in a term neonate, this is considered a pathological condition. The premature baby shows a delay in the remodelling process of the tunica media layer and is less responsive to oxygen, probably as a result of the immaturity of the structures [16, 17].

Since the ductus has a predominant muscular layer, its occlusion is influenced by a number of different constrictor and relaxing factors. Relaxing factors are prostaglandins, nitric oxide and bradycinin, which cause liberation of prostaglandins and nitric oxide. Constrictive factors are oxygen, high doses of bradycinin and the autonomic nervous system, both sympathetic and parasympathetic [14]. The vasoconstrictive effect is dose-dependent to several neurotransmitters, such as acetylcholine, histamine, serotonin and cathecolamins. With the increase in gestational age, the ductus becomes less sensitive to the dilating effects and more sensitive to constrictive factors [14, 18, 19]. Production of prostaglandins is dependent of two enzymes, which act in different states, cyclo-oxygenase-1 (COX-1), expressed endogenously, and cyclo-oxygenase-2 (COX-2), locally induced during inflammatory processes [7, 20].

Prostaglandins have been extensively studied, with clear demonstration of its potent vasodilating action upon the ductus arteriosus. However, in the last years new substances with constrictive and dilating effects on the ductus arteriosus have been described. The dilating action of 3- and 5- phosphodiesterase inhibitors upon fetal and neonatal ductus arteriosus in rodents have been reported [21, 22]. This effect was shown to be more potent in fetuses than in neonates, suggesting that these substances could be useful in primary and secondary fetal ductal constriction, especially in preterm fetuses when compared to term fetuses [23]. Other substances with dilating effect on the ductus were described, based on the knowledge of the role of endothelin receptors as messengers of postnatal ductal constriction [9, 24, 25]. It was shown that antagonists of endothelin receptors cause potent in vitro inhibition of the constrictive effect of cyclo-oxygenase inhibitors during fetal life, and of the postnatal physiological ductal constriction induced by oxygen [26, 27].

Among the substances with known constrictive effect upon the ductus arteriosus, indomethacin, a cyclo-oxygenase inhibitor used in the treatment of premature labor, is one of the most extensively studied [28-30]. Fetal ductal constriction may occur a few hours after maternal administration and its action may last for several weeks. For this reason, the absence of signs of ductal constriction after 24 to 72 hours of usage does not exclude the diagnosis [28, 29, 31-33]. Ductal sensitivity to indomethacin increases with gestational age, occurring in 5-10% of fetuses with less than 27 weeks, but reaching nearly 100% after 34 weeks of gestation [34, 35]. In addition to indomethacin, it has been shown that several other non-steroidal anti-inflammatory drugs (NSAID), such as nimesulide [36], diclofenac [37], aspirin, matamizole, ibuprofen [38] and many others also have the potential to cause constriction of ductus arteriosus. Selective cyclo-oxygenase-2 inhibitors, such as rofecoxib [20, 38, 39], have also shown a constrictive ductal effect on rat and sheep fetuses [40-42]. Sulindac, another prostaglandin inhibitor drug utilized in premature labor, was demonstrated to have a milder and more transient constrictive effect on fetal ductus than indomethacin [33]. Glucocorticoids also show effects upon the ductus arteriosus patency [43, 44], but the pathophysiologic mechanism involved in the alteration of ductal tonus does not seem to be the same. There is apparent reduction in the ductal sensitivity to prostaglandin E2, which may be consequent to inhibition of the enzymatic liberation of arachidonic acid from phospholipids, a step in prostaglandin synthesis preceding cyclo-oxygenase [45]. Similar to other anti-inflammatory drugs, the ductal effect of glucocorticoid is dose-dependent [46]. Moreover, if associated with selective or non selective NSAID, glucocorticoids have a synergistic action which increases the frequency and severity of ductal constriction; its incidence may double, possibly due to glucocorticoid's ability to decrease the ductal sensitivity to prostaglandin [20, 30]. Other experimentally tested substances with proven constrictive action on rat fetuses are retinoic acid [20, 30, 34, 47], antagonists of prostanoid EP4 receptors [21, 48, 49] and inhibitors of nitric oxide synthesis (L-name) [50-53], the latter with proven effects in humans. Recently, a novel mechanism for sustaining postnatal ductal constriction induced by oxygen has been described, based on activation of the enzyme Rho-kinase [54].

The action of NSAID results from inhibition of prostaglandin synthesis, by inactivation of cyclo-oxygenases. COX-1 and COX-2 are enzymes involved in prostaglandin, prostacyclin and thromboxane biosynthesis[7]. This inhibitory mechanism interferes with the synthesis of prostaglandin G_2, which is a precursor of prostaglandin E_2 e F_2 [28, 29]. The use of anti-inflammatory drugs during pregnancy for the treatment of premature labor, pre-eclampsia or intrauterine growth restriction through prostaglandin biosynthesis inhibition has allowed the study of the relation between ductal constriction and cyclo-oxygenase inhibitors. Indomethacin is the drug with prostaglandin inhibiting action most widely reported in the literature. Its inhibitor effect on cyclo-oxygenase is reversible, persisting until the drug is excreted [32, 55]. The drug passage through the placentary barrier occurs freely during the second half of pregnancy, being minimal in early gestation [56]. The response to indomethacin is individual in each fetus, and even in a twin pregnancy only one fetus could be affected, which suggests differences in ductus maturation [57]. The ductus arteriosus becomes more sensitive to indomethacin as gestational age increases, ductal constriction occurring in 5-10% in fetuses with less than 27 weeks, 15-20% in fetuses between 27 and 31 weeks, 50% at the 32nd week and near 100% above 34 weeks. The occurrence of ductal constriction before the 27th week is uncommon, but there are reports of cases with 22 weeks [58].

As already mentioned, many other non-steroidal anti-inflammatory compounds besides indomethacin are potentially involved in ductal constriction, such as nimesulide [36], diclofenac [37], aspirin, metamizole, ibuprofen [38], and others [59]. An experimental study in rats has suggested a gradation in the magnitude of the action of NSAID upon the fetal ductus, being the constrictive dose-dependent effect [60].

Glucocorticoids are synthetic hormones which mimic endogenous cortisol actions, a hormone produced by the glomerular zone of the adrenal gland. Glucocorticoids also act on ductal patency. As occurs with the majority of other anti-inflammatory substances, this effect is dose-dependent [46]. There is enzymatic liberation of arachidonic acid, blocking prostaglandin synthesis [45], and apparent reduction in sensitivity of the ductus to prostaglandin E_2. Despite the tendency to premature closure of ductus arteriosus, the mechanism of action seems to be related to a primary alteration of the vessel, decreasing vascular reactivity to the relaxing effects of prostaglandin E_2, without altering its synthesis [40, 61]. The association of corticosteroids with indomethacin has shown a synergistic effect [62], and the incidence of ductal constriction doubles when these drugs are taken together, even though other studies have shown that the incidence of ductal constriction with glucocorticoid in isolation was similar to that of a control group [30].

2. Repercussion, Diagnosis and Management of Premature Ductus Arteriosus Constriction

Premature constriction of ductus arteriosus is followed by fetal hemodynamic repercussion. The higher resistance in the ductus generates blood flow turbulence, with increase in systolic and diastolic velocities and decrease in ductal pulsatility index. As a result, there is dilation of the pulmonary artery, right atrium and right ventricle, right to left bulging of the interventricular septum, tricuspid and pulmonary insufficiency and systolic and diastolic ventricular dysfunction [36, 63].

It has been demonstrated in a study in fetuses from 28 to 32 weeks of gestation after indomethacin administration that the drug shows a reversible constrictive effect on the ductus with significant reduction of pulsatility index and association with secondary disturbances, mainly in the right ventricle, as a result of the increase in afterload, observed after about 4 hours, and normalization 24 hours after withdrawal of the substance. It was suggested that the hemodynamic alterations secondary to ductal constriction are right ventricular dilation and signs of heart failure, followed by concentric hypertrophy, decrease in the right ventricular chamber caused by mass increase and left ventricular compromise. These ventricular repercussions were more prominent in the presence of tricuspid regurgitation [64, 65]. Flow redirected through the foramen ovale results in left chambers volumetric overload [65-67]. The aortic isthmus shows a rapid increase in its sectional area in response to local increased flow [68]. This redistribution keeps peripheral perfusion and may explain the findings from clinical experience that show that severe ductal constriction is well tolerated for some days in the human fetus.

Past experimental studies used to speculate that constriction of the ductus arteriosus resulted in an increase of the tunica media layer of pulmonary arteries and generates a secondary increase in intrauterine vascular pulmonary resistance [69]. The hemodynamic alterations in ductal constriction may be related to pulmonary vascular alterations. In the vast majority of studies directed to increase the knowledge about fetal and neonatal pulmonary arterial hypertension, fetal ductal constriction is the experimental model of choice. In a classical study, administration of indomethacin to fetal lambs was followed by fetal ductal constriction and pulmonary hypertension [70]. Blocking of prostaglandin biosynthesis probably has a direct effect in pulmonary arterioles in mammalian fetuses [71, 72]. The sustained increase in right ventricular afterload is capable of producing morphological, functional and hemodynamic modifications, with chronic histological and degenerative alterations of the right ventricular myocardium [73]. Severe ductal constriction may interfere with placentary flow and myocardial performance, and may lead to fetal death. If ductal constriction is less severe or chronical, fetal pulmonary arterial hypertension is a consequence of excessive development of the arteriolar smooth muscular layer and constriction of the pulmonary arterioles. Predominance of the increased thickness of the muscular layer and of the aerial pathway mass is a feature less described in neonatal pulmonary hypertension consequent to other causes [74, 75]. In cases related to maternal drug usage, ventricular dysfunction may reverse after its suspension. However, if this picture is not treated, it may be followed by endocardial ischemia and right ventricular papillary muscles dysfunction, and later on by heart failure, hydrops and potentially death [58]. Intrauterine ductal constriction may cause transient or permanent tricuspid regurgitation and neonatal myocardial ischemia [69, 76].

In clinical practice, in cases with severe ductal constriction after prostaglandin inhibitory drugs, the suspension of its usage may result in a decrease of ductal velocities and an increase in the pulsatility index within 24 hours, with posterior normalization of hemodynamic consequences [55]. Mild cases may be approached with just a decrease in the administered substance concentration, but in every fetus serial echocardiographic follow-up is recommended [28].

The evidence of fetal cardiac dysfunction was described as a characteristic feature of fetal closure of ductus arteriosus [77]. In severe cases, interruption of pregnancy may be indicated, with neonatal cardiopulmonary resuscitation. The clinical course after birth depends on the severity of intrauterine right ventricular cardiac insufficiency and to the response to elevation in pulmonary vascular resistance [78].

Long-term prognosis is still uncertain, but when early evolution is favorable, there are usually no late complications. After the occurrence of fetal heart failure, right ventricular functional abnormalities may persist throughout the neonatal period, even in those patients with a benign outcome.

Utilization of echocardiographic and Doppler techniques has allowed that the diagnosis of fetal ductal constriction, formerly possible only in necropsy, could be made in prenatal life [79]. Fetuses at risk for development of premature constriction of ductus arteriosus could be monitorized and submitted to early intervention when necessary.

Echocardiographic diagnosis of fetal ductal constriction is based on the presence, at color Doppler, of turbulent flow in the ductus (figures 2 and 3), with increased systolic velocity [SV] (higher than 1.4 m/s), increased diastolic velocity [DV] (higher than 0.30 m/s) and decreased pulsatility index [PI] (below 2.2). In the first publications, the cutoff point for the pulsatility index was described as 1.9 [80], but more recent studies have considered a somewhat higher limit [81, 82]. The PI is independent of the ultrasound angle and is useful in the differential diagnosis when there is increased ductal flow without concomitant constriction. This situation may occur when the increased SV is caused by an increase in right ventricular output. The PI does not change with gestational age and should be used to define the diagnosis [83]. When there is total occlusion of the ductus arteriosus, absence of transductal flow is considered diagnostic. With the increase in afterload secondary to ductal constriction, the fetal heart shows initially proliferative growing and, at later stages, hyperplasia is substituted to apoptosis and hypertrophic response [84]. There is characteristically an increase in right to left diameters ratio, an increase in pulmonary artery to aorta ratio with the interventricular septum bulging toward the left ventricle [33] (figure 4).

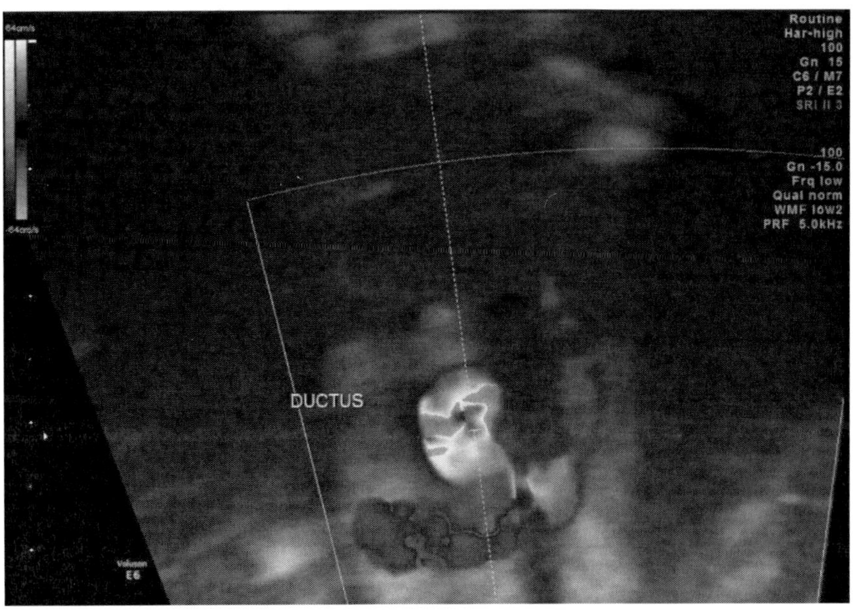

Figure 2. Echocardiographic image with color flow mapping in a 29-week-old fetus showing ductal constriction. There is important flow turbulence and narrowing of the sinuous ductus.

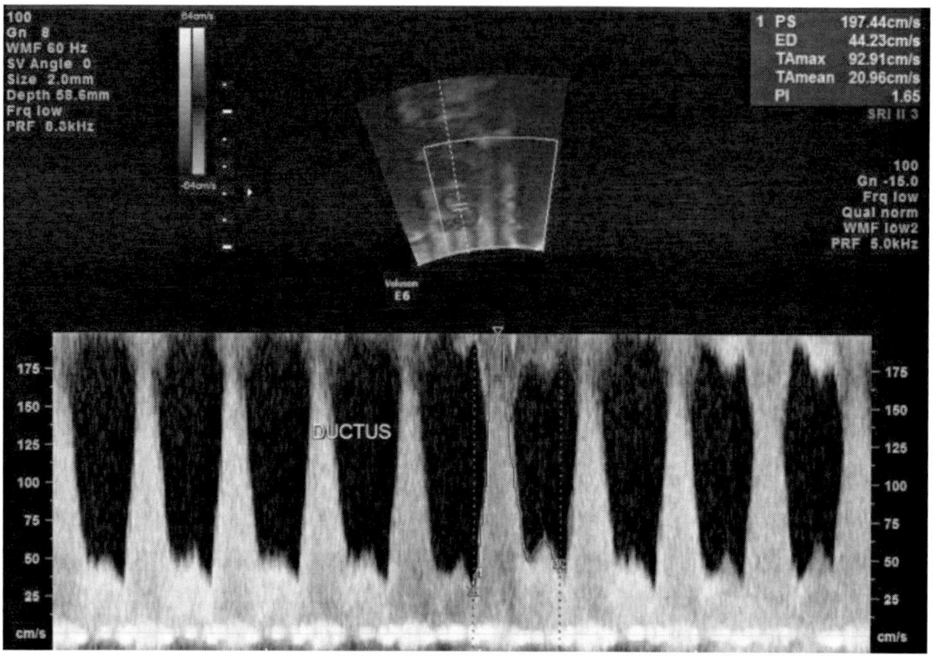

Figure 3. Pulsed Doppler tracing of the same fetus of Figure 2, showing increased systolic and diastolic velocities (1.97 and 0.44 m/s, respectively). The pulsatility index is decreased (1.65).

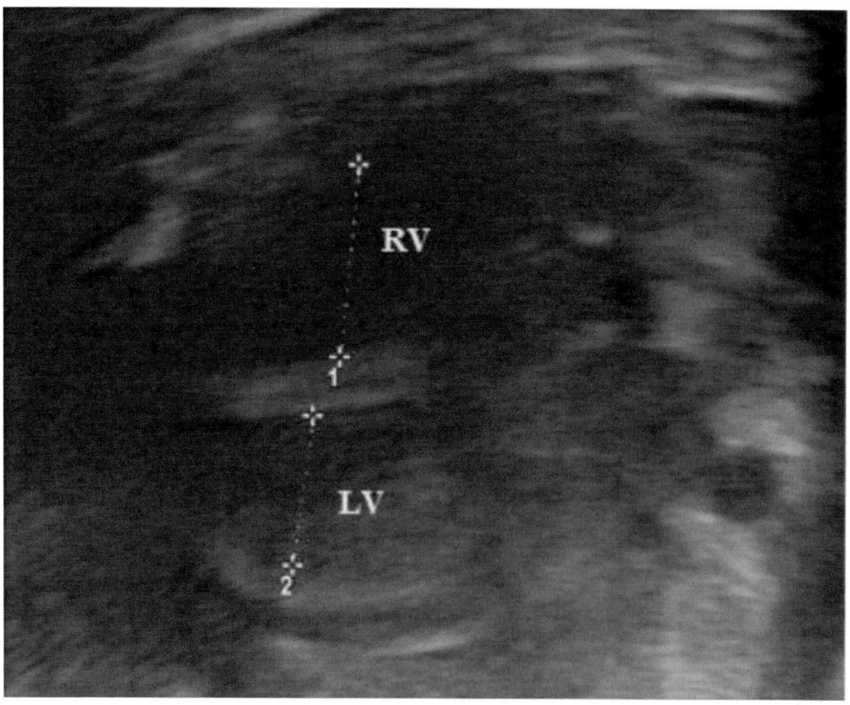

Figure 4. 2D echocardiographic image in a four chambers view (same fetus of Figures 2 and 3). There is marked right to left ventricular disproportion secondary to ductal constriction.

Right ventricular systolic and diastolic functions are impaired in fetuses with ductal constriction, assessed by different methods [73, 79, 85]. The hemodynamic compromise is considered mild when there is mild or no tricuspid and/or pulmonary regurgitation, with normal chambers diameters; moderate in the presence of tricuspid regurgitation with right ventricular dilation without hypertrophy and/or impaired contractility, and severe when the tricuspid and/or pulmonary insufficiency is important or there is functional pulmonary atresia, right ventricular dilation with ventricular parietal hypertrophy and alteration in right ventricular contractile function. The compromise is also considered severe when there is total ductal occlusion or, alternatively, in the presence of a PI lower than 1.0, associated to any degree of hemodynamic repercussion [23, 79]. Since the constrictive effect upon the ductus arteriosus is predominantely dose-dependent [60], it is usual the resolution of hemodynamic alterations after suspension of the causing substances without development of fetal or neonatal cardiac dysfunction [33, 34, 86-88]. Even in the presence of a severe ductal constriction after maternal utilization of drugs with prostaglandin inhibiting effect, withdrawal of their use may show reversal of the increased SV and DV within 24 hours, with improvement of the hemodynamic alterations [33]. In some more severe cases, interruption of pregnancy may be necessary, sometimes with immediate cardiopulmonary neonatal resuscitation. Despite not having established the association between the duration of fetal ductal constriction and the prevalence and severity of neonatal pulmonary hypertension [19], it is obviously important to remove the cause as soon as possible, in order to allow early recovery.

The decision to interrupt pregnancy should take into account fetal pulmonary maturity, the severity of clinical and echocardiographic manifestations of ductal constriction and the presence or not of a progressive pattern. In the immediate neonatal period, the physiologic ductal closure associated to hemodynamic changes usual to this period allow normalization of the cardio-circulatory alterations secondary to the increased right ventricular overload. However, as already mentioned, the prolonged increase in right ventricular pressure, when transmitted to the lungs, may cause a reactive pulmonary arteriolar vasoconstriction with secondary pulmonary artery hypertension, which will need intensive treatment [89]. Since persistent pulmonary hypertension of the neonate without cardiac abnormalities occurs in approximately 1/1000 liveborns, and around 23% of the cases do not have a known definitive etiology, very probably many of these cases are secondary to undetected fetal premature constriction of ductus arteriosus [90]. Thus, ductal constriction should always be considered an etiological possibility in "idiopathic" neonatal persistent pulmonary hypertension. This disorder carries a bad prognosis and is characterized by postnatal persistence of increased pulmonary vascular resistance, cyanosis due to right-to-left shunts through the foramen ovale and ductus, decreased pulmonary blood flow and severe hypoxemia [91, 92]. Persistent pulmonary hypertension of the newborn has been associated to antenatal exposure to NSAID [19, 93-102], even though a recent case-control study could not confirm this risk [103]. In fetal lambs, mechanical occlusion of the fetal ductus arteriosus reproduces the hemodynamic and structural features of persistent pulmonary hypertension of the newborn. Experimental prenatal exposition to NSAID has demonstrated alterations similar to those found in ductal constriction, with increased thickness of the smooth muscle layer of the pulmonary arterial vasculature [29, 104-106].

3. Anti-Inflammatory and Antioxidant Actions of Polyphenols

Polyphenols are chemical structures present in all the superior vegetal organisms. More than 8000 structures are known, and they act on pigmentation, growing, reproduction and resistance of plants against diseases [107]. There are flavonoid and non-flavonoid polyphenols.

Flavonoids represent the major family and are the basic structures of tannins or proanthocyanidins. Tannins and its flavonoids are the most well-known polyphenols in alimentation, because of their presence in beer and wine, but a wide variety of polyphenols are present in a great number of foods and beverages. Many studies have investigated the cynetic and extension of absorption of polyphenols by mensuration of plasma concentration and urinary or plasmatic excretion [108].

Flavonoids are the most abundant polyphenols in the human diet and its consumption has triggered the interest of consumers and food industries for many reasons, but mainly because of their biological activity in systems relevant to human health [109]. This biological activity is related to anti-inflammatory and antioxidant effects [110], based on its interference in the inflammatory cascade, with inhibition of prostaglandin synthesis and mediation of nitric oxide synthetase [111, 112].

Polyphenols with greater importance and literature references are catechins mainly in green and black tea, resveratrol in wine and black grape, chlorogenic acid in coffee and teas and flavonoids present in fruits and vegetables [113].

The principal alimentary sources with higher concentration in polyphenols are herbal teas, mate tea, dark chocolate, fruits, natural juices, vegetables, olive and soy oils and red wine. Among fruits, the highest concentration of flavonoids is orange, red and purple grape, strawberry and other berries, black prune and its derivatives. Vegetables with higher polyphenol purple onion concentration are purple onion, green spices, tomato and derivatives. These foods show a concentration above 30 mg of flavonoids per 100g of food, representing an amount above the 75th percentile of the USDA database [113].

In recent years, many investigational studies have been trying to ascertain the real therapeutic effect of substances found in nature and commonly used by the general population. Several of these substances presently have their anti-inflammatory and antioxidant effects [114, 115] scientifically and unequivocally demonstrated upon the chain of production of oxidative stress related to inflammatory mediators such as COX-2 and prostaglandin E2, metal proteinases and others. Substances rich in polyphenols are among the most widely used for a variety of reasons, even during pregnancy. The anti-inflammatory and antioxidant effects of these substances are secondary to inhibition of the metabolic route of prostaglandin, especially of cyclooxygenase-2, preventing the transformation of arachidonic acid into prostaglandin [20, 39, 59]. The literature reports on the mechanism of antioxidant and anti-inflammatory action of polyphenols, which are beneficial to a large portion of the population, and the scientific evidence of their ethnomedicinal effect, show that a large number of molecules derived from functional foods and plants have been isolated and even introduced successfully in the international pharmaceutical industry [116]. It has been demonstrated unambiguously that the polyphenols decrease oxidative stress (including in pregnancy) [117], plasma triglycerides and cholesterol levels [118], blood pressure [119],

[120, 121], the consequences of gastric hypersecretion [122], the development of some neoplasms [123-125] and atherosclerosis [126, 127], the manifestations of aging [128] and Alzheimer's disease [129], and various other health problems. Polyphenols such as quercitin and kaempferol, among many others, are present in many foods and their anti-inflammatory and antinociceptive activities have been shown to be as or more powerful than those of indomethacin [129-131].

Green tea, for example, is a compound of young leaves from the plant *Camellia sinensis* [132]. Approximately 30-40% of the leaves´ solid extract is composed of polyphenols, mainly catechins. Among the most important catechins present in green tea are epicatechin, gallate-3.epicatechin, epigallocatechin and, predominantely, gallate-3-epigallocatechin, with contains 7g per 100g of dry leaves. Several *in vitro* studies, both in animals and in humans, have demonstrated their antioxidant, anticarcinogenic, anti-inflammatory, probiotic and antimicrobial *actions secondary to inhibition of the endogenous inflammatory response, dependent on the interference on the prostaglandin synthesis pathway* [133-136]. Black tea has also showed to be rich in catechins, and the tea compound involving theaflavin has been shown to act on nitric oxide and on the liberation of arachidonic acid. It has already been clearly demonstrated that tea drinkers could benefit from the protective cardiovascular effects exerted by this polyphenol-rich substance [137, 138].

Resveratrol, a polyphenol compound found in grape rind, grape juice and red wine, is known by its antioxidant, antithrombotic anti-inflammatory and anticarcinogenic actions [139]. Several studies have demonstrated the effect of resveratrol upon the nervous system, as well as on the liver and the cardiovascular system. One of the possible mechanisms that explain its biological activity is related to a decrease in liberation of arachidonic acid, thus affecting induction of COX-2, with a consequent reduction in prostaglandin synthesis [140, 141].

Mate tea, a typical regional beverage very rich in polyphenols, widely consumed in South America, mainly Paraguay, Brazil, Argentina and Uruguay, is obtained from the dried and minced leaves of *Ilex paraguariensis*. Many studies have demonstrated its potent antineoplasic, anti-inflammatory and antioxidant effects, due to the action of its polyphenolic compounds [142].

Orange juice has been shown to have important antioxidant activity as a result of a high content of flavonoids, especially quercitin, and the ability of the phytochemical substance to interact with biomembranes. It was speculated that the daily consumption of orange juice might be useful in providing additional protection against cellular oxidation *in vivo* [143].

Dark chocolate shows high concentration of flavonoids and has anti-inflammatory properties. It has been demonstrated to have an inverse association with C-reactive protein, in amounts as low as 20g every 3 days, suggesting that the regular intake of dark chocolate may reduce inflammatory processes [144]. Since flavonoids modify the production of pro-inflammatory cytokines, the synthesis of eicosanoids, the activation of platelets and nitric oxide-mediated mechanisms, a growing body of evidence is available to support the potential action of cocoa flavonoids in inflammation [145].

Many other substances rich in polyphenols present in nature commonly used in daily routine by the general population also have shown definite anti-inflammatory effects secondary to inhibition of the prostaglandin synthesis pathway. Examples are boldine, with anti-inflammatory and antithermic activities [146], propolis, with anti-inflammatory action in asthmatic patients [147], passion fruit, with cytotoxic, anti-inflammatory and scar-promoting effects [147-149], tomato and ginseng, also with anti-inflammatory action on COX-2 [150] salvia, with anti-inflammatory effects on acute and chronic processes [151, 152], chamomile, with moderate antioxidant and animicrobial activity and significant *in vitro* antiplatelet actions [153-155], and many others, with variable concentrations of polyphenol substances presenting anti-inflammatory and antioxidant effects, all of them by interfering with prostaglandin synthesis.

A number of foods and beverages such as herbal teas, grapes and derivatives, orange, chocolate, fruits and many others, with high concentrations of polyphenols, are freely consumed throughout gestation. Despite the positive effects of polyphenols in general health, as discussed in the previous sections, other studies from our group and others point toward the indication that maternal consumption of polyphenol-rich foods in late pregnancy, specifically in the third trimester, may be harmful to fetal health, as a result of the anti-inflammatory and antioxidant effects of these substances upon the ductus arteriosus, due to the inhibition of prostaglandin synthesis [81, 156-162]. These findings will be discussed in the next topics.

4. Role of Maternal Intake of Polyphenol-Rich Substances upon Fetal Ductus Arteriosus

As stated, constriction of fetal ductus arteriosus is a risk factor for pulmonary hypertension in the newborn period, with its known severe consequences. We have already suggested that maternal ingestion of polyphenol-rich foods in late pregnancy, such as herbal teas, orange and grape juice, dark chocolate, coffee, berries, olive and soy oils and many others, could be associated to fetal ductal constriction. The rationale for understanding the behavior of fetal ductal arteriosus flow dynamics after maternal ingestion of polyphenols in late pregnancy is that these substances have definite anti-inflammatory and antioxidant effects, largely reported in the literature, based on the inhibition of cyclooxygenase-2 or other components of the metabolic cascade resulting in prostaglandins biosynthesis. These actions are similar to that involved in prostaglandin inhibition caused by NSAID.

The following sections intend to show the summary of the ongoing research dealing with this issue. The majority of these experimental and clinical studies have been published and are quoted in the references.

4.1. Experimental Studies

Experimental studies to assess the fetal ductal effects of maternal consumption of polyphenol-rich foods utilized ewes in the last third of pregnancy (more than 120 days), corresponding to the third trimester of human gestation.

The first study has shown that fetuses of ewes submitted to an experimental diet of mate tea or green tea as the only source of liquid for one week developed ductal constriction, with unequivocal histological signs: right ventricular enlargement, right ventricular hypertrophy and increased avascular zone thickness at the ductal wall [163].

The second study demonstrated that maternal exposure of green tea for one week was followed by fetal constriction, with an increase in mean systolic velocity and mean diastolic velocity, decrease of pulsatility index and increase of mean right ventricular/left ventricular diameter ratio. Morphological repercussion was shown by dilated and hypertrophic right ventricles and increased ductal lumen avascular zone in the group exposed to green tea, but not in those of the control group, whose mothers received only water [159].

An experimental study recently submitted for publication tested the hypothesis that maternal exposure to a diet with a high content of polyphenols is followed by fetal ductal constriction and by alteration of endogenous inflammatory and oxidant mediators. Six pregnant sheep with more than 120 days of gestational age were fed for two weeks with a standardized amount of polyphenol-rich foods (basal intake + 3100 mg/day). A significant increase of ductal systolic and diastolic velocities and a decrease in pulsatility index was shown after 14 days of intervention when compared to the basal state, indicating fetal ductal constriction. Total urinary polyphenol excretion increased significantly after intervention. It showed a decrease in lipid peroxidation, determined by plasma thiobarbituric acid reactive substances (TBARS) and by non-protein reduced thiols after treatment. There was an increase in enzymes catalase and glutathione peroxidase after dietary intervention. The vasoconstrictor and anti-inflammatory effects were demonstrated by a decrease in nitric oxide after polyphenol consumption. Oxidative stress was associated with echocardiographic parameters of ductal constriction. Moreover, ductal systolic velocity was correlated with catalase and a ductal flow pulsatility index inversely with glutathione peroxidase. Ductal constriction was also negatively associated with inflammatory parameters, being systolic and diastolic velocities correlated with nitric oxide, and likewise ductal pulsatility index. In addition, both anti-inflammatory and antioxidant mechanisms (nitric oxide with glutathione peroxidase, and nitric oxide with catalase) were correlated, confirming that both effects could be attributed to polyphenols. In conclusion, elevated experimental maternal polyphenol consumption in ewes induced fetal ductal constriction with increased urinary excretion of total polyphenols and alterations in biomarkers of oxidative stress, characterizing the antioxidant and anti-inflammatory actions of polyphenols [164, 165].

4.2. Clinical Studies

4.2.1. Development and Validation of a Food Frequency Questionnaire for Consumption of Polyphenol-Rich Foods in Pregnant Women

All clinical studies were performed to evaluate the effects of maternal intake of polyphenol-rich foods after the third trimester of pregnancy on fetal ductus arteriosus depend on the adequate assessment of its concentration, and there were no validated instruments to quantify total polyphenols in pregnant women. Thus, the aim of this study was to evaluate the reproducibility and validity of a food frequency questionnaire (FFQ) with 52 items, to assess the intake of polyphenol-rich foods in pregnant women in Brazil. This cross-sectional study included 120 pregnant women who participated in two-minute nutritional interviews. The intake of polyphenols estimated by the developed FFQ was compared with the average of two 24-h recalls (24HR), with the average intake measured by a 3-day food diary (D3days) and with the urinary excretion of total polyphenols. Analysis of the reproducibility between the FFQ showed a very high correlation. A low but significant association was observed between the FFQ and urinary excretion, as usual in this kind of comparison. The association between the dietary survey methods varied from moderate to very high. In conclusion, this questionnaire showed reproducibility and validity for the quantification of consumption of total polyphenols in pregnant women[160].

4.2.2. Maternal Consumption of Polyphenol-Rich Foods in Late Pregnancy and Fetal Ductus Arteriosus Flow Dynamics

We hypothesized that polyphenols or flavonoids present in food and beverages commonly consumed by pregnant women could influence ductal flow dynamics, probably by inhibition of prostaglandin synthesis, and thus be a risk factor for ductal constriction. With that in mind, we compared ductal flow behavior and right ventricular size in third-trimester fetuses exposed, and not exposed, to polyphenol-rich foods and beverages via maternal consumption, to test the hypothesis that maternal consumption of polyphenol-rich foods during the third trimester interferes with fetal ductal dynamics. In a prospective analysis, Doppler ductal velocities and right-to-left ventricular dimensions ratio of 102 normal fetuses exposed to polyphenol-rich foods (daily estimated maternal consumption above the 75th percentile, or 1089 mg, as previously determined) were compared with 41 normal unexposed fetuses (polyphenol ingestion below the 25th percentile, or 127 mg). In the exposed fetuses, ductal velocities were higher and right-to-left ventricular ratio was higher than in unexposed fetuses. We concluded that since it was shown that polyphenol-rich foods intake in late gestation may trigger alterations in fetal ductal dynamics, changes in perinatal dietary orientation should be recommended, with the purpose to decrease maternal polyphenol ingestion [157].

4.2.3. Reversal of Fetal Ductal Constriction after Maternal Restriction of Polyphenol-Rich Foods: An Open Clinical Trial

The purpose of this study was to test the hypothesis that fetuses with constriction of ductus arteriosus and no history of maternal ingestion of NSAID, but whose mothers have used polyphenol-rich foods (PRF) in the third trimester, show complete reversal of the ductal constrictive effect and its hemodynamics consequences after maternal dietary intervention aimed at restriction of these substances. A controlled clinical trial of 51 third trimester fetuses with ductal constriction with no history of NSAID intake was designed. All mothers were submitted to a food frequency questionnaire and were oriented to withdraw polyphenol-rich foods, being reassessed after 3 weeks. A control group of 26 third trimester normal fetuses, with no ductus arteriosus constriction, in which no dietary intervention was offered, was reviewed after 3 weeks. After discontinuation of PRF for three weeks or more, by means of a detailed nutritional intervention, with adequate substitution of essential nutrients, 48/51 fetuses (96%) showed complete reversal of ductal constriction, with decrease in mean ductal systolic velocity, mean diastolic velocity, mean right to left ventricular dimension ratio and increase in mean ductal pulsatility index. Median daily maternal consumption of polyphenol-rich foods was 286 mg per day and decreased after orientation to 0 mg per day. In the control group, there was no significant differences in median daily maternal consumption of PRF, mean ductal systolic velocity, diastolic velocity, pulsatility index and right ventricular to left ventricular diameter ratio. This behavior is similar to that already widely reported upon the withdrawal of NSAID in fetuses with constriction of ductus arteriosus caused by those pharmacological agents, when there is habitual regression of the disorder. The original conclusion of this controlled clinical trial was that reduction of maternal polyphenol intake during pregnancy, especially in the third trimester, is followed by complete reversal of ductal constriction, which may reduce the risk of neonatal hypertension and influence maternal dietary habits in late pregnancy [81].

4.2.4. Restriction of Polyphenols and Fetal Ductal Flow in Normal Pregnancies: An Open Clinical Trial

Since we had have demonstrated reversal of fetal ductal constriction after dietary maternal restriction of polyphenol-rich foods, due to its inhibitory action on prostaglandin synthesis, we tested the hypothesis that normal third trimester fetuses also improve ductus arteriosus dynamics after maternal restriction of polyphenols. We designed a controlled clinical trial with 46 fetuses with gestational age equal to or above 28 weeks submitted to two Doppler echocardiographic studies with an interval of at least two weeks, being the examiners blinded to maternal dietary habits. A validated food frequency questionnaire was applied and a diet based on polyphenol-poor foods (less than 30mg/100mg) was recommended. A control group of 26 third trimester fetuses was submitted to the same protocol. Mean daily maternal estimated polyphenol intake (DMPI) decreased after dietary orientation. Significant decreases in systolic (SV) and diastolic [166] ductal velocities, and RV/LV diameters ratio, as well as an increase in ductal pulsatility index (PI) were observed. In the control group there were no significant differences in DMPI, mean SV, DV, PI and RV/LV ratio.

This study demonstrated that, as already reported for fetuses with ductal constriction, dietary intervention for restricting the intake of foods rich in polyphenols by pregnant women in the third trimester for a period of two weeks or more improves ductus arteriosus flow dynamics and decreases the right ventricle size in normal fetuses. Ductal constriction is a non-categorical, "yes or no" phenomenon, but rather a continuous spectrum with increasing severity related to the clinical manifestations of right ventricular overload, tricuspid and/or pulmonary regurgitation and Doppler-echocardiographic findings of increased systolic and mainly diastolic ductal flow velocities, as well as a decrease of the ductal pulsatility index. Therefore, it seems logical to consider that the initial changes, even though still not filling in the classic criteria of constriction, can develop into more serious forms, exceeding the established diagnostic cutoff points. The sample assessed in this study was composed of normal fetuses, with exclusion of those who already had a diagnosis of ductal constriction, in order to demonstrate how the nutritional guidance can decrease the potential risk for development of the disease. This data can influence obstetric monitoring and guidance of the eating habits of pregnant women at late pregnancy [156].

4.2.5. Other Studies Relating Maternal Polyphenol Ingestion to Ductal Constriction

Several studies in the international literature have discussed the relationship between idiopathic prenatal ductal constriction and maternal consumption of polyphenol-rich foods in late pregnancy, in the absence of exposure to non-steroidal anti-inflammatory drugs [167, 168]. Case reports have shown the association of severe ductal constriction with hemodynamic repercussion (hydrops, enlarged right atrium and right ventricle) to maternal ingestion of polyphenols, such as violet vegetable juice, prune berry [169] and chamomile herbal tea [162].

Kapadia, V., et al reported a case of fetal ductal constriction related to maternal consumption of a juice blend containing the cyclooxygenase and nitric oxide synthase inhibitors anthocyanins and proanthocyanidins for one week in late pregnancy. After birth, the newborn developed persistent neonatal pulmonary hypertension, needing oxygen for a prolonged period [161].

Conclusion

When the level of evidence regarding the recommendation of avoidance of polyphenol-rich substances by pregnant women, at the third trimester, is critically analyzed, an important question naturally arises: why not perform a randomized clinical trial to obtain the strongest possible evidence of this action, at the apex of the pyramid? Such a study, in simple terms, would try to resolve the research problem of the value of nutritional intervention (restriction of polyphenols in the maternal diet) against no intervention, in the presence of fetal ductal constriction without history of prenatal exposure to NSAID. In this hypothetical trial, the study factor would be the restriction of maternal intake of polyphenol-rich foods in fetuses with ductal constriction in late pregnancy and the outcome the improvement of fetal echocardiographic signs of ductal constriction - decrease is systolic and diastolic ductal velocities, increase in pulsatility index, decrease in right to left ventricular diameters ratio and pulmonary artery to aorta dimensions ratio, of flow turbulence, septal bulging and tricuspid regurgitation. Would there be equipoise in a randomized clinical trial with the proposed intervention and outcomes [170-174]? In other words, would it be ethical to perform a randomized clinical trial to assess the benefit of polyphenol restriction in the maternal diet at the third trimester in the presence of ductal constriction? The answer to that question, considering the conceptual model to obtain a state of equipoise, is "no"! Such a state of equipoise needs the triangular interrelationship of the 3 points: 1) definite benefit of the study to society; 2) doubt of the investigator about the intervention effectivity; 3) safety of all the subjects in the two arms of the clinical trial [172, 175-178]. Even though there is a clear benefit to society in defining if maternal nutritional intervention decreasing maternal intake of polyphenols in late pregnancy improves fetal ductal constriction, the two remaining points of the triangle of the conceptual model of equipoise are not fulfilled. The uncertainty about the effectivity of maternal restriction of polyphenols is no longer present, based on the previous published studies herein disclosed and, most importantly, safety in the two arms of a randomized clinical trial in which one of them would not receive a clearly effective intervention cannot be established. The deleterious effects of ductal constriction upon fetal hemodynamics and the risk of pulmonary arterial hypertension secondary to this functional disorder are well known. There are no reports in the literature of spontaneous reversal of ductal constriction, without removal of the causal factor. How to submit the control group to the risk of keeping the ductus constricted, with all its potential complications? In summary, a randomized clinical trial to assess the effect of maternal dietary intervention in fetuses with ductal constriction, with the level of evidences today accumulated, do not fulfill the equipoise principles, and for this reason cannot be considered ethical.

The number of evidences already available recommend (Class II, level A) a note of caution with regard to the consumption by women in the third trimester of pregnancy of foods with high concentrations of polyphenols, as well as non-steroidal anti-inflammatory drugs, in order to avoid triggering constriction of ductus arteriosus, with its potential harmful consequences, such as fetal and neonatal heart failure and pulmonary arterial hypertension of the newborn.

In the presence of fetal ductal constriction unrelated to exposure of NSAID, it is essential to apply a food frequency questionnaire to assess maternal daily consumption of polyphenols, in order to program the necessary nutritional intervention.

All the information disclosed in this chapter have been discussed in a review article recently published by the same authors [179].

References

[1] Bergwerff, M., M.C. DeRuiter, and A.C. Gittenberger-de Groot, Comparative anatomy and ontogeny of the ductus arteriosus, a vascular outsider. *Anat Embryol* (Berl), 1999. 200(6): p. 559-71.

[2] Ho, S.Y. and R.H. Anderson, Anatomical closure of the ductus arteriosus: a study in 35 specimens. *J Anat,* 1979. 128(Pt 4): p. 829-36.

[3] Yajima, I., et al., A subpopulation of smooth muscle cells, derived from melanocyte-competent precursors, prevents patent ductus arteriosus. *PLoS One,* 2013. 8(1): p. e53183.

[4] Tada, T., et al., Human ductus arteriosus. A histological study on the relation between ductal maturation and gestational age. *Acta Pathol Jpn,* 1985. 35(1): p. 23-34.

[5] Slomp, J., et al., Formation of intimal cushions in the ductus arteriosus as a model for vascular intimal thickening. An immunohistochemical study of changes in extracellular matrix components. *Atherosclerosis,* 1992. 93(1-2): p. 25-39.

[6] de Reeder, E.G., et al., Distribution of prostacyclin synthase, 6-keto-prostaglandin F1 alpha, and 15-hydroxy-prostaglandin dehydrogenase in the normal and persistent ductus arteriosus of the dog. *Am J Pathol,* 1989. 135(5): p. 881-7.

[7] Majed BH, K.R., Molecular mechanisms regulating the vascular prostacyclin pathways and their adaptation during pregnancy and in the newborn. *Pharmacological Reviews,* 2012.

[8] Slomp, J., et al., Differentiation, dedifferentiation, and apoptosis of smooth muscle cells during the development of the human ductus arteriosus. *Arterioscler Thromb Vasc Biol,* 1997. 17(5): p. 1003-9.

[9] Hong, Z., et al., Role of dynamin-related protein 1 (Drp1)-mediated mitochondrial fission in oxygen sensing and constriction of the ductus arteriosus. *Circ Res,* 2013. 112(5): p. 802-15.

[10] Obladen, M., History of the ductus arteriosus: 1. Anatomy and spontaneous closure. *Neonatology,* 2011. 99(2): p. 83-9.

[11] Coceani, F., Oxygen sensing in the ductus arteriosus: endothelin still a player. *Circ Res,* 2013. 112(11): p. e154.

[12] Michelakis, E.D., et al., Hypoxic pulmonary vasoconstriction: redox regulation of O2-sensitive K+ channels by a mitochondrial O2-sensor in resistance artery smooth muscle cells. *J Mol Cell Cardiol,* 2004. 37(6): p. 1119-36.

[13] Coceani, F. and B. Baragatti, Mechanisms for ductus arteriosus closure. *Semin Perinatol,* 2012. 36(2): p. 92-7.

[14] Heymann, M.A. and A.M. Rudolph, Control of the ductus arteriosus. *Physiol Rev,* 1975. 55(1): p. 62-78.

[15] Brezinka, C., A.C. Gittenberger-de Groot, and J.W. Wladimiroff, The fetal ductus arteriosus, a review. *Zentralbl Gynakol,* 1993. 115(10): p. 423-32.

[16] Tynan, M., The ductus arteriosus and its closure. *N Engl J Med,* 1993. 329(21): p. 1570-2.

[17] Stoller, J.Z., et al., Current Perspectives on Pathobiology of the Ductus Arteriosus. J Clin Exp Cardiolog, 2012. 8(1).

[18] Levin, M., et al., ATP depletion and cell death in the neonatal lamb ductus arteriosus. *Pediatr Res,* 2005. 57(6): p. 801-5.

[19] Tarcan, A., et al., Persistent pulmonary hypertension in a premature newborn after 16 hours of antenatal indomethacin exposure. *J Perinat Med,* 2004. 32(1): p. 98-9.

[20] Takami, T., K. Momma, and S. Imamura, Increased constriction of the ductus arteriosus by dexamethasone, indomethacin, and rofecoxib in fetal rats. *Circ J,* 2005. 69(3): p. 354-8.

[21] Momma, K., et al., In vivo constriction of the fetal and neonatal ductus arteriosus by a prostanoid EP4-receptor antagonist in rats. *Pediatr Res,* 2005. 58(5): p. 971-5.

[22] Ichikawa, Y., et al., Inhibition of phosphodiesterase type 3 dilates the rat ductus arteriosus without inducing intimal thickening. *Circ J,* 2012. 76(10): p. 2456-64.

[23] Toyoshima, K., et al., In vivo dilatation of the fetal and postnatal ductus arteriosus by inhibition of phosphodiesterase 3 in rats. *Biol Neonate,* 2006. 89(4): p. 251-6.

[24] Coceani, F., et al., Deletion of the endothelin-A-receptor suppresses oxygen-induced constriction but not postnatal closure of the ductus arteriosus. *J Cardiovasc Pharmacol,* 2000. 36(5 Suppl 1): p. S75-7.

[25] Baragatti, B., et al., Cytochrome P-450 3A13 and endothelin jointly mediate ductus arteriosus constriction to oxygen in mice. *Am J Physiol Heart Circ Physiol,* 2011. 300(3): p. H892-901.

[26] Momma, K., T. Nakanishi, and S. Imamura, Inhibition of in vivo constriction of fetal ductus arteriosus by endothelin receptor blockade in rats. *Pediatr Res,* 2003. 53(3): p. 479-85.

[27] Takizawa, T., et al., Effects of TAK-044, a nonselective endothelin receptor antagonist, on the spontaneous and indomethacin- or methylene blue-induced constriction of the ductus arteriosus in rats. *J Vet Med Sci,* 2000. 62(5): p. 505-9.

[28] Norton, M.E., Teratogen update: fetal effects of indomethacin administration during pregnancy. *Teratology,* 1997. 56(4): p. 282-92.

[29] Sharpe, G.L., K.S. Larsson, and B. Thalme, Studies on closure of the ductus arteriosus. XII. In utero effect of indomethacin and sodium salicylate in rats and rabbits. *Prostaglandins,* 1975. 9(4): p. 585-96.

[30] Levy, R., et al., Indomethacin and corticosteroids: an additive constrictive effect on the fetal ductus arteriosus. *Am J Perinatol,* 1999. 16(8): p. 379-83.

[31] Dudley, D.K. and M.J. Hardie, Fetal and neonatal effects of indomethacin used as a tocolytic agent. *Am J Obstet Gynecol,* 1985. 151(2): p. 181-4.
[32] Gordon, M.C. and P. Samuels, Indomethacin. *Clin Obstet Gynecol,* 1995. 38(4): p. 697-705.
[33] Rasanen, J. and P. Jouppila, Fetal cardiac function and ductus arteriosus during indomethacin and sulindac therapy for threatened preterm labor: a randomized study. *Am J Obstet Gynecol,* 1995. 173(1): p. 20-5.
[34] Moise, K.J., Jr., et al., Indomethacin in the treatment of premature labor. Effects on the fetal ductus arteriosus. *N Engl J Med,* 1988. 319(6): p. 327-31.
[35] Vermillion, S.T., et al., The effect of indomethacin tocolysis on fetal ductus arteriosus constriction with advancing gestational age. *Am J Obstet Gynecol,* 1997. 177(2): p. 256-9; discussion 259-61.
[36] Paladini, D., M. Marasini, and P. Volpe, Severe ductal constriction in the third-trimester fetus following maternal self-medication with nimesulide. *Ultrasound Obstet Gynecol,* 2005. 25(4): p. 357-61.
[37] Auer, M., et al., Prenatal diagnosis of intrauterine premature closure of the ductus arteriosus following maternal diclofenac application. *Ultrasound Obstet Gynecol,* 2004. 23(5): p. 513-6.
[38] Schiessl, B., et al., Prenatal constriction of the fetal ductus arteriosus--related to maternal pain medication? *Z Geburtshilfe Neonato*l, 2005. 209(2): p. 65-8.
[39] Toyoshima, K., et al., Constriction of the ductus arteriosus by selective inhibition of cyclooxygenase-1 and -2 in near-term and preterm fetal rats. *Prostaglandins Other Lipid Mediat,* 2006. 79(1-2): p. 34-42.
[40] Clyman, R.I., et al., Glucocorticoids alter the sensitivity of the lamb ductus arteriosus to prostaglandin E2. *J Pediatr,* 1981. 98(1): p. 126-8.
[41] Karadas, B., et al., Comparison of effects of cyclooxygenase inhibitors on myometrial contraction and constriction of ductus arteriosus in rats. *Eur J Pharmacol,* 2004. 485(1-3): p. 289-98.
[42] Takahashi, Y., et al., Cyclooxygenase-2 inhibitors constrict the fetal lamb ductus arteriosus both in vitro and in vivo. *Am J Physiol Regul Integr Comp Physiol*, 2000. 278(6): p. R1496-505.
[43] Clyman, R.I., et al., Prenatal administration of betamethasone for prevention of patient ductus arteriosus. *J Pediatr,* 1981. 98(1): p. 123-6.
[44] Azancot-Benisty, A., et al., Constriction of the fetal ductus arteriosus during prenatal betamethasone therapy. *Obstet Gynecol,* 1995. 85(5 Pt 2): p. 874-6.
[45] Hassid, A., Regulation of prostaglandin biosynthesis in cultured cells. *Am J Physiol,* 1982. 243(5): p. C205-11.
[46] Momma, K., S. Nishihara, and Y. Ota, Constriction of the fetal ductus arteriosus by glucocorticoid hormones. *Pediatr Res,* 1981. 15(1): p. 19-21.
[47] Wu, G.R., et al., The effect of vitamin A on contraction of the ductus arteriosus in fetal rats. *Pediatr Res,* 2001. 49(6): p. 747-54.
[48] Chen, J.X., et al., Isoprostanes as physiological mediators of transition to newborn life: novel mechanisms regulating patency of the term and preterm ductus arteriosus. *Pediatr Res,* 2012. 72(2): p. 122-8.
[49] Fenling Fan, A.M.a., Youfei Guan, Jianhua Huo, Zhi Hu, Hongyan Tian, Lihong Chen, Sen Zhu, Lihong Fan, Effect of PGE2 on DA tone by EP4 modulating Kv channels

with different oxygen tension between preterm and term. *International Journal of Cardiology,* 2009.

[50] Keller, R.L., et al., Combined treatment with a nonselective nitric oxide synthase inhibitor (l-NMMA) and indomethacin increases ductus constriction in extremely premature newborns. *Pediatr Res,* 2005. 58(6): p. 1216-21.

[51] Takizawa, T., T. Kihara, and A. Kamata, Increased constriction of the ductus arteriosus with combined administration of indomethacin and L-NAME in fetal rats. *Biol Neonate,* 2001. 80(1): p. 64-7.

[52] Reese J, O.M.P., Poole SD, Brown N, Tolentino C, Eckman DM, Aschner JL., Regulation of the fetal mouse ductus arteriosus is dependent on interaction of nitric oxide and COX enzymes in the ductal wall. *Prostaglandins & Other Lipid Mediators,* 2009.

[53] Hsu, J.H., et al., Nitric oxide alterations following acute ductal constriction in the fetal lamb: a role for superoxide. *Am J Physiol Lung Cell Mol Physiol,* 2010. 298(6): p. L880-7.

[54] Kajimoto, H., et al., Oxygen activates the Rho/Rho-kinase pathway and induces RhoB and ROCK-1 expression in human and rabbit ductus arteriosus by increasing a mitochondria-derived reactive oxygen species: a newly recognized mechanism for sustaining ductal constriction. *Circulatio*n, 2007. 115(13): p. 1777-88.

[55] Vogel M, W.-H.L., McElhinney DB, Marshall AC, Benson CB, Silva V, Tworetzky W., Reversible ductus arteriosus constriction due to maternal indomethacin after fetal intervention for hypoplastic left heart syndrome with intact/restrictive atrial septum. *Fetal Diagnosis and Therapy,* 2011.

[56] Moise, K.J., Jr., et al., Placental transfer of indomethacin in the human pregnancy. *Am J Obstet Gynecol,* 1990. 162(2): p. 549-54.

[57] Hallak, M., et al., Indomethacin for preterm labor: fetal toxicity in a dizygotic twin gestation. *Obstet Gynecol,* 1991. 78(5 Pt 2): p. 911-3.

[58] Moise, K.J., Jr., Effect of advancing gestational age on the frequency of fetal ductal constriction in association with maternal indomethacin use. *Am J Obstet Gynecol,* 1993. 168(5): p. 1350-3.

[59] Koren, G., et al., Nonsteroidal antiinflammatory drugs during the third trimester and the risk of premature closure of the ductus arteriosus: a meta-analysis. *Ann Pharmacother,* 2006. 40(5): p. 824-9.

[60] Momma, K., H. Hagiwara, and T. Konishi, Constriction of fetal ductus arteriosus by non-steroidal anti-inflammatory drugs: study of additional 34 drugs. *Prostaglandins,* 1984. 28(4): p. 527-36.

[61] Cooper, C.L. and K.U. Malik, Effect of glucocorticoids on vascular reactivity to vasoactive hormones in rat isolated kidney: lack of relationship to prostaglandins. *Br J Pharmacol,* 1984. 82(3): p. 679-88.

[62] Wasserstrum, N., et al., Betamethasone and the human fetal ductus arteriosus. *Obstet Gynecol,* 1989. 74(6): p. 897-900.

[63] Mushiake K, M.F., Kinoshita Y, Nakagawa A, Ito M., Severe heart failure due to ductal constriction caused by maternal indomethacin. *Pediatrics Internacional,* 2002.

[64] Eronen, M., et al., The effects of indomethacin and a beta-sympathomimetic agent on the fetal ductus arteriosus during treatment of premature labor: a randomized double-blind study. *Am J Obstet Gynecol,* 1991. 164(1 Pt 1): p. 141-6.

[65] Eronen, M., The hemodynamic effects of antenatal indomethacin and a beta-sympathomimetic agent on the fetus and the newborn: a randomized study. *Pediatr Res,* 1993. 33(6): p. 615-9.
[66] Harlass, F.E., et al., Hydrops fetalis and premature closure of the ductus arteriosus: a review. *Obstet Gynecol Surv,* 1989. 44(7): p. 541-3.
[67] Fyfe, D.A. and C.H. Kline, Fetal echocardiographic diagnosis of congenital heart disease. *Pediatr Clin North Am,* 1990. 37(1): p. 45-67.
[68] Momma, K. and M. Ando, In situ morphology of fetal aortic isthmus following ductal constriction in rats. *Fetal Diagn Ther,* 1994. 9(1): p. 53-61.
[69] Levin, D.L., et al., Fetal hypertension and the development of increased pulmonary vascular smooth muscle: a possible mechanism for persistent pulmonary hypertension of the newborn infant. *J Pediatr,* 1978. 92(2): p. 265-9.
[70] Levin, D.L., L.J. Mills, and A.G. Weinberg, Hemodynamic, pulmonary vascular, and myocardial abnormalities secondary to pharmacologic constriction of the fetal ductus arteriosus. A possible mechanism for persistent pulmonary hypertension and transient tricuspid insufficiency in the newborn infant. *Circulation,* 1979. 60(2): p. 360-4.
[71] Cassin, S., et al., Pulmonary and systemic vascular responses of perinatal goats to prostaglandins E1 and E2. *Am J Physiol,* 1979. 236(6): p. H828-32.
[72] Starling, M.B. and R.B. Elliott, The effects of prostaglandins, prostaglandin inhibitors, and oxygen on the closure of the ductus arteriosus, pulmonary arteries and umbilical vessels in vitro. *Prostaglandins,* 1974. 8(3): p. 187-203.
[73] Harada, K., et al., Doppler echocardiographic evaluation of ventricular diastolic filling in fetuses with ductal constriction. *Am J Cardiol,* 1997. 79(4): p. 442-6.
[74] Murphy, J.D., et al., The structural basis of persistent pulmonary hypertension of the newborn infant. *J Pediatr,* 1981. 98(6): p. 962-7.
[75] Murphy, J.D., G.F. Vawter, and L.M. Reid, Pulmonary vascular disease in fatal meconium aspiration. *J Pediatr, 1*984. 104(5): p. 758-62.
[76] Levin, D.L., et al., Morphological development of the pulmonary vascular bed in fetal lambs. *Circulation,* 1976. 53(1): p. 144-51.
[77] Macones, G.A. and C.A. Robinson, Is there justification for using indomethacin in preterm labor? An analysis of neonatal risks and benefits. *Am J Obstet Gynecol,* 1997. 177(4): p. 819-24.
[78] Hofstadler, G., et al., Spontaneous closure of the human fetal ductus arteriosus--A cause of fetal congestive heart failure. *Am J Obstet Gynecol,* 1996. 174(3): p. 879-83.
[79] Harada, K., et al., Two-dimensional echocardiographic evaluation of ventricular systolic function in human fetuses with ductal constriction. *Ultrasound Obstet Gynecol,* 1997. 10(4): p. 247-53.
[80] Huhta, J.C., et al., Detection and quantitation of constriction of the fetal ductus arteriosus by Doppler echocardiography. *Circulation,* 1987. 75(2): p. 406-12.
[81] Zielinsky, P., et al., Reversal of fetal ductal constriction after maternal restriction of polyphenol-rich foods: an open clinical trial. *J Perinatol,* 2012. 32(8): p. 574-9.
[82] Mielke, G. and N. Benda, Reference ranges for two-dimensional echocardiographic examination of the fetal ductus arteriosus. *Ultrasound Obstet Gynecol,* 2000. 15(3): p. 219-225.
[83] Tulzer, G., et al., Doppler echocardiography of fetal ductus arteriosus constriction versus increased right ventricular output. *J Am Coll Cardiol,* 1991. 18(2): p. 532-6.

[84] van den Hoff, M.J., et al., Increased cardiac workload by closure of the ductus arteriosus leads to hypertrophy and apoptosis rather than to hyperplasia in the late fetal period. *Naunyn Schmiedebergs Arch Pharmacol,* 2004. 370(3): p. 193-202.

[85] Mori, Y., et al., Evaluation of systolic and diastolic ventricular performance of the right ventricle in fetuses with ductal constriction using the Doppler Tei index. *Am J Cardiol,* 2001. 88(10): p. 1173-8.

[86] Mari, G., et al., Doppler assessment of the pulsatility index of the middle cerebral artery during constriction of the fetal ductus arteriosus after indomethacin therapy. *Am J Obstet Gynecol,* 1989. 161(6 Pt 1): p. 1528-31.

[87] Respondek, M., S.R. Weil, and J.C. Huhta, Fetal echocardiography during indomethacin treatment. *Ultrasound Obstet Gynecol,* 1995. 5(2): p. 86-9.

[88] Rudolph, A.M., The effects of nonsteroidal anti-inflammatory compounds on fetal circulation and pulmonary function. *Obstet Gynecol,* 1981. 58(5 Suppl): p. 63S-7S.

[89] Coceani, F., Control mechanisms for the ductus arteriosus and the perinatal pulmonary circulation. *J Lipid Mediat,* 1993. 6(1-3): p. 473-6.

[90] Van Marter, L.J., et al., Persistent pulmonary hypertension of the newborn and smoking and aspirin and nonsteroidal anti-inflammatory drug consumption during pregnancy. *Pediatrics,* 1996. 97(5): p. 658-63.

[91] Abman, S.H., Abnormal vasoreactivity in the pathophysiology of persistent pulmonary hypertension of the newborn. *Pediatr Rev,* 1999. 20(11): p. e103-9.

[92] Walsh-Sukys, M.C., Persistent pulmonary hypertension of the newborn. The black box revisited. *Clin Perinatol,* 1993. 20(1): p. 127-43.

[93] Manchester, D., H.S. Margolis, and R.E. Sheldon, Possible association between maternal indomethacin therapy and primary pulmonary hypertension of the newborn. *Am J Obstet Gynecol,* 1976. 126(4): p. 467-9.

[94] Csaba, I.F., E. Sulyok, and T. Ertl, Relationship of maternal treatment with indomethacin to persistence of fetal circulation syndrome. *J Pediatr,* 1978. 92(3): p. 484.

[95] Goudie, B.M. and J.F. Dossetor, Effect on the fetus of indomethacin given to suppress labour. *Lancet,* 1979. 2(8153): p. 1187-8.

[96] Rubaltelli, F.F., et al., Effect on neonate of maternal treatment with indomethacin. *J Pediatr,* 1979. 94(1): p. 161.

[97] Besinger, R.E., et al., Randomized comparative trial of indomethacin and ritodrine for the long-term treatment of preterm labor. *Am J Obstet Gynecol,* 1991. 164(4): p. 981-6; discussion 986-8.

[98] Wilkinson, A.R., A. Aynsley-Green, and M.D. Mitchell, Persistent pulmonary hypertension and abnormal prostaglandin E levels in preterm infants after maternal treatment with naproxen. *Arch Dis Child,* 1979. 54(12): p. 942-5.

[99] Turner, G.R. and D.L. Levin, Prostaglandin synthesis inhibition in persistent pulmonary hypertension of the newborn. *Clin Perinatol,* 1984. 11(3): p. 581-9.

[100] Norton, M.E., et al., Neonatal complications after the administration of indomethacin for preterm labor. *N Engl J Med,* 1993. 329(22): p. 1602-7.

[101] Alano, M.A., et al., Analysis of nonsteroidal anti-inflammatory drugs in meconium and its relation to persistent pulmonary hypertension of the newborn. *Pediatrics,* 2001. 107(3): p. 519-23.

[102] Hernández-Díaz S, V.M.L., Werler MM, Louik C, Mitchell AA., Risk factors for persistent pulmonary hypertension of the newborn. *Pedatrics,* 2007.

[103] Van Marter, L.J., et al., Nonsteroidal anti-inflammatory drugs in late pregnancy and persistent pulmonary hypertension of the newborn. *Pediatrics,* 2013. 131(1): p. 79-87.

[104] Heymann, M.A. and A.M. Rudolph, Effects of acetylsalicylic acid on the ductus arteriosus and circulation in fetal lambs in utero. *Circ Res,* 1976. 38(5): p. 418-22.

[105] Levin, D.L., et al., Morphologic analysis of the pulmonary vascular bed in infants exposed in utero to prostaglandin synthetase inhibitors. *J Pediatr,* 1978. 92(3): p. 478-83.

[106] Lock, J.E., et al., Indomethacin-induced pulmonary vasoconstriction in the conscious newborn lamb. *Am J Physiol,* 1980. 238(5): p. H639-51.

[107] Y. S. Velioglu , G.M., L. Gao , and B. D. Oomah, Antioxidant Activity and Total Phenolics in Selected Fruits, Vegetables, and Grain Products. *Journal of Agricultural and Food Chemistry,* 1998.

[108] Bravo, L., Polyphenols: chemistry, dietary sources, metabolism, and nutritional significance. *Nutr Rev,* 1998. 56(11): p. 317-33.

[109] Scalbert, A. and G. Williamson, Dietary intake and bioavailability of polyphenols. *J Nutr,* 2000. 130(8S Suppl): p. 2073S-85S.

[110] Majewska, M., et al., Evaluation of antioxidant potential of flavonoids: an in vitro study. *Acta Pol Pharm,* 2011. 68(4): p. 611-5.

[111] Fukumoto, L.R. and G. Mazza, Assessing antioxidant and prooxidant activities of phenolic compounds. *J Agric Food Chem,* 2000. 48(8): p. 3597-604.

[112] Nijveldt, R.J., et al., Flavonoids: a review of probable mechanisms of action and potential applications. *Am J Clin Nutr,* 2001. 74(4): p. 418-25.

[113] USDA, Database for the Flavonoid Content of Selected Foods Release Available at: http://www.nal.usda.gov/fnic/foodcomp/Data/Flav/Flav02-1.pdf, 2007.

[114] Heijnen, C.G., et al., Peroxynitrite scavenging of flavonoids: structure activity relationship. *Environ Toxicol Pharmacol,* 2001. 10(4): p. 199-206.

[115] Chun, O.K., D.O. Kim, and C.Y. Lee, Superoxide radical scavenging activity of the major polyphenols in fresh plums. *J Agric Food Chem,* 2003. 51(27): p. 8067-72.

[116] Akkol, E.K., et al., The treatment of inflammation, pain, and Fever using medicinal plants. *Adv Pharmacol Sci,* 2012. 2012: p. 476985.

[117] Chen, B., et al., Pomegranate juice and punicalagin attenuate oxidative stress and apoptosis in human placenta and in human placental trophoblasts. *Am J Physiol Endocrinol Metab,* 2012. 302(9): p. E1142-52.

[118] Andujar, I., et al., Cocoa polyphenols and their potential benefits for human health. *Oxid Med Cell Longev,* 2012. 2012: p. 906252.

[119] Mathew, A.S., et al., Acute effects of pomegranate extract on postprandial lipaemia, vascular function and blood pressure. *Plant Foods Hum Nutr,* 2012. 67(4): p. 351-7.

[120] Hodgson, J.M., et al., Black tea lowers the rate of blood pressure variation: a randomized controlled trial. *Am J Clin Nutr*, 2013. 97(5): p. 943-50.

[121] Hodgson, J.M., et al., Short-term effects of polyphenol-rich black tea on blood pressure in men and women. *Food Funct,* 2013. 4(1): p. 111-5.

[122] D'Argenio, G., et al., Apple polyphenol extracts prevent aspirin-induced damage to the rat gastric mucosa. *Br J Nutr,* 2008. 100(6): p. 1228-36.

[123] Khan, H.Y., et al., A prooxidant mechanism for the anticancer and chemopreventive properties of plant polyphenols. *Curr Drug Targets*, 2012. 13(14): p. 1738-49.
[124] Hadi, S.M., et al., Oxidative breakage of cellular DNA by plant polyphenols: a putative mechanism for anticancer properties. *Semin Cancer Biol,* 2007. 17(5): p. 370-6.
[125] Malik, A., et al., DNA degradation by water extract of green tea in the presence of copper ions: implications for anticancer properties. *Phytother Res,* 2003. 17(4): p. 358-63.
[126] Widmer, R.J., et al., Beneficial effects of polyphenol-rich olive oil in patients with early atherosclerosis. *Eur J Nutr,* 2013. 52(3): p. 1223-31.
[127] Romain, C., et al., Vineatrol and cardiovascular disease: beneficial effects of a vine-shoot phenolic extract in a hamster atherosclerosis model. *J Agric Food Chem*, 2012. 60(44): p. 11029-36.
[128] Andrade, J.P. and M. Assuncao, Protective effects of chronic green tea consumption on age-related neurodegeneration. *Curr Pharm Des,* 2012. 18(1): p. 4-14.
[129] Valls-Pedret, C., et al., Polyphenol-rich foods in the Mediterranean diet are associated with better cognitive function in elderly subjects at high cardiovascular risk. *J Alzheimers Dis,* 2012. 29(4): p. 773-82.
[130] Kupeli, E., et al., Estimation of antinociceptive and anti-inflammatory activity on Geranium pratense subsp. finitimum and its phenolic compounds. *J Ethnopharmacol,* 2007. 114(2): p. 234-40.
[131] Kupeli, E., et al., Bioassay-guided isolation of anti-inflammatory and antinociceptive glycoterpenoids from the flowers of Verbascum lasianthum Boiss. ex *Bentham. J Ethnopharmacol,* 2007. 110(3): p. 444-50.
[132] Lorenzi, H.M., F. J. A, Plantas medicinais no Brasil: nativas e exóticas. Nova Odessa: *Instituto Plantarum de Estudo da Flora,* 2002: p. 512.
[133] Chen, P.C., et al., A green tea-derived polyphenol, epigallocatechin-3-gallate, inhibits IkappaB kinase activation and IL-8 gene expression in respiratory epithelium. *Inflammation,* 2002. 26(5): p. 233-41.
[134] Di Paola, R., et al., Green tea polyphenol extract attenuates lung injury in experimental model of carrageenan-induced pleurisy in mice. *Respir Res,* 2005. 6: p. 66.
[135] Smith, D.M. and Q.P. Dou, Green tea polyphenol epigallocatechin inhibits DNA replication and consequently induces leukemia cell apoptosis. *Int J Mol Med,* 2001. 7(6): p. 645-52.
[136] Zhang, G., Y. Miura, and K. Yagasaki, Suppression of adhesion and invasion of hepatoma cells in culture by tea compounds through antioxidative activity. *Cancer Lett,* 2000. 159(2): p. 169-73.
[137] Duffy, S.J., et al., Short- and long-term black tea consumption reverses endothelial dysfunction in patients with coronary artery disease. *Circulation,* 2001. 104(2): p. 151-6.
[138] Duffy, S.J., et al., Effect of acute and chronic tea consumption on platelet aggregation in patients with coronary artery disease. *Arterioscler Thromb Vasc Biol*, 2001. 21(6): p. 1084-9.
[139] Kris-Etherton, P.M., et al., Bioactive compounds in foods: their role in the prevention of cardiovascular disease and cancer. *Am J Med,* 2002. 113 Suppl 9B: p. 71S-88S.

[140] Martinez, J. and J.J. Moreno, Effect of resveratrol, a natural polyphenolic compound, on reactive oxygen species and prostaglandin production. *Biochem Pharmacol,* 2000. 59(7): p. 865-70.

[141] Subbaramaiah, K., et al., Resveratrol inhibits cyclooxygenase-2 transcription and activity in phorbol ester-treated human mammary epithelial cells. *J Biol Chem,* 1998. 273(34): p. 21875-82.

[142] Bixby, M., et al., Ilex paraguariensis extracts are potent inhibitors of nitrosative stress: a comparative study with green tea and wines using a protein nitration model and mammalian cell cytotoxicity. *Life Sci,* 2005. 77(3): p. 345-58.

[143] Ito, H., et al., Polyphenol levels in human urine after intake of six different polyphenol-rich beverages. *Br J Nutr,* 2005. 94(4): p. 500-9.

[144] di Giuseppe R, D.C.A., Centritto F, Zito F, De Curtis A, Costanzo S, Vohnout B, Sieri S, Krogh V, Donati MB, de Gaetano G, Iacoviello L., Regular consumption of dark chocolate is associated with low serum concentrations of C-reactive protein in a healthy Italian population. *The Journal of Nutrition,* 2008.

[145] Selmi, C., et al., Chocolate at heart: the anti-inflammatory impact of cocoa flavanols. *Mol Nutr Food Res,* 2008. 52(11): p. 1340-8.

[146] Backhouse, N., et al., Anti-inflammatory and antipyretic effects of boldine. *Agents Actions,* 1994. 42(3-4): p. 114-7.

[147] Khayyal, M.T., et al., A clinical pharmacological study of the potential beneficial effects of a propolis food product as an adjuvant in asthmatic patients. *Fundam Clin Pharmacol,* 2003. 17(1): p. 93-102.

[148] Silva, J.R., et al., [Extract of Passiflora edulis in the healing process of gastric sutures in rats: a morphological and tensiometric study]. *Acta Cir Bras,* 2006. 21 Suppl 2: p. 52-60.

[149] Montanher, A.B., et al., Evidence of anti-inflammatory effects of Passiflora edulis in an inflammation model. *J Ethnopharmacol*, 2007. 109(2): p. 281-8.

[150] Jin, U.H., et al., Inhibitory effect of Panax notoginseng on nitric oxide synthase, cyclo-oxygenase-2 and neutrophil functions. *Phytother Res,* 2007. 21(2): p. 142-8.

[151] Bozin, B., et al., Antimicrobial and antioxidant properties of rosemary and sage (Rosmarinus officinalis L. and Salvia officinalis L., Lamiaceae) essential oils. *J Agric Food Chem,* 2007. 55(19): p. 7879-85.

[152] Celik, I. and I. Isik, Determination of chemopreventive role of Foeniculum vulgare and Salvia officinalis infusion on trichloroacetic acid-induced increased serum marker enzymes lipid peroxidation and antioxidative defense systems in rats. *Nat Prod Res,* 2008. 22(1): p. 66-75.

[153] Della Loggia, R., et al., The role of flavonoids in the anti-inflammatory activity of Chamomilla recutita. *Prog Clin Biol Res,* 1986. 213: p. 481-4.

[154] Pozharitskaya, O.N., et al., Separation and evaluation of free radical-scavenging activity of phenol components of green, brown, and black leaves of Bergenia crassifolia by using HPTLC-DPPH* method. *J Sep Sci,* 2007. 30(15): p. 2447-51.

[155] Pozharitskaya, O.N., et al., Separation and evaluation of free radical-scavenging activity of phenol components of Emblica officinalis extract by using an HPTLC-DPPH* method. *J Sep Sci,* 2007. 30(9): p. 1250-4.

[156] Zielinsky, P., et al., Maternal restriction of polyphenols and fetal ductal dynamics in normal pregnancy: an open clinical trial. *Arq Bras Cardiol,* 2013. 101(3): p. 217-225.

[157] Zielinsky, P., et al., Maternal consumption of polyphenol-rich foods in late pregnancy and fetal ductus arteriosus flow dynamics. *J Perinatol,* 2010. 30(1): p. 17-21.
[158] Zielinsky, P., et al., New insights on fetal ductal constriction: role of maternal ingestion of polyphenol-rich foods. *Expert Rev Cardiovasc Ther,* 2010. 8(2): p. 291-8.
[159] Zielinsky, P., et al., Fetal ductal constriction caused by maternal ingestion of green tea in late pregnancy: an experimental study. *Prenat Diagn,* 2012. 32(10): p. 921-6.
[160] Vian, I., et al., Development and validation of a food frequency questionnaire for consumption of polyphenol-rich foods in pregnant women. *Matern Child Nutr,* 2013.
[161] Kapadia, V., et al., Prenatal closure of the ductus arteriosus and maternal ingestion of anthocyanins. *J Perinatol,* 2010. 30(4): p. 291-4.
[162] Sridharan, S., N. Archer, and N. Manning, Premature constriction of the fetal ductus arteriosus following the maternal consumption of camomile herbal tea. *Ultrasound Obstet Gynecol,* 2009. 34(3): p. 358-9.
[163] Zielinsky, P.M., J. L. L. ; Piccoli JR, Antônio L. ; Areias, J. C. N. ; Nicoloso, Luiz Henrique ; Menezes, H. S. ; Frajdlich, R. ; Busato, A. ; Petracco, R. ; Hagemann, L. ; Moraes, M. ; Silva, J. S. ; Aliev, M. ; Centeno, P, Experimental study of the role of maternal consumption of green tea, mate tea and grape juice on fetal ductal constriction. 17th World Congress on Ultrasound in Obstetrics and Gynecology, 2007 - *Ultrasound in Obstetrics and Gynecology,* 2007. 30: p. 515.
[164] Bubols, G., et al., Inflammation and oxidative stress are involved in the polyphenol-induced ductus arteriosus constriction in pregnant sheep. *in press,* 2013.
[165] Zielinsky, P., et al., Experimental Assessment of Ductus Arteriosus Flow, Oxidative Stress and Polyphenol Excretion After Maternal Polyphenol-Rich Diet in Late Pregnancy. 22nd World Congress on Ultrasound in Obstetrics and Gynecology, 2012, *Copenhagen - Ultrasound in Obstetrics & Gynecology* (Print), 2012. 40: p. 16.
[166] Mercanti, I., et al., Ibubrofen in the treatment of patent ductus arteriosus in preterm infants: what we know, what we still do not know. *Curr Pharm Des,* 2012. 18(21): p. 3007-18.
[167] Shima, Y., et al., Idiopathic severe constriction of the fetal ductus arteriosus: a possible underestimated pathophysiology. *Eur J Pediatr,* 2011. 170(2): p. 237-40.
[168] Enzensberger, C., et al., Idiopathic constriction of the fetal ductus arteriosus: three cases and review of the literature. *J Ultrasound Med,* 2012. 31(8): p. 1285-91.
[169] Tanaka, M., et al., Functional foods for the fetus? *Acta Obstet Gynecol Scand,* 2011. 90(10): p. 1172-3.
[170] Sheehan, M., et al., Position statement on ethics, equipoise and research on charged particle radiation therapy. *J Med Ethics,* 2013.
[171] Petticrew, M., et al., In search of social equipoise. *BMJ,* 2013. 347: p. f4016.
[172] Freedman, B., Equipoise and the ethics of clinical research. *N Engl J Med,* 1987. 317(3): p. 141-5.
[173] Hellman, S. and D.S. Hellman, Of mice but not men. Problems of the randomized clinical trial. *N Engl J Med,* 1991. 324(22): p. 1585-9.
[174] Joffe, S. and F.G. Miller, Equipoise: asking the right questions for clinical trial design. *Nat Rev Clin Oncol,* 2012. 9(4): p. 230-5.
[175] Adibe, O.O. and S.D. St Peter, Equipoise, ethics, and the necessity of randomized trials in surgery. *Arch Surg,* 2012. 147(10): p. 899-900.

[176] Gifford, F., Pulling the plug on clinical equipoise: a critique of Miller and Weijer. *Kennedy Inst Ethics J,* 2007. 17(3): p. 203-26; discussion 227-46.

[177] van der Graaf R, v.D.J., On what we will lose in giving up on clinical equipoise: A reply to Miller. *Clinical Trials,* 2012.

[178] van der Graaf R, v.D.J., Equipoise should be amended, not abandoned. *Clinical Trials,* 2011.

[179] Zielinsky, P. and S. Busato, Prenatal effects of maternal consumption of polyphenol-rich foods in late pregnancy upon fetal ductus arteriosus. *Birth Defects Res C Embryo Today,* 2013. 99(4): p. 256-74.

In: Congenital Heart Diseases
Editor: Raúl Cayré and José Milei
ISBN: 978-1-61122-003-2

Chapter 6

Fetal Cardiac Arrhythmias: Diagnosis and Treatment

Pedro O. Weisburd*[*] *and Esteban Vázquez
Institution: Department of Cardiology. Children's Hospital Superiora Sor María Ludovica of La Plata. Buenos Aires, Argentina

Abstract

Fetal cardiac arrhythmias (FCAs) detected during a routine clinical obstetric or ultrasonography examination constitute, in our experience, a relatively frequent finding and generate a marked anxiety in the family and the obstetrician. At least 2% of all pregnancies this problem is presented.

In our 25-year experience (1988-2013) a total 203 FCAs was detected. 8 patients (p) (3,9%) with premature ventricular contractions; 53p (26,1%) with flutter or atrial fibrillation; 66p (32,5%) with supraventricular tachycardia; and only 2p (0.98%) with ventricular tachycardia; 5p (4,5%) sustained sinusal bradycardia; 1p (0,5%) second-degree heart block and 68p (33,5%) with complete atrioventricular block (CAVB).

They manifest at any gestational age, as early as 13th week of gestation until the term.

The association with cardiac malformations was more frequently in patients with complete congenital heart block 31 of 68 p (45.5%). The tachycardias we found were associated in 6 of 129p (4, 6%).

The aim of the present chapter is to help to recognize the different FACs, carry out a correct analysis, perform an adequate diagnosis and choose the best therapeutic behavior and follow-up. We will therefore describe the different methods of analysis of the fetal cardiac rhythm (FCR), revise their disorder patterns, and describe their therapeutic options and responses.

Conclusion: FCAs impose an emergency for the cardiologist since they generate a marked anxiety in both the family and the obstetrician. In flutter and fibrillation as well as in SVT the association of hydrops and/or cardiac malformation does not imply a bad

[*] E-mail: pedro.weisburd@gmail.com.

prognosis sign. Hospital admission should be limited to the presence of hydrops or prematurity before 26th week of gestation according to our criteria.

In CAVB, the presence of hydrops, FCF< 50 bpm and/or the association to cardiopathies are of very bad prognosis. In the cases without malformation with maternal positive antibodies, the treatment with corticoids must be performed promptly after maternal blood extraction. Fetal-maternal Doppler of umbilical and middle cerebral arteries gives us the possibility of ruling out hypoxic component, and it must only be taken into account that cerebral/umbilical resistance index relation must be >1 whatever the gestational age. Doppler of ductus venosus, suprahepatic veins and umbilical veins must be controlled since they may allow distinguishing fetuses with higher risk of developing hydrops.

Introduction

Fetal cardiac arrhythmias (FCAs) detected during a routine clinical obstetric or ultrasonography examination constitute, in our experience, a relatively frequent finding in at least 2% of all pregnancies. [1] Though most of them are benign, obstetricians and parents are faced to an important anxiety state. They are consequently urged to have a specialized cardiologic consultation in order to characterize the type of arrhythmia present and determine the eventual cardiac malformation.

They represent almost 15% of the specific reasons of referrals in our case studies. Less that 10% of detected FCAs can be under potential risk to develop certain degree of fetal heart failure (FHF), therefore, it is important to diagnose the specific type of arrhythmia, rule out any structural malformative association and determine the need for a type of intrauterine treatment if necessary as well as the conditions for a follow-up.

The Table 1 shows our 25-year experience (1988-2013) of all FCAs we detected. In the total number neither supraventricular extrasystoles (SVEs) nor transient sinus bradycardias (TSBs) are included since they are considered of low risk. They were only taken into account when associated to supraventricular tachycardias (SVTs) and only pointed out when a malformative association is reported. Normal fetal heart rate (FHR) ranges from 100 to 180 bpm during all gestation on a regular basis. We define FCAs as an alteration of the fetal cardiac rhythm manifested by: 1) the presence of irregular beats, 2) FHR greater than 180 bpm sustained or not, 3) FHR lower than 180 bpm in a sustained way. They manifest at any gestational age as early as week 13 until the term, not related to pregnancy delivery or uterine contractions. We firstly cite those most frequently diagnosed arrhythmias and then follow a decreasing order: Transient Sinus Bradycardias (TSBs) and supraventricular extrasystoles (SVEs), supraventricular tachycardias of atrial origin such as flutter and fibrillation, and, in a lesser frequency, chaotic atrial tachycardias (CATs). You will find those using accessory pathways of anterograde or retrograde flow between atria and ventricles, either inside the atrioventricular (AV) node or through the AV ring, thus generating a reentry mechanism with a same atrial and ventricular frequency named as junctional supraventricular tachycardias (JSVTs). Persistent bradycardias are rarely shown such as the CAVB, atrioventricular block of second grade, and very uncommonly permanent sinus bradycardia (PSB). Finally, tachycardias of ventricular origin (VT) are observed.

The aim of the present chapter is to help recognize the different FACs, carry out a correct analysis, perform an adequate diagnosis and choose the best therapeutic behavior and follow-up.

Table 1. Experience 1988-2013: PAC, Premature Atrial Contraction is not included in this statistic.; PVC, Premature Ventricular Contraction;, F, Flutter; AF, Atrial Fibrilation; SVT, Supraventicular Tachycardia;, VT, Ventricular Tachycardia; SSB, Sustained Sinus Bradycardia; AVB Atrio-Ventricular Block; SGHB, Second Degree Heart Block; CAVB, Complete Atrio-Ventricular Block; CM, Cardiac Malformations; FD, Fetal death

Fetal Cardiac Arrhythmias (1988-2013)N= 203

	n	CM	HYDROPS	F D
PAC	9			
PVC	8 (3,9 %)	1		
F and AF	53 (26,1 %)		21 (39,6%)	
SVT	66 (32,5 %)	4	30 (45,4%)	
VT	2 (0.98 %)	1		
SSB	5 (4,5 %)			
SDHB	1 (0.5 %)			
CAVB	68 (33,5 %)	31	25/68 (36,7%)	36/68 (53%)

We will therefore describe the different methods of analysis of the fetal cardiac rhythm (FCR), revise their disorder patterns, and describe their therapeutic options and responses. We will also stress the importance of arterial and venous maternal-fetal Doppler for its evolutional follow-up.

Analysis of the FCR

The analysis of the cardiac rhythm is performed with the surface record (ECG) in the neonate obtaining the electric sequence of each beat, what makes it possible to exactly determine events such as the atrial electric activation (P wave) and ventricular electric activation (QRS complex).

Echocardiography was established as the main technique available for the detection, diagnosis and follow-up of FCAs. [2-4] The Movement Mode or M Mode and the Pulsed Doppler enable the simultaneous record of the mechanical phenomena and arterial and venous flows which will be mainly used for their relative simplicity as an important complement for the assessment of the aforementioned arrhythmias.

The study of fetal PR (fPR) interval with the use of the intracardiac Doppler Method is of great importance in the follow-up of pregnancies of mothers bearing connective tissue diseases and/or with history of children with CAVB, as well as for the analysis of sustained sinus bradycardias (SSB).

Magnetocardiography is the instrument used at present to detect and record the electromagnetic signals related to electric phenomena of fetal heart. [5-7] This diagnostic instrument is currently available in a few centers.

Movement Mode (M Mode)

The M Mode allows the simultaneous record of the atrial and ventricular wall, thus extrapolating the mechanical sequence of the atrial contraction (AC) and ventricular contraction (VC) in real time with P wave and QRS of surface ECG respectively. This allows the determination of an AC/VC relationship (AC/VC R) which will help define the types and behaviors of the different FCAs.

Their obtaining is simple and is performed from a cross section of the four-chambers view (4ch), placing the line of MM so as to simultaneously cross an atrium and the contralateral ventricle, thus obtaining both contractions and its sequence (Figure 1). The use of a short-axis view cross of great vessels is another possibility of obtaining this sequence; AC is obtained followed by the aortic opening as VC. We prefer to routinely obtain the analysis from the 4ch for its simplicity and reproducibility.

Simultaneous Venous and Arterial Doppler

The time is obtained through the simultaneous spectral Doppler record of the inlet flow of the left ventricle and the aortic ejection.

For the Pulmonary Vein/Pulmonary Artery record we recommend to place the sample volume with a size of at least 4 mm, outside the left atrium in the portion proximal to the lung, what is facilitated by the use of the Color Doppler. AC is identified in the venous flow as the most profound notch (near 0 line) immediately before the appearance of the arterial flow corresponding to VC (Figure 2 a and b)

Doppler of Superior Vena Cava (SVC)/Aortic flows are obtained from a longitudinal or transverse cross, locating the sample volume of the size including SVC and ascending aorta (AAo). Breathing and/or fetal movements impede correct measurements due to the variation of venous flows; therefore, we prefer to use MM for its interpretation.

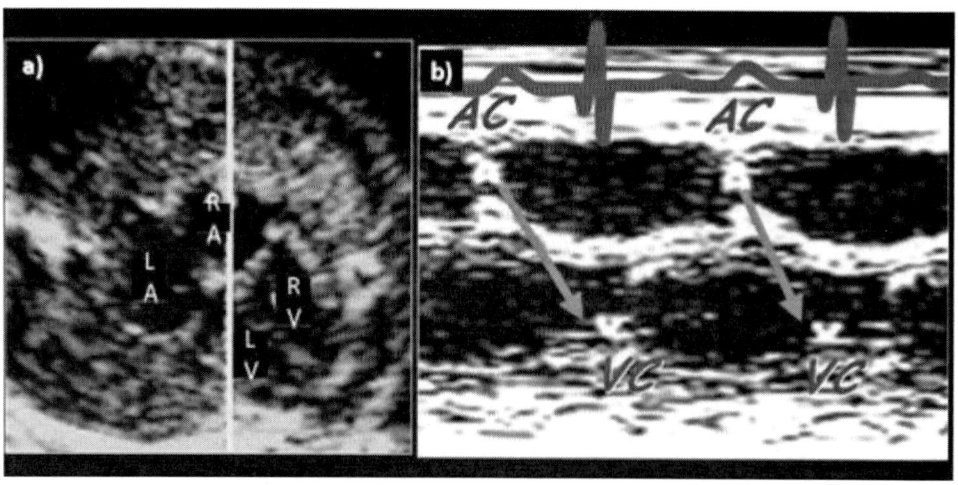

Figure 1. a) 4 chambers view and Mode line; b) M mode; Atrial Contraction (AC): and Ventricular Contraction (VC). Correlation with EKG.

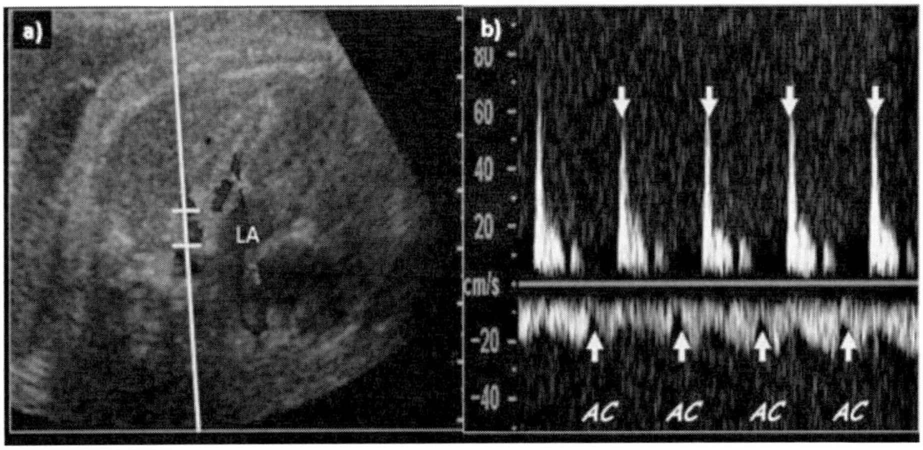

Figure 2. a) Doppler volume in fetal thorax, near the Left Atrium (LA). b) Arterial and Venous Doppler. VC, Ventricular Contractions in the pulmonary artery; AC, Atrial Contractions in the pulmonary vein.

Fetal PR:

PR is referred to as the time interval of the cardiac cycle corresponding to the delay of atrial-ventricular conduction between the P wave and the onset of QRS of surface ECG. This time is obtained from the spectral record of left ventricular inlet and aortic ejection flow. The pulsed Doppler sample volume is placed inside the ventricular cavity near the interventricular septum on the aortic outflow tract (Figure 3 a and b). Spectral Doppler shows the mitral flow followed by the aortic ejection. Time measurement is performed placing the caliper at the notch formed by the end of E wave and the onset of A wave until the aortic ejection (Figures 3 and 4).

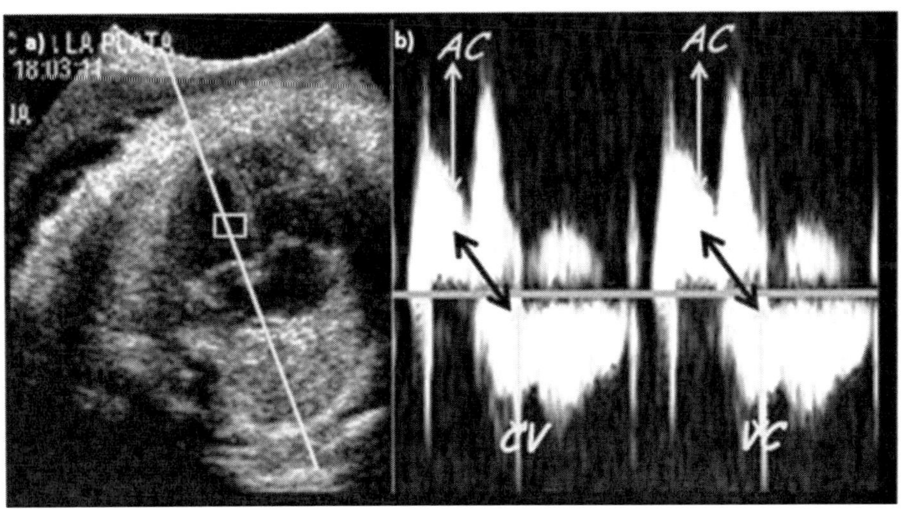

Figure 3. a) Pulsed Doppler volume into the left ventricle. b) Mitral and Aortic flow. CA; Atrial Contraction, VC; Ventricular Contraction. Block arrows marks the beginning and the end of PR fetal interval.

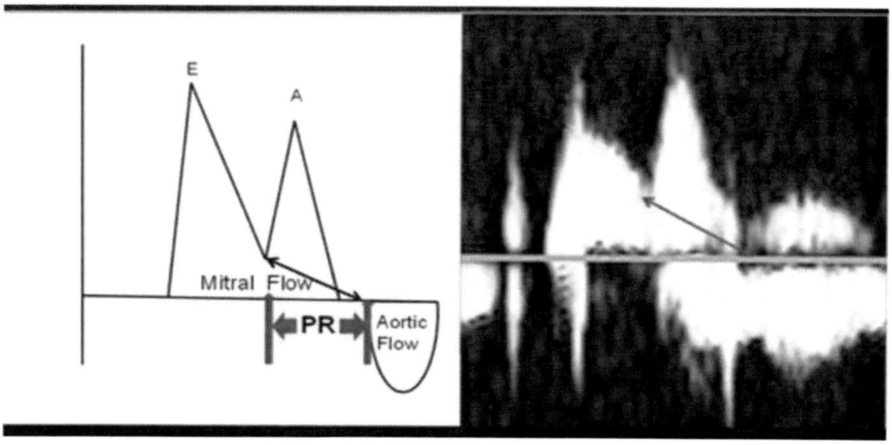

Figure 4. Transmital flow compared with pulsed Doppler PR interval.

The value thus obtained is of 122 +/- 10 ms with an increase of 0.4 ms for each week of gestational age (GA) evolution and an increase of its value of 1.4 ms each 5 beats per minute of the increase of fetal cardiac frequency (FCF). No significant differences were found with relation to the inter sex variability.

We suggest the fPR monitoring for special cases in order to precociously detect its prolongation, establish a convenient treatment and avoid its evolution to CAVB.

Fetal Cardiac Arrhythmias

Fetal Cardiac Arrhythmias: Diagnosis, Evaluation and Treatment

For their study, the fetal cardiac arrhythmias are divided into three groups:

1) Extrasystolic
   - Supraventricular (SVE)
   - Ventricular (VE)
2) Tachycardias:
   - Flutter and Atrial fibrillation (AF)
   - Supraventricular or junctional (JSVT)
   - Ventricular (VT)
3) Bradycardias:
   - Transient Sinus Bradycardia (TSB)
   - Sustained Sinus Bradycardia (SSB)
   - Complete Atrioventricular Block (CAVB)

Extrasystoles

Supraventricular Extrasystoles (SVEs):

It is one of most frequent derivation causes generally on healthy heart, and less than 2% is associated to cardiopathies. During the examination, an intake of stimulants is manifested such as caffeine, cigarettes, alcohol and even substances namely mateine, cola-flavored drinks and phenols included in aromatic compounds. Fetal hypoxia can occasionally origin these arrhythmias [8].

Most of these arrhythmias sometimes disappear spontaneously when these substances are no longer used, as pregnancy progresses or in the first hours after birth. SVE is defined as the presence of a premature contraction of atrial origin (PAC) that generates a regular or irregular alteration of FCF, generally self-limited, and even transient bradycardia of scarce duration in some cases.

AC/VC R can be regular or not depending on the PAC precocity and the moment of the refractory period when it is produced. When PAC is presented in an absolute refractory period, its block is generated what may cause bradycardia in high frequency cases. The passage depending on the frequency and types of PACs (bigeminated or trigeminated) together with different degrees of block can generate regular or irregular cardiac arrhythmias.

Sometimes it is very difficult to differentiate PACs from extrasystoles of ventricular origin, though the latter are much less frequent.

The diagnosis is performed in M Mode to demonstrate the premature movement of the atrial wall, followed or not by a VC. For its correct interpretation M Mode should be utilized as previously pointed out. (Figure 5)

After a conducted PAC takes place, a fall of stroke volume develops shown through the arterial Doppler as well as in those cases where non-conducted PACs generate an increase of stroke volume produced by an accompanying compensating pause. Only in cases where they are very irregular and frequent, they should be closely controlled since sometimes they can cause SVT exceptions that should be treated.

Figure 6 depicts a fixed bigeminated SVE that generates a ventricular bradycardia with a ventricular FCF of 74 bpm due to the block of the PAC.

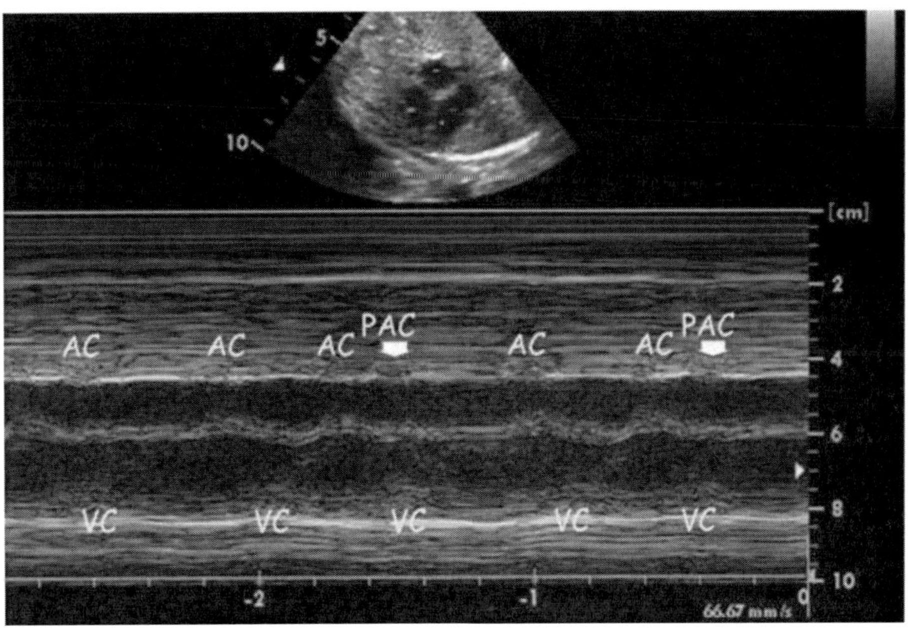

Figure 5. M Mode. Regular PAC, Premature Atrial Contraction; AC, Atrial Contraction; VC, Ventricular Contraction.

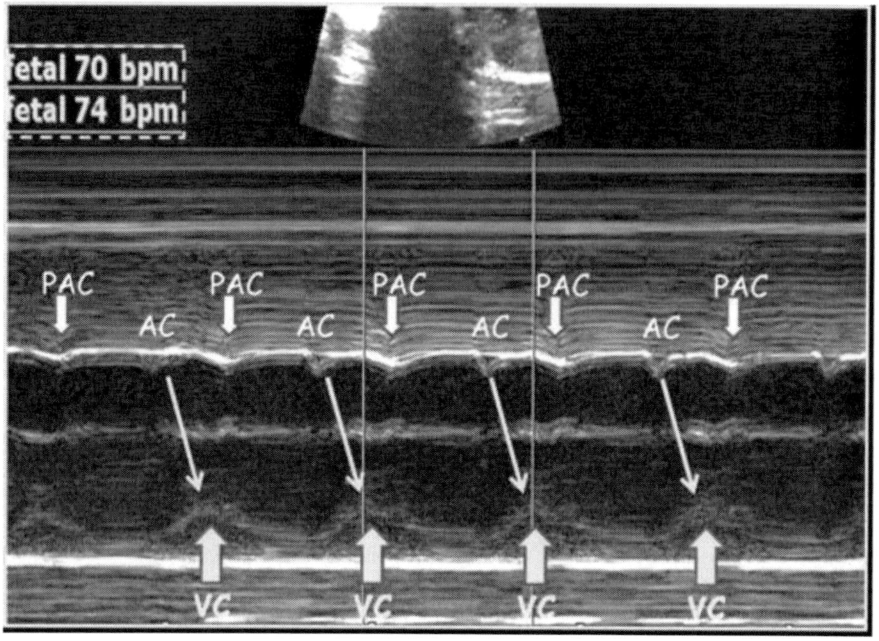

Figure 6. M Mode Blocked premature atrial contractions can cause ventricular Bradycardia PAC. Premature Atrial Contraction; AC, Atrial Contraction; VC, Ventricular Contraction.

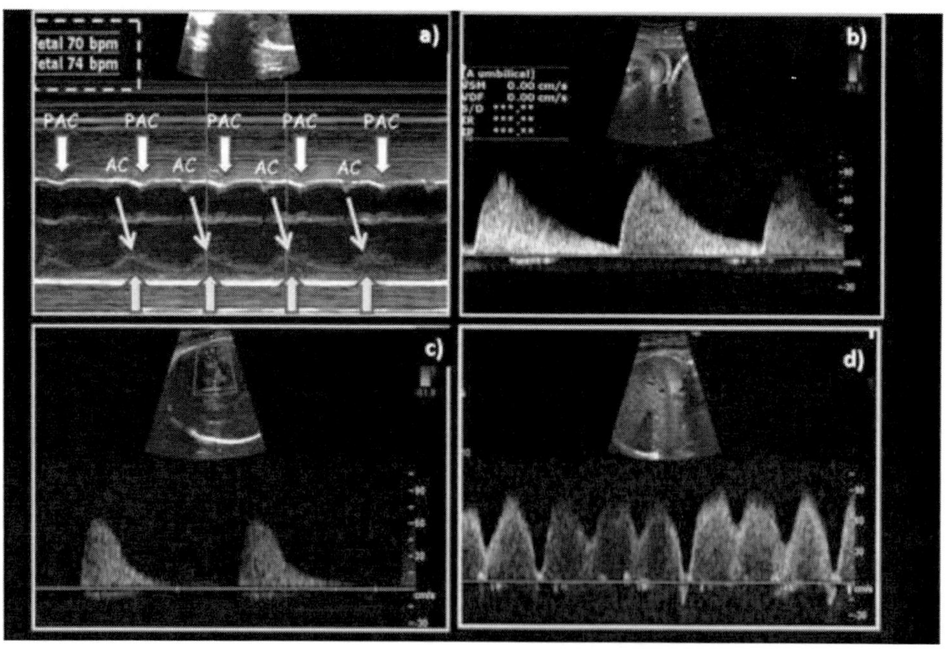

Figure 7. a) M Mode: Blocked PAC cause Ventricular Bradycardia; b) Doppler Umbilical Artery; c) Middle Cerebral Artery; d) Ductus Venosus, PAC; Premature Atrial Contraction, AC; Atrial Contraction; VC; Ventricular Contraction.

Figure 7 makes it possible to observe the effect of this arrhythmia over the flows of the umbilical and middle fetal arteries and over the ductus venosus. The patient continued until the term normalizing FCF at birth.

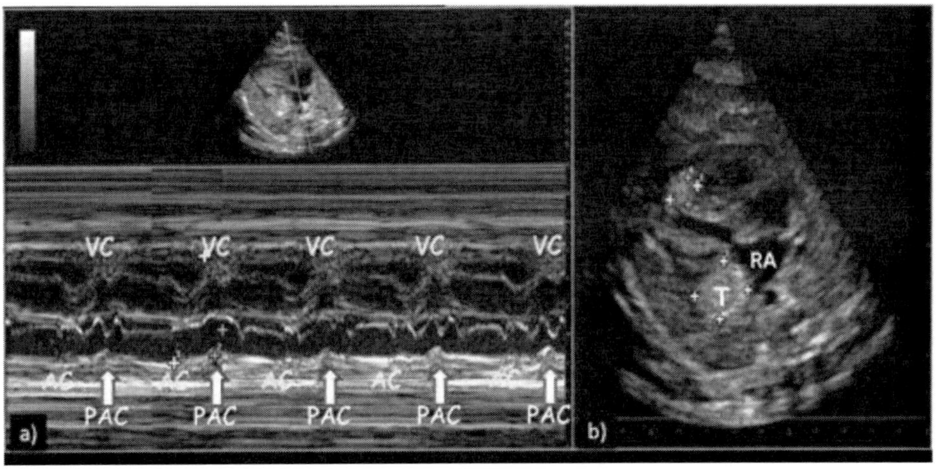

Figure 8. a) M Mode blocked Premature Atrial Contraction bigeminy in a fetus with a tumor located in the Right Atrium; b) Tumor located in the Right Atrium.

Only in 2 % (9 patients) of all cases we have detected PAC association with cardiac structural malformation, mainly complex cardiopathies; and in one case ventricular septal defect (VSD) was found, one associated to Pulmonary Stenosis (PS) and the other to Aortic Coarctation (AoCo) and the rest with complex cardiopathies.

In two cases we detected cardiac tumors in association to bigeminy PAC what induced an apparent sustained bradycardia with FCF less than 85 bpm. These tumors were rhabdomyomas and were placed at the roof of the right atrium and ventricle. (Figure 8, a and b). Arrhythmia disappeared immediately after birth.

9 patients manifesting polymorphic SVE before week the 16th week of gestation with frequent 2-second pauses showed extracardiac malformations without cardiopathies (5 patients with diaphragmatic hernia, 2 patients with omphalocele, and 2 patients with anomalies of the systemic venous return (persistency of right umbilical vein to SVC and another umbilical vein to the coronary sinus). The follow-up for these patients is performed together with the ultrasound scanner technician, evaluating the growth (usually not affected) and through a maternal-fetal Doppler in order to rule out the presence of disorders of the placental flow. Fetal hypoxia might cause some of these arrhythmias, therefore the evaluation of the flows of the umbilical and middle cerebral arteries should be performed systematically. The relationship between both resistance indices known as cerebral/umbilical relationship (c/u R) should be greater than 1 independent of the gestational age [9-12]. If inverted, there is evidence of the presence of hypoxic phenomena by cerebral vasodilation, known as phenomenon of cerebral redistribution. Then values should always be taken in the waves posterior to the post-extrasystolic wave. Venous flows such as Ductus Venosus (DV), Inferior Vena Cava (IVC) or Suprahepatic Veins can be performed but they will only be irregularly affected and do not generate special patterns.

Ventricular Extrasystoles (VEs)

VEs are very uncommon and difficult to diagnose, sometimes they can be confused as of supraventricular origin. They are characterized by a premature ventricular contraction (PVC) without respecting the normal atrioventricular (AV) sequence.

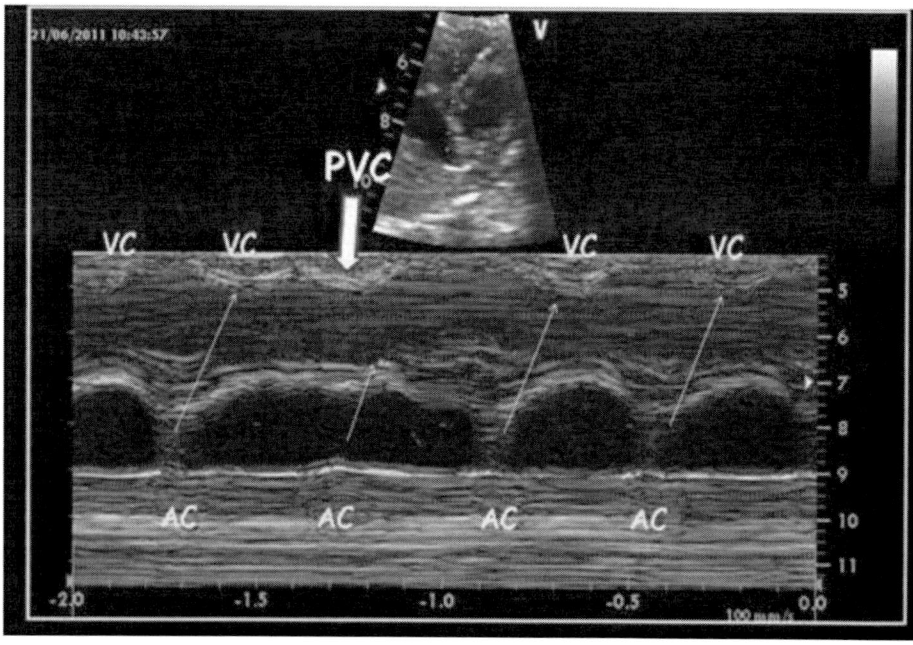

Figure 9. PVC; premature ventricular contraction. (AC), Atrial Contraction is regular.

M Mode detects an AC with regular frequency and isolated PVC (Figure 9). Pulsed Doppler does not add any help in the diagnosis since it fails to reliably detect AC.

To differentiate VE from ventricular tachycardia, we should take into account that VEs are isolated and do not show warm-up phenomenon.

In 8 patients where this disorder was detected, there was no association to structural cardiopathy. None of our patients had any complications and at birth VE disappeared spontaneously.

Tachycardias

Tachycardias are defined as the presence of a FCF greater than 180 bpm that can be sustained or not and may show an abrupt onset and end. They can be regular or irregular depending on the conduction at the AV node.

Generally they manifest on a healthy heart, their association to cardiopathies is very uncommon and can potentially present risk of systemic failure and fetal death. Their association to the development of hydrops is frequent (near 40% of our cases) not only in the Flutter but also in JSVT.

Flutter and Atrial Fibrillation

It is characterized by the presence of an atrial frequency of 300 to 500 bpm with a variable ventricular frequency in accordance with the conduction through the AV node to the ventricles, either regular (eg.: 2/1, 3/1) or irregular.

Flutter tends to show a more stable ventricular frequency than fibrillation. This is due to the fact that its mechanism is usually the persistence of an intraatrial circular circuit, generating an incessant but regular tachycardia (Figure 10). It can cease spontaneously (Figure 11).

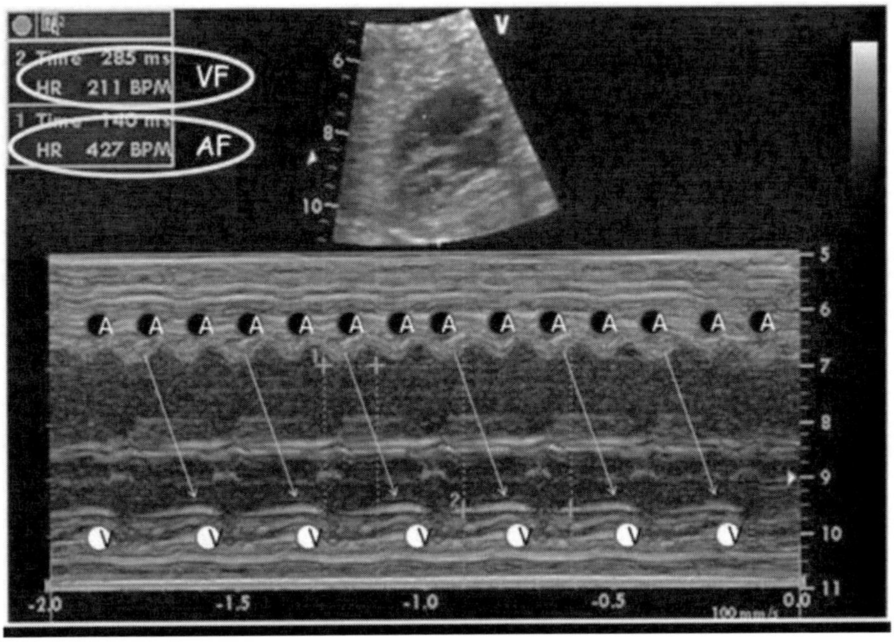

Figure 10. Atrial Flutter: Atrial Frecuency (AF) is more than 427 bpm; the Ventricular Frecuency (VF) is 211 bpm.

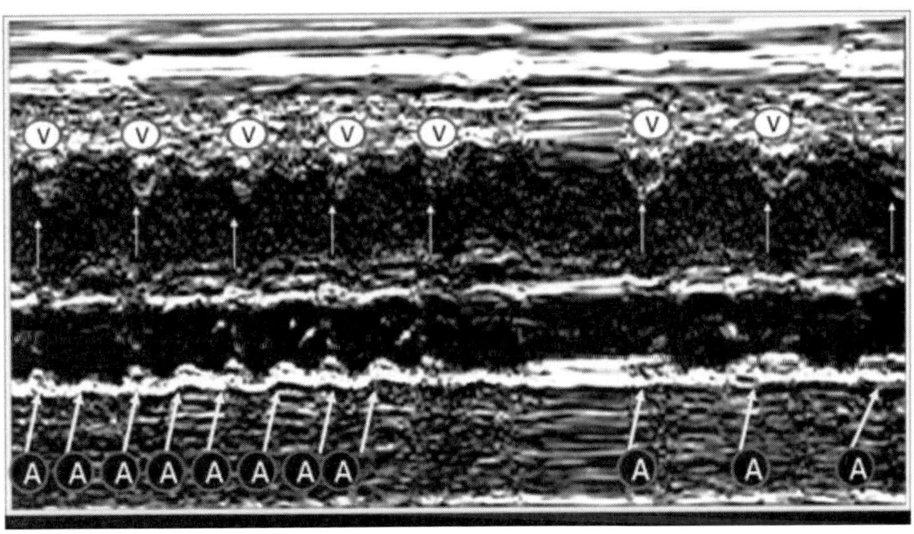

Figure 11. M Mode recording the spontaneous stopped in a Atrial Flutter (A) and reverted to normal sinus rhythm.

On the contrary, fibrillation generally involves the presence of different excitation focuses that activate chaotically, generating a disorganization of the AC and different types of blocks at the AV node which generates an irregular ventricular frequency.

The presence or development of fetal hydrops is frequent due to the disorganization of the venous flow, generated by the increase of the intraatrial pressure. This generates a retrograde A wave that reaches 0 line or retrograde in the ductus venosus and in the superior and inferior caval veins.

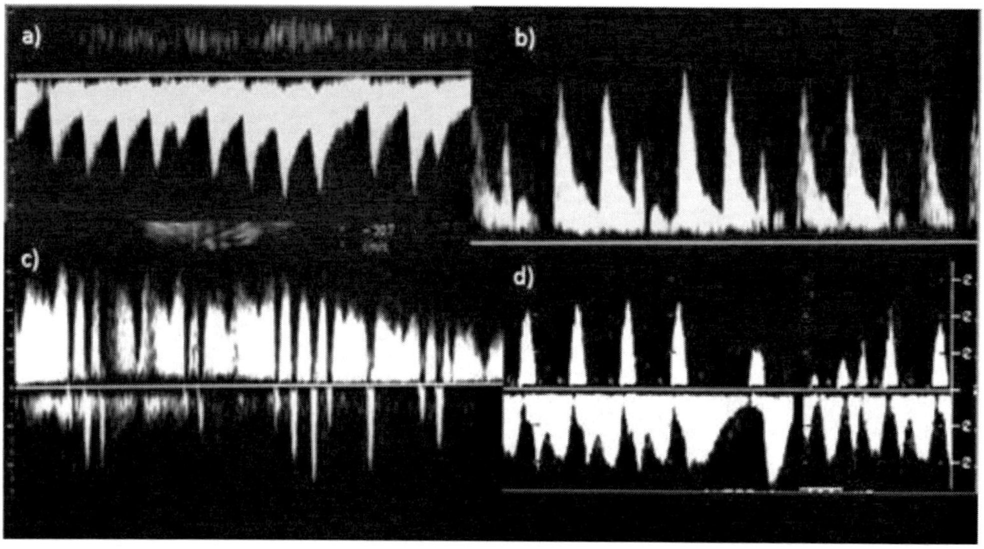

Figure 12. Arterial and venous Dopplee in an atrial fibrillation. Note the chaotic Venous flow. Indicate high risk to develop fetal hydrops.

The treatment can be indicated orally provided that at the diagnosis time hydrops or marked cardiomegaly is not presented. In such a case hospitalization and endovenous treatment (EV) are indicated.

In hydropic patients a premature delivery can be induced after reversing the arrhythmia, due to the sudden absorption of the liquid of the third fetal space, and the consequent generation of a sudden polyhydramnios. This leads us to think of increasing the attack dose of the anti-arrhythmic drugs.

Its association with cardiac malformations is uncommon.

When analyzing the resistance of the flows of the umbilical and fetal cerebral arteries, their values should not be related to gestational age and Cerebral/Umbilical Relationship (Rc/u) should only be calculated in order to rule out fetal hypoxia signals. Figure 12 shows its effect on the different fetal flows. The disorders produced on the venous flows are mainly the origin of the potential development of hydrops fetalis.

Junctional Supraventricular Tachycardia (JSVT)

These are characterized by the presence of an identical Atrial and Ventricular frequency (AC/VC 1:1). They are generally greater than 220 bpm until lesser than 280 bpm. Its onset and disappearance are sudden and can be frequently associated to extrasytoles, especially if they are polymorphic. (Figure 13)

Its onset can be as early as week 14th week of gestational age. Figure 14 shows a SVT in a 14-week fetus that required a treatment that only responded to Flecainide, after having been treated with Digoxin, Sotalol and Amiodarone. The mechanism of origin is the anterograde or retrograde reentry by the AV node or by accessory pathways. Most of them are on a healthy heart.

To determine the type of reentry the times ranging from AC to VC and from VC to AC should be compared. When the time from AC to VC is greater than that of VC to AC, the presence of an antidromic pathway is determined. The slower atrial impulse travels through the AV node, whereas the ventricular impulse is faster from an accessory pathway. The appearance of extrasystoles might evidence its mechanism of re-entry and generate its interruption.

Figure 15 shows a VC-AC time lesser than AC-VC. It has a high incidence of hydrops and generally a good response to the treatment with only one drug at high doses.

The same as in Flutter and fibrillation, we only indicate hospitalization when it is associated or develops ascites or hydrops during the treatment or at the moment of diagnosis.

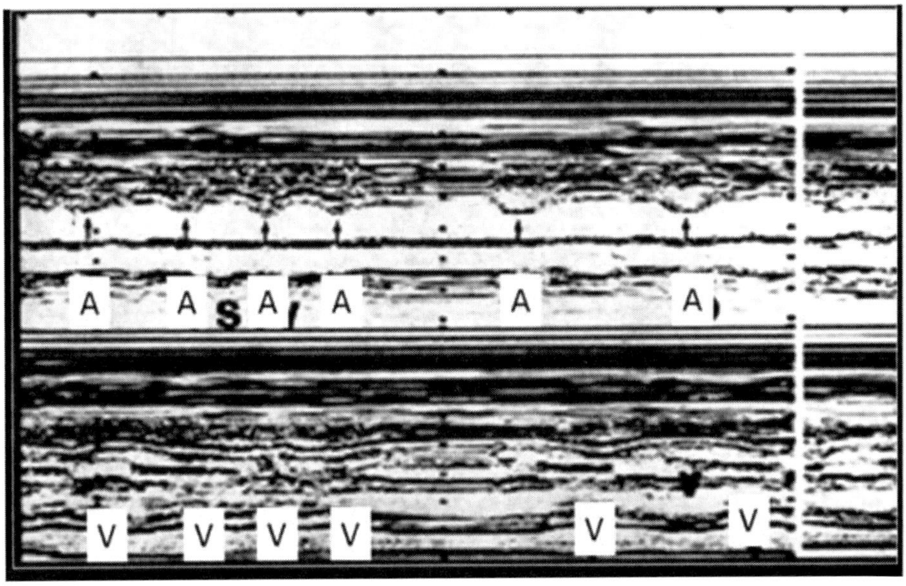

Figure 13. M Mode: SVT and spontaneous reversion to normal frequency.

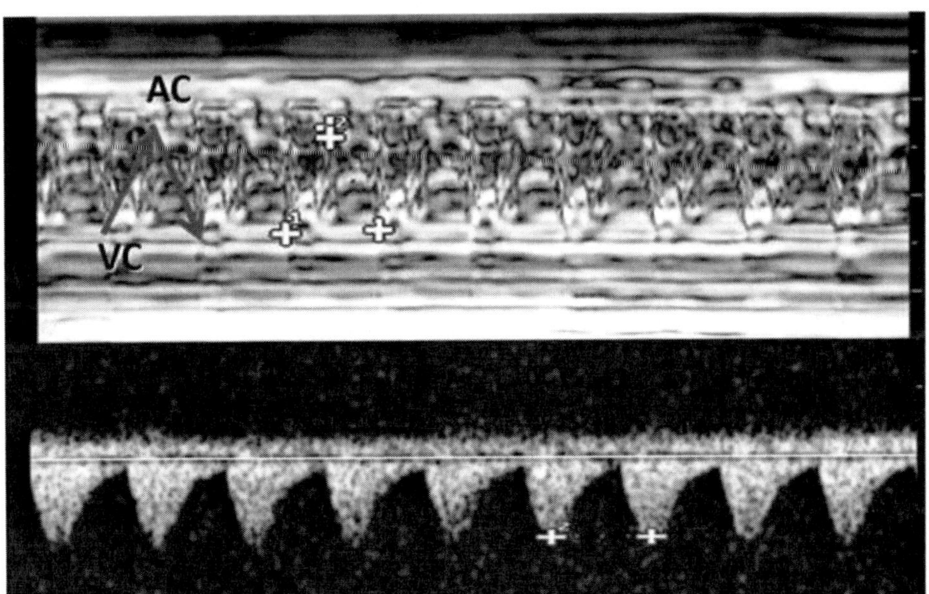

Figure 14. a) M Mode of Supraventricular tachycardia in a fetus of 14th weeks of gestation. The time VC-AC is 120 ms; the time AV-VC is 153 ms, b) Doppler Umbilical Artery at 250 bpm.

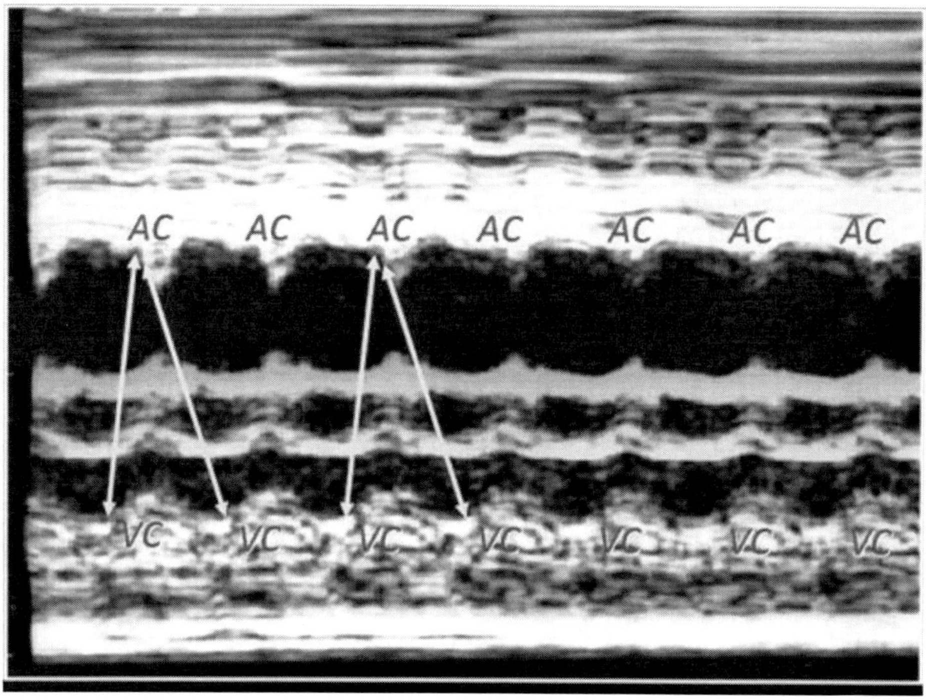

Figure 15. M Mode to SVT: the time VC-AC than Ac-VC.

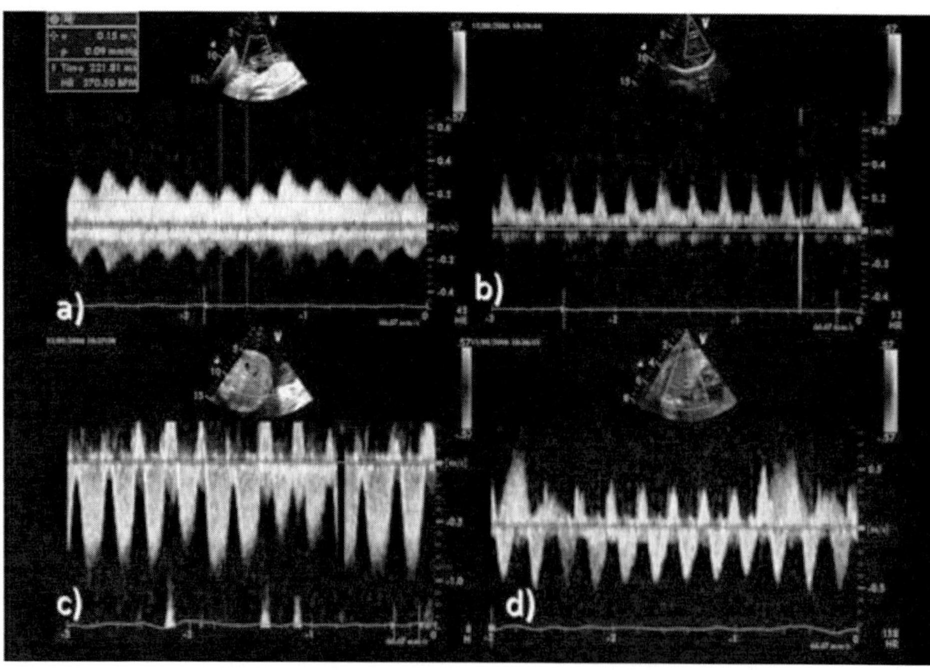

Figure 16. Doppler Flow in a) Umbilical Artery; b) Middle Cerebral Artery; c) Ductus Venosus and d) Suprahepatic vein during Supraventricular Tachycardia.

Figures 16 and 17 show the arterial and fetal venous Doppler during SVT, and its normalization after reversion.

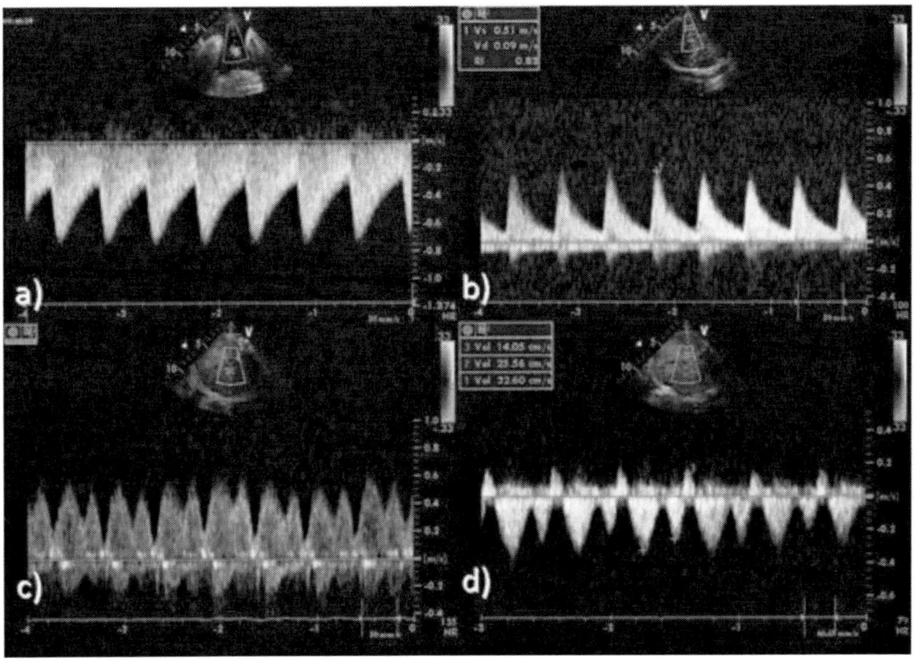

Figure 17. Doppler Flow after reversion of SVTin a) Umbilical Artery; b) Middle Cerebral Artery c) Ductus Venosus and d) Suprahepatic vein.

Ventricular Tachycardia

They are the most uncommon tachycardias, and we could only diagnose them in two opportunities. They are very hard to differentiate from supraventricular ones.

Atrial frequency is normal, and an increase of the ventricular frequency of scant beats is only observed, characterized by the reduction of the time between each ventricular beat as a warm-up mechanism, typical of this arrhythmia.

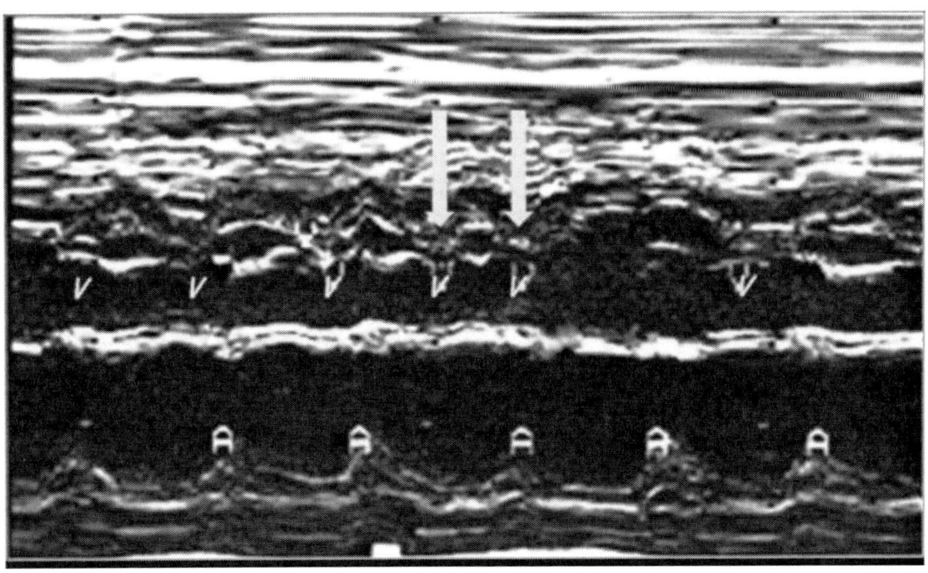

Figure 18. Ventricular tachycardia (V), regular atrial contraction (a).

Figure 18 shows a normal auricular frequency (AF) sequence until the appearance of 3 VC with time shortening among them. A VT case of postnatal spontaneous disappearance was associated to a Critical Pulmonary Stenosis that required Percutaneous Balloon Valvuloplasty after birth.

This arrhythmia may be accompanied by the presence of a prolonged QT Syndrome (pQTS), therefore the treatment with B-Blockers to the mother (Propranolol 80 mg 2 per day) is indicated until birth.

Treatment and Follow-up of Tachycardias

Before the presence of one of these arrhythmias the following items should be taken into account: 1) Fetal hemodynamic state at the moment of the diagnosis; 2) the choice of the pathway, the response and tolerance to drugs; 3) gestational age; 4) its malformative association; 5) Ultrasonography diagnosis follow-up and fetal monitoring; and 6) Arterial and Venous maternal-fetal Doppler evaluation.

Fetal Hemodynamic State

Independently of the gestational age the fetus may be compensated or with signs of fetal cardiac failure (FCF). We understand FCF as the presence or development of liquid in abdomen (ascites), thorax, subcutaneous or generalized tissue (hydrops) as well as isolated cardiomegaly, present or not at the moment of derivation or its development during the follow-up.

The follow-up with fetal-maternal Doppler of the umbilical and fetal middle cerebral arteries (UA and MCA) should be performed. The calculation of the resistance index cerebral/umbilical relationship must be >1 (c/u R>1). As described by Pourcelot [13] and Wladimiroff [14], it must be performed in all these fetuses since it allows ruling out the presence of fetal hypoxia signs. We indicate the carrying out of this calculation since it remains unmodified whatever the estimated FCF.

The analysis of the venous flows must be taken into account for each patient since due to its disorganization it may allow identifying those with high risk to develop hydrops due to the increase of the reversal flow during ACs.

Choice of Pathway, Response and Tolerance:

Oral administration (OA) is our first alternative at the onset of the treatment with the most elevated dose available according to the specific arrhythmia.

In our opinion hospitalization is compulsory under the following conditions:

Presence of fetal edema of any type at the moment of diagnosis or its development during the follow-up, especially with marked hydrops fetalis. When the reversal of the arrhythmia is accomplished, the reabsorption of the fetal edema may induce a sudden polyhydramnios, thus going into a premature labor. This was the cause of preterm birth in three of our patients.

Resistance to treatment by OA after at least 2 or 3 weeks of the onset and with two or more drugs without having obtained a manifested improvement or at least periods without arrhythmia, forcing the passage to Way IV.

Recurrence of arrhythmia after having been detected by either fetal echocardiography or transabdominal fetal monitoring (in case of gestational ages over week 33)

Gestational Age

We consider that it is always possible to attempt first the intrauterine treatment by any pathway, at any gestational age even near term as long as there are no FCF signs and/or hypoxic suffering.

Malformative Association

Its association with cardiopathies is very uncommon. In our experience most of them associated lesions with those of left pathologies, aortic stenosis with double outlet of right ventricle (DORV) for instance.

Ultrasonography Follow-up and Fetal Monitoring

The ultrasonography follow-up must be performed each 48 hours in all cases until reversal is accomplished, then continuing on a weekly basis. Conventional ultrasonographies must be carried out each 2 weeks in order to evaluate fetal growth and vitality and until the term of pregnancy.

The performance of the fetal monitoring (FM), that is the transabdominal record of FCR, is of great utility since it allows the record of at least 30 minutes or more. If the patient is hospitalized this can be done three or more times per day, and after reversal an ambulatory control can be achieved each 48 or 72 hours.

In Figure 19 it is observed a FM record of an ambulatory patient where a tachycardia was detected after two weeks of ambulatory treatment, forcing a dose increase.

Caesarean Section is limited to those arrhythmias that did not revert with development of hydrops or by another obstetric indication.

Arrhythmias and Anti-Arrhythmic Medication

The decision on the physician on both the drugs and the arrhythmias.

Table 2 shows the doses, the estimated transplacentary passage and some of their adverse effects.

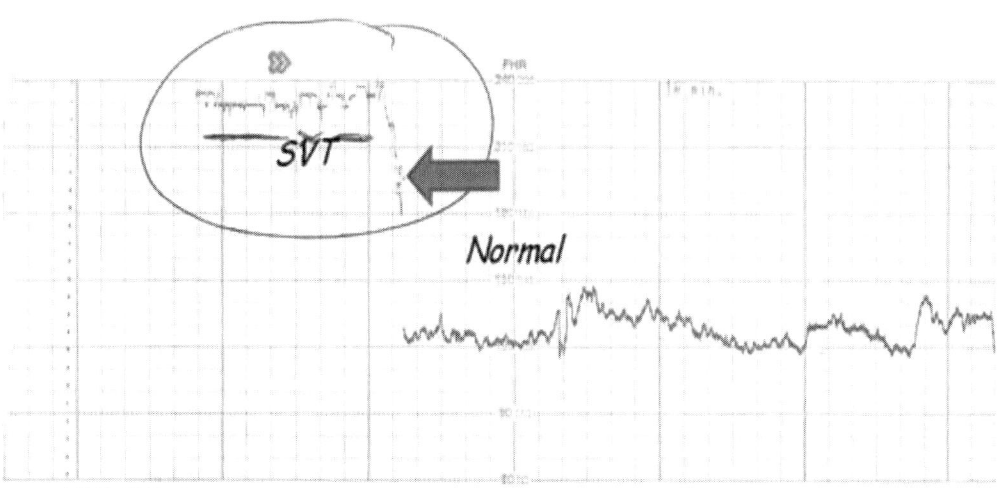

Figure 19. Monitoring of fetal heart rate. A superventricular tachycardia stopping at the arrow.

Table 2. Antiarrythmics drugs.: LD Loading Doses, MD Maintenance Doses

Drugs	Dose range	M/F Transfer*	Adverses effects
Digoxin	LD: 1,5-2 gm PO o IV MD: 0,25-0,5 / d PO	80-100%	Nausea and/or Vomiting Sinus Bradycardia or AV Block
Amiodarone	LD: 1200-1800 mg PO o IV IV 1/2 dose in the first 6 hs MD: 200-400 mg/d. PO	25-40 %	Maternal and fetus BAV Maternal or neonatal thyroid dysfunction Fetal Sinus Bradycardia
Sotalol	LD: 160- 480 mg/d PO MD: 80 mg/d	80-100%	Maternal QT Control Proarrythmics events Nausea and or vomiting
Flecainide	LD 100-300 mg/ d PO MD: 100 mg/d	80 %	Proarrythmics maternal effects Bundle branch block
Propanolol	LD 40-240 mg/d PO	40 - 100%	Fatigue, Hypotension; Bradycardia Noenatal Hipoglucemia; IUGR
≠Dexamethasone	LD 4-8 mg PO PO 4 mg/d		Similar others corticosteroids IUGR ?

* Maternal/Fetal placental transfer.
*≠ indication for fetal Complete Atrioventricular Block.

Flutter and Fibrillation

We firstly administered Digoxin at high doses (2 gm per day for 48 to 72 hours), accomplishing its reversal in almost 45% of our patients. In the event of persistence or appearance of maternal signs of bad tolerance, we have used Amiodarone OA or intravenously (IV) with excellent results. The longest time period of the treatment at high doses (1000 mg OA per day) was of ten days.

In fetuses with hydrops the firstly chosen drug was Amiodarone, starting with 1600 mg p/day IV until obtaining periods without arrhythmias recorded by the FM of at least 30 minutes during hospitalization. From then onwards 200 mg/each 48 h are reduced on a regular basis until reaching the maintenance dose, passing on to OA.

In 40% of the cases, 2 or more drugs were required. In 38% of the cases, hydrops were manifested at the moment of diagnosis, reducing in all the cases and provoking a premature delivery in 2 patients as aforementioned

In AF Amiodarone was the first choice drug according to the previously described dose and treatment administration. Almost 50% required a second drug, coinciding with the postnatal presence of a Chaotic Atrial Tachycardia. Ascites was present in more than 40% of the cases at the moment of diagnosis. In all the cases it was achieved a reversal of the prenatal arrhythmia, without fetal or neonatal deaths.

SVT: In SVT the first drug of choice is generally Digoxin, followed by Amiodarone or Flecainide. (8, 15-18) Amiodarone was in most of the cases the first choice drug especially with the presence of hydrops. More recently and in ambulatory ways without hydrops, Sotalol was the first drug of choice, reverting SVT in less than 24 h. Its dose was of 80 mg each 8 h as attack dose, with ECG control for assessment of maternal QT. The Digoxin-Amiodarone association was the most frequently used, followed by Flecainide as third choice. In some cases we associated Amiodarone and Flecainide if the arrhythmia was persistent.

Echocardiographic control is performed each 24 hrs. until reversion of the arrhythmia, dose reduction must be slow, especially if 2 or more drugs were required, since arrhythmia recurrence after its reversal and during dose reduction induced dose increase and/or the addition of a second or third drug apart from the already administered one.

In a case associated to cardiac tumors, SVT was present until the age of four years under medical treatment.

No fetal death was reported for all the cases and no adverse events with relation to their toxicity were found. There were only two cases of premature delivery with hydrops and already solved arrhythmia.

Bradycardias

Transient Sustained Sinus Bradycardia (TSSB)

TSSB is of no relevance and may take place at any gestational age. Due to their benign condition they do not require any treatment or follow-up, though this characteristic does not minimize the important anxiety generated by the family.

This is one of the most frequent causes of consultation, generally they are produced at the onset or during a routine echocardiographic study, characterized by the deceleration of FCF with less than 100 bpm even at pauses lasting no more than 3 seconds. They immediately recover when the mother is lateralized, placing her lateral decubitus or simply reducing the transducer pressure on the abdomen.

Sustained Sinus Bradycardia (SSB)

It is defined as the presence of a constant FCF lesser than 100 bpm until the end of pregnancy with a normal fPR, stressing a low sinus frequency. Although in some cases they can be associated to infections or disorders caused by anesthesia.

The diagnosis in M Mode shows a normal atrial-ventricular sequence (AC/VC; 1/1) and pulsed Doppler registering the inlet of left ventricle and aortic ejection, which evidence a normal fPR, thus indicating that the sequence of atrioventricular conduction is found within normal values. (Figure 20)

It is not associated to maternal collagenopathy or any malformative pathology.

Bradycardia is detected by means of a routine ultrasound scanning, has a permanent condition and no recovery despite the reduction of the transducer pressure or the modification of the maternal position as in the case of SB. Generally this frequency remains stable until the end of the pregnancy, forcing the delivery by cesarean section because of the impossibility of performing an adequate fetal monitoring.

In our experience we have observed that bradycardia spontaneously disappeared in all the cases, observing HR recovery to normal values. Because some authors state that these patients are under risk of manifesting prolonged QT syndrome, an electrocardiographic control is suggested in newborns. None of our patients reported the present or another electric anomaly after over a three-year follow-up.

The Figure 21 shows the changes of maternal-fetal Doppler flows. None of them showed fetal hypoxia since c/u R was always superior to 1.

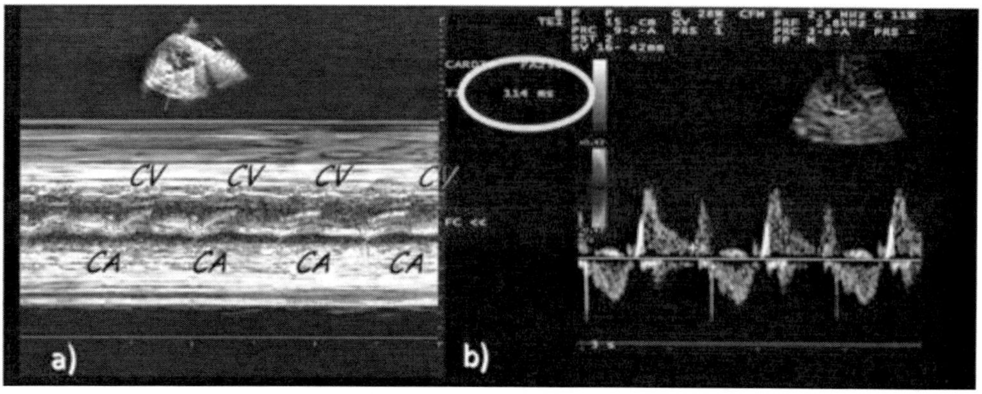

Figure 20. Sustained Sinus Bradycardia a) M Mode shows a normal atrial-ventricular sequence; b) Pulsed Doppler with a normal FPR indicating normal atrio-ventricular conduction.

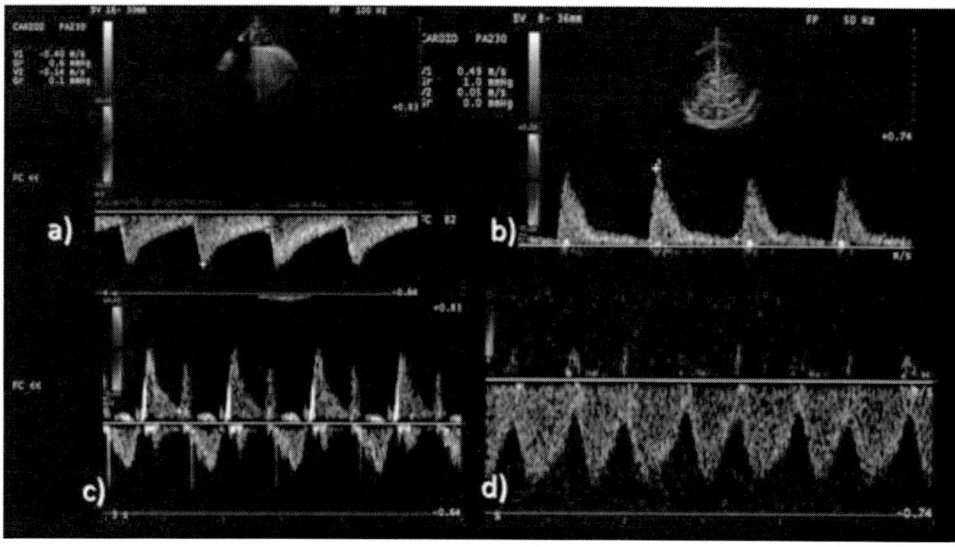

Figure 21. Doppler Flow in Sustained Sinus Bradycardia a) Umbilical Artery; b) Middle Cerebral Artery c) FPR and d) Ductus Venosus.

Atrioventricular (AV) Block

AV block can be classified according to its severity in three types: AV block of first and second-degree (incomplete ways) and third-degree or complete (CAVB). CAVB is characterized by a complete dissociation of AC of the ventricular ones, that is to say, there is no transmission of any stimulus from the atrium to the ventricle conditioning a normal atrial frequency but a low ventricular one. Figure 22 Therefore, the ventricle is in charge of the escape or idioventricular pacemaker with a FCF generally lesser than 80 bpm.

The diagnosis is performed with the M Mode, observing a regular AC and greater than VC, with a 3/1 relation generally. The dissociation between AC and VC stresses the presence of CAVB. Figure 23

CAVB is a type of irreversible bradyarrhythmia because the injury of the AV node is irredeemable. It occurs approximately in one of 22,000 [19] alive newborns, with greater incidence in prenatal life.

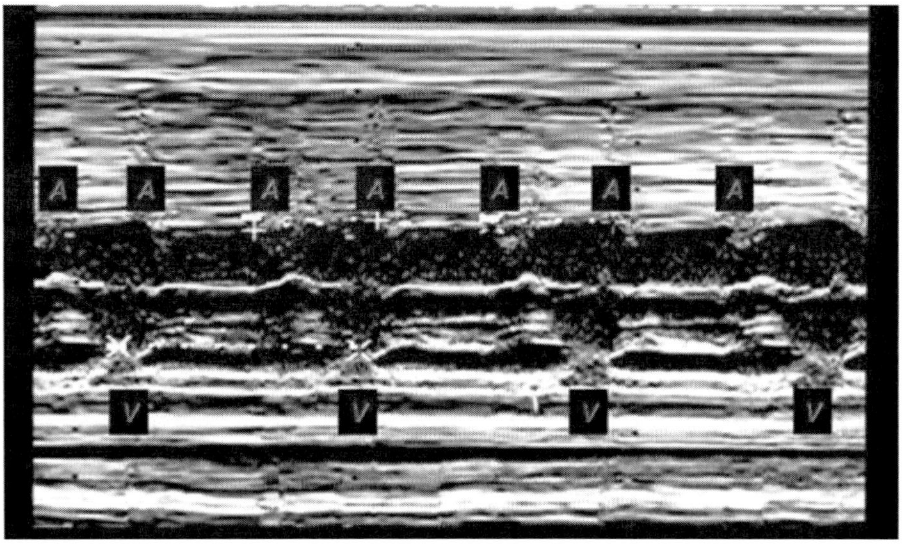

Figure 22. A Complete Atrioventricular Block with dissociation of auricular contractions (A) of the ventricular ones (V).

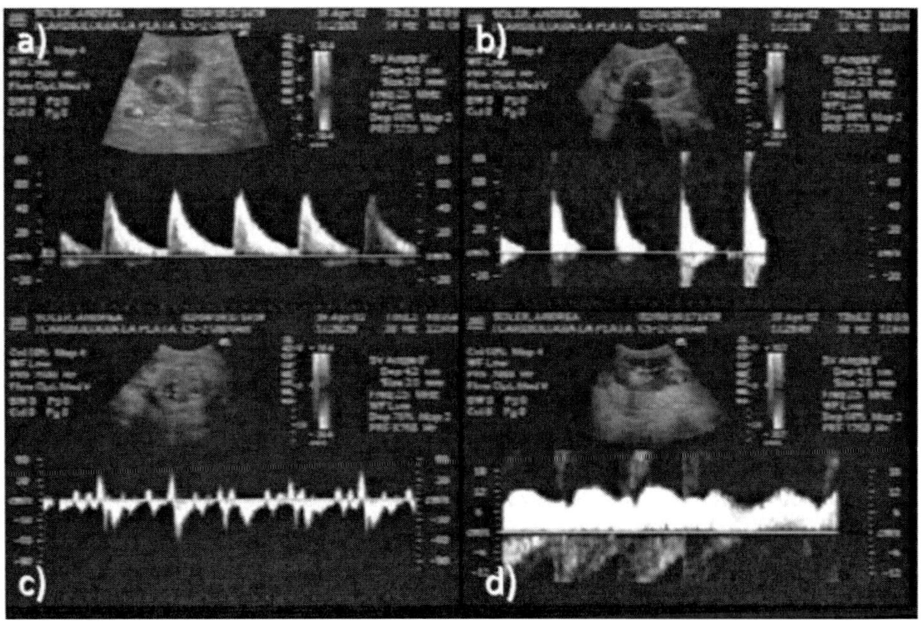

Figure 23. Doppler Flow in Complete Atrioventricular Block a) Umbilical Artery; b) Middle Cerebral Artery c) Ductus Venosus and d) Umbilical.

The cardiac output is reduced due to the lack of synchronicity of beats and bradycardia, what more often than not is translated into cardiomegaly, fetal cardiac failure and hydrops due to the lack of synchronicity between AC and VC stresses the disorders on the venous flow.

It is frequently associated to cardiac malformations or immune diseases of the maternal connective tissue with the presence of antibodies anti RO/SSa and La/SSb. Its origin still remains strikingly unknown.

CAVB and Malformations

31 of 68 patients (45.5%) manifested cardiac malformations associated to block: Disorders with dextro and levo-isomerism together with univentricular hearts with severe anomalies of the vessels, Complete Atrioventricular Canal with Aortic and pulmonary Stenosis, Congenitally corrected transposition of the great vessels (CCTGV) with Pulmonary Stenosis and IVC and only 3 patients with isolated CCTGV.

Intrauterine mortality or within the neonatal period was of 90% within the present group. Only 3 (10%) manifesting CCTGV without IVC or PS with dextrocardia survived.

CAVB without Malformations

The presence of a CAVB without structural malformations was more frequent, 37 of 68 patients (54.5%). 35 of the 37 patients (94.5%) were associated to the presence of antibodies anti Ro/SSA and La/SSB in the maternal serum, despite the absence of symptoms or history of maternal auto-immune diseases (Systemic Lupus Erythematosus, Sjogren's Syndrome or another Collagenopathy). Only in 2 patients (5.5%) its etiology could not be shown or its association with the prolonged QT syndrome at birth.

The injury of the system of immunomediated conduction as a result of transplacental passage of maternal anti Ro/SSA and La/SSB antibodies would trigger the inflammation of AV node and the myocardium of those susceptible fetuses of mothers bearing inflammatory diseases of the connective tissue. The molecular mechanism leading to the block still remains unknown. CAVB development takes place only in 1-2% of pregnancies with anti Ro/SSA and La/SSB antibodies what indicated the presence of other factors that determine the development of the block. Most mothers are nonsymtomatic bearers at the moment of diagnosis of fetal CAVB.

We have not reported AV blocks of first or second degree which may have evolved toward CAVB, though this was observed by other authors.

As a consequence of the fibrosis in the AV node, leading to complete Block, endocardial fibroelastosis, and dilated cardiomyopathy. This would explain the improvement achieved by the administration of corticoids (dexametasone) to the mother, evidencing in four cases the reversal of hydrops and the reduction of fetal cardiomegaly.

CAVB has appeared as early as week 18.

The first-degree block would precede the development of CAVB and its early detection through the follow-up of fetal PR would allow preventing the development of the injury of AV node by means of the administration of a steroid therapy, though there is no concluding evidence.

Treatment with Corticoids

When CAVB is detected and after the maternal blood extraction for the search of antibodies, the administration of dexametasone should be performed orally. The present therapy could improve the survival of affected fetuses. Doses are found in table II.

During the treatment we could reverse hydrops in 4 patients with FCF> 65 bpm. No positive response was found when FCF was < 50 bpm.

Intrauterine mortality was produced in 8 patients (21.6%) of the present group, all of them showing FCF < 50 bpm and/or hydrops. 2 patients (5.5%) died during the neonatal period despite the placing of transient pacemakers.

Conclusion

FCAs impose an emergency for the cardiologist since they generate a marked anxiety in both the family and the obstetrician.

SVE and TB do not represent any risk.

In Flutter and Fibrillation as well as in SVT the association of hydrops and/and cardiac malformation does not imply a bad prognosis sign. The treatment with drugs must start with high doses, either OA or IV. Hospital admission should be limited to the presence of hydrops or prematurity before week 26 according to our criteria.

In CAVB hydrops, FCF< 50 bpm and/or the association to cardiopathies is of very bad prognosis. In the cases without malformation with maternal positive antibodies, the treatment with corticoids must be performed immediate to after maternal blood extraction.

Fetal-maternal Doppler of Umbilical and fetal medium cerebral arteries gives us the possibility of ruling out hypoxic component, and it must only be taken into account that c/u R must be >1 whatever the gestational age.

Doppler of Ductus Venosus, suprahepatic veins and Umbilical veins must be controlled since they may allow distinguishing fetuses with higher risk of developing hydrops fetalis.

References

[1] Hornberger LK, Sahn DJ. Rhythm abnormalities of the fetus. *Heart* 2007 October; 93: 1294-300. doi: 10.1136/hrt.2005.069369

[2] Allan LD, Anderson RH, Sullivan ID, Campbell S, Holt DW, Tynan M. Evaluation of fetal arrhythmias by echocardiography. *Br. Heart J.* 1983; 50: 240-45.

[3] Simpson J. Fetal arrhythmia. In Snider AR, Serwer GA, Ritter SB (eds). Echocardiography in pediatric heart disease. St. Louis, *Mosby Year Book* 1997: 93-98.

[4] Simpson J. Fetal arrhythmias. In Allan L, Hornberger LK, Sharland G (eds). *Textbook of fetal cardiology*. London, Greenwich Medical Media 2000: 423-437.

[5] Kahler C, Grimm B, Schleussner E et al. The application of fetal magnetocardiography (FMCG) to investigate fetal arrhythmias and congenital heart defects (CHD). *Prenat. Diagn.* 2001; 21: 176-182.

[6] Quartero HW, Stinstra JG, Golbach EG, Meijboom EJ, Peters MJ. Clinical implications of fetal magnetocardiography. *Ultrasound Obstet. Gynecol.* 2002; 20: 142–153.

[7] Wakai RT, Strasburger JF, Li Z, Deal BJ, Gotteiner NL. Magnetocardiographyc rhythm patterns at initiation and termination of fetal supraventricular tachycardia. *Circulation* 2003; 107: 307-312.

[8] Hornberger LK, Sahn DJ. Rhythm abnormalities of the fetus. *Heart* 2007; 93: 1294–1300. doi: 10.1136/hrt.2005.069369
[9] Arbeille P, Roncin A, Berson M, Patat F, Pourcelot L. Exploration of the fetal cerebral blood flow by duplex Doppler linear array system in normal and pathological pregnancies. *Ultrasound Med. Biol.* 1987; 13: 329-37.
[10] Bonnin P, Guyot O, Bailliart O, Benard C, Blot P, Martineaud JP. Relationship between umbilical and fetal cerebral flow velocity waveforms and umbilical venous blood gases. *Ultrasound Obstet. Gynecol.* 1992; 2: 18-22.
[11] Arbeille P, Carles G, Bousquet F, Body G, Lansac J (1998). Fetal vascular changes during pregnancy complicated by malaria. *J. Ultrasound Med.* 1998; **17:** 223–29.
[12] Salihagic-Kadic A, Medic M, Jugovic D, Kos M, Latin V, Kusan Jukic M, Arbeille P. Fetal cerebrovascular response to chronic hypoxia—implications for the prevention of brain damage. *The journal of maternal-fetal and neonatal medicine* 2006; 19: 387-96 doi: 10.1080/14767050600637861
[13] Pourcelot L. Applications cliniques de l'examen Doppler transcutane. In Peronneau P ed. *Velocimetre Ultrasonore Doppler*. Seminaire INSERM, Paris 1974; 34: 213-240.
[14] Wladimiroff JW, Tonge HM, Stewart PA. Doppler ultrasound assessment of cerebral blood flow in the human fetus. *Br. J. Obstet. Gynaecol.* 1986; 93: 471-75.
[15] Tan HL, Lie KI. Treatment of tachyarrhythmias during pregnancy and lactation. *Eur. Heart J.* 2001; 22: 458-64.
[16] Simpson JM. Fetal arrhythmias. *Ultrasound Obstet. Gynecol.* 2006; 27: 599-06.
[17] Maeno Y, Hirose A, Kanbe T, Hori D. Fetal arrhythmia: Prenatal diagnosis and perinatal management. *J. Obstet. Gynaecol. Res.* 2009; 35: 623–29.
[18] Shah A, Moon, Bhogal N et al. Effectiveness of sotalol as first-line therapy for fetal supraventricular tachyarrhythmias. *Am. J. Cardiol.* 2012; 109: 1614-18.
[19] Kertesz NJ, Fenrich AL, Friedman RA. Congenital complete atrioventricular block. *Tex. Heart Inst. J.* 1997; 24: 301-07.

In: Congenital Heart Diseases
Editor: Raúl Cayré and José Milei
ISBN: 978-1-61122-003-2

Chapter 7

Pulmonary Hypertension and Congenital Heart Diseases

Gabriel Fernando Díaz Góngora *
Department of Pediatrics
Universidad Nacional De Colombia, Colombia

Abstract

This chapter is an actualized review of different aspects related to pulmonary hypertension associated with congenital heart disease. The main message that we try to convey to the readers is the importance of early diagnosis and treatment of congenital heart disease, to avoid pulmonary vascular disease; this means, the importance of prevention of pulmonary vascular disease. Considering that left to right shunts are the more frequent congenital heart disease associated with pulmonary hypertension, this topic is analyzed in wide form, from physiopathology until treatment, emphasizing the importance of a clinical approach for early detection of Congenital Heart Disease. I propose a pyramidal approach to the diagnosis and treatment of congenital heart disease associated with pulmonary hypertension.

We emphasize that it is not correct to extrapolate the result of studies made in adults and apply it to children. I mention that the Dana Point Classification (with the Update of Nice) is difficult to apply to children; for this reason I see that it is more applicable to use in pediatric patients the, Panama Classification: Classification of pulmonary vascular disease in children.

I give special importance to two topics: The adult with congenital heart disease and Pulmonary Hypertension, including the Eisenmenger Syndrome, and pulmonary hypertension associated with congenital heart disease at altitude. This last topic is very important, considering that a great population lives at high altitudes (more than 140,000,000 people); on the other hand, hypobaric hypoxia gives a special characteristic to pulmonary hypertension at high altitude, which influences biopathogenesis, clinical aspects, diagnostic approach and treatment.

* E-mail: gfdiazg50@gmail.com.

Introduction

The understanding pulmonary hypertension (PH) has been transformed largely in the last two decades, after a growing interest and great advances made in different aspects, supported by a better understanding of the etiopathogenesis and biopathogenesis of this condition. This is very different from the "shadows " that existed few years ago, as confirmed with the update on this topic written by Marlene Rabinovitch in 1997 in which she referred to this pathology as "a mysterious disease" [1].

It is important to note that most PH studies have been carried out in adults at sea level in developed countries. Furthermore, the results of these studies have been extrapolated to children, without regard to important aspects, such as those related to the different ages of the patients or the altitude above sea level. This last aspect is important because more than 140,000,000 people in the world live over 2,500 meters above sea level (masl) [2] and a large percentage of patients with PH live in developing countries.

Within the different types of pulmonary hypertension, pulmonary hypertension associated to congenital heart defects is included. In this group of patients it is important to note, aside from those already mentioned, other considerations specific to the different congenital heart defects. This has an influence in different age groups, from the neonate to the adult, since with the passage of time and the advances in cardiovascular surgery, the chapter of congenital heart defects in the adult is growing and in this context, pulmonary hypertension has an important implication.

So far, it has been established that pulmonary hypertension is an irreversible disease but in the last fifteen years there have been major therapeutic advances that have not only improved the quality of life of these patients but also prolonged it. This is very different from just over eleven years ago, when once diagnosed with idiopathic PH, life expectancy was 2.8 years for adults and 10 months for children [3].

It is important to differentiate between pulmonary hypertension and pulmonary vascular disease. In patients with pulmonary hypertension, the prevention of pulmonary vascular disease is fundamental (see Pathophysiology), and this implies early detection. Therefore, within the process of approaching pulmonary hypertension, there should be a progressively growing and evolving chapter: *the prevention of pulmonary vascular disease.*

Definition

The current definition of PH, which has not undergone many changes since the Congress of Venice (2003) is: a mean pulmonary artery pressure above 25 mm Hg with a wedge pressure or left atrial pressure less than 15 mm Hg. This implies that for the correct diagnosis, catheterization is required [4]. If only these values are considered, in patients with large left to right shunt, pulmonary pressures over these values are frequently found, without any pulmonary vascular disease. In these cases, the patient could be sent to surgery because the patient has hyperkinetic pulmonary hypertension. This means that it is essential to take into account the value of pulmonary resistance. For the definition of PH in children we follow the consensus of the Pulmonary Vascular Research Institute (PVRI) pediatric taskforce held in Panama City in 2011. This consensus establishes criteria for the diagnosis of PH: a mean pulmonary artery pressure greater than 25 mm Hg with increased pulmonary resistance above 3 WU/m^2 for biventricular heart and an index of pulmonary vascular resistance greater than 3 WU/m^2 or a transpulmonary gradient of 6 mm Hg for cavopulmonary shunts [5].

Classification

Pulmonary hypertension classification has recently undergone modifications. The 2008 Dana Point classification, shown in Table 1, is currently used [4].

Table 1. Clinical Classification of Pulmonary Hypertension. Dana Point 2008. J Am Coll Cardiol, 2009; Jun 30; 54(1 Suppl):S43-54

1. Pulmonary arterial hypertension (PAH)
1.1 Idiopathic PAH
1.2 Heritable
1.2.1 BMPR2
1.2.2 ALK1, endoglin (with or without hereditary hemorrhagic telangiectasia)
1.3 Drug- and toxin-induced
1.4 Associated with
1.4.1 Connective tissue diseases
1.4.2 HIV infection
1.4.3 Portal hypertension
1.4.4 Congenital heart diseases
1.4.5 Schistosomiasis
1.5 Persistent pulmonary hypertension of the newborn
1' Pulmonary veno-occlusive disease (PVOD) and/or pulmonary capillary hemangiomatosis (PCH)
2 Pulmonary hypertension owing to left heart disease
2.1 Systolic dysfunction
2.2 Diastolic dysfunction
2.3 Valvular disease
3 Pulmonary hypertension owing to lung diseases and/or hypoxia
3.1 Chronic obstructive pulmonary disease
3.2 Interstitial lung disease
3.3 Other pulmonary diseases with mixed restrictive and obstructive pattern
3.4 Sleep-disordered breathing
3.5 Alveolar hypoventilation disorders
3.6 Chronic exposure to high altitude
4 Chronic thromboembolic pulmonary hypertension (CTEPH)
5 Pulmonary hypertension with unclear multifactorial mechanisms
5.1 Hematologic disorders
5.2 Systemic disorders
5.3 Metabolic disorders
5.4 Others: tumoral obstruction, fibrosing mediastinitis.

Recently modifications were made in Nice in 2013 that have not yet been published. However, this classification is not fully applicable to pulmonary hypertension in children. For this reason, in the taskforce previously mentioned, a classification of pulmonary vascular disease in children was developed [5], as summarized in Table 2.

Table 2. Classification of Pediatric Pulmonary Hypertensive Vascular Disease (PHVD) Pulmonary Circulation 2011; 1 (2), 286-298

1. Prenatal or developmental PHVD
2. Perinatal pulmonary vascular maladaptation
3. Cardiovascular disease
4. Bronchopulmonary dysplasia
5. Isolated PHVD
6. Multifactorial PHVD in congenital malformation syndromes
7. Lung disease
8. Thromboembolic disease
9. Hypobaric hypoxia exposure
10. PHVD with systemic disorders

For the purposes of this text, only pulmonary hypertension associated with congenital heart defects will be analyzed.

Congenital Heart Defects with Associated Pulmonary Hypertension

Overview

Since 1935, [6] the severe histological changes secondary to CHD at a pulmonary vascular level are known, which gave origin to two classical classifications (see below). This means that the first knowledge of PH was based on histological studies. This knowledge has recently been supplemented with much research, such as the study related to the role of elastase in the remodeling of the pulmonary vascular bed [7] and the increase of the Von Willebrand antigen component of the factor VIII originating in endothelial cells [8]. Another factor to consider in patients with PH is the decreased number of pulmonary arterioles.

Several classifications based on the hemodynamic situation and the natural history have been proposed for pulmonary hypertension associated with congenital heart defects and specifically for those with left to right shunts [9, 10].

There are five major groups of heart conditions that originate PH as seen in Table 3.

A) Left to Right Shunts

Left to right shunts are the most common heart defect group and can be divided into pre-tricuspid (e.g. ASD) and post tricuspid (e.g. VSD, ductus arteriosus, aortopulmonary window). This division is important due to the impact each of these has on pulmonary pressure, the post tricuspid defects being much more aggressive [11] (see below); nevertheless, the defect with the highest risk for developing pulmonary hypertension is the total atrioventricular septal defect (complete AV canal). The more severe effects on the pulmonary vascular tree due to increased pulmonary flow have been known since 1897 when Eisenmenger described the syndrome that bears his name [12, 13].

Table 3. Congenital Heart Defects Associated With Pulmonary Hypertension

a) Left to right shunts.
b) Cyanotic congenital heart defects with increased blood flow: TGA, Truncus Arteriosus.
c) CHD originating venocapilar pulmonary hypertension: -Obstructions to the systemic blood flow: Aortic coarctation, severe aortic stenosis, etc. -Obstructions to the pulmonary venous drainage: Obstructed pulmonary venous drainage, pulmonary vein stenosis, cor triatriatum etc. -Pathologies of the mitral valve: mitral valve stenosis, etc. -Obstructions at left ventricular or atrial level: Obstructive hypertrophic cardiomyopathy, cor triatriatum, mitral supravalvular ring, etc.
d) Heart defects with pulmonary circulation of systemic origin: Pulmonary branch originated in aorta, scimitar syndrome, etc.
e) Complex CHD as univentricular heart and double outlet ventricle without pulmonary stenosis, etc.

Pathophysiology

Two aspects of PH need to be considered regarding the pathophysiology:

1. The direct effect of the flow per se on the pulmonary pressure considering the equation: Pressure = Flow x Resistance. This indicates that the higher the flow, the greater the pressure will be, resulting in pulmonary hypertension (PH) without necessarily causing pulmonary vascular damage; in these cases, hyperkinetic pulmonary hypertension is referred to.
2. Pulmonary hypertension secondary to pulmonary vascular disease (PVD). At this point we make reference to PH secondary to high resistance associated with pulmonary vascular disease, a result of increased flow on the pulmonary arterioles. It is important to remark upon the difference between pretricuspid and post tricuspid defects. In the latter group, besides the influence of the increased flow, the effect of systemic pressure is added, in which the shear stress gradually rises up to produce structural damage in the arteriolar wall as can be seen in VSD, ductus arteriosus and aortopulmonary window. The pulmonary vascular remodeling that ensues, affects resistance arterioles mainly (100 to 300 mmcrs). On the other hand, in pre-tricuspid defects (e.g. ASD), flow depends on right ventricular compliance and is not influenced by systemic pressure. This is why the vascular damage is much slower, generally appearing significantly after the second decade of life.

The histological changes related with left to right shunts were analyzed by *Heath and Edwards* in 1958 and were the basis of their classification of 6 stages [14]. Above stage 3, the Eisenmenger syndrome ensues with irreversibility as the principal characteristic. This emphasizes the need for early detection and treatment of these defects. Another classification used is that of Rabinovitch [7, 15], which classifies the vascular damage in three levels and, as Haworth and Reid, takes into account the extent of smooth muscle distally [16].

The severity of PH is related to increased flow and therefore with the defect size [17,18]. Initially, the increased flow creates a hyperkinetic state but gradually pulmonary vascular disease develops. The progression to PH and pulmonary vascular disease is also influenced by genetic factors, altitude over sea level and by the genetically determined hyper-reactivity of the pulmonary vascular tree. Even in postnatal life, in infants with large defects, the histological changes that normally occur after birth can be altered [19]. It is important to take into account that in patients with Down syndrome pulmonary vascular disease develops early, but the evidence is still controversial [20].

From the pathophysiological point of view, the balance between vasoconstrictor and vasodilator substances should be considered when pulmonary hypertension is developed, with a predominance of vasoconstrictor substances, such as endothelin [21, 22].

Diagnosis

In general, early clinical diagnosis of PH is not easy, because initially it is a "silent" disease. For the diagnosis it is very important to differentiate between pulmonary hypertension and pulmonary vascular disease, making clear that all pulmonary vascular disease involves pulmonary hypertension, but not all pulmonary hypertension implies pulmonary vascular disease. In the context of these patients, it is essential to evaluate how compromised the pulmonary vascular bed is.

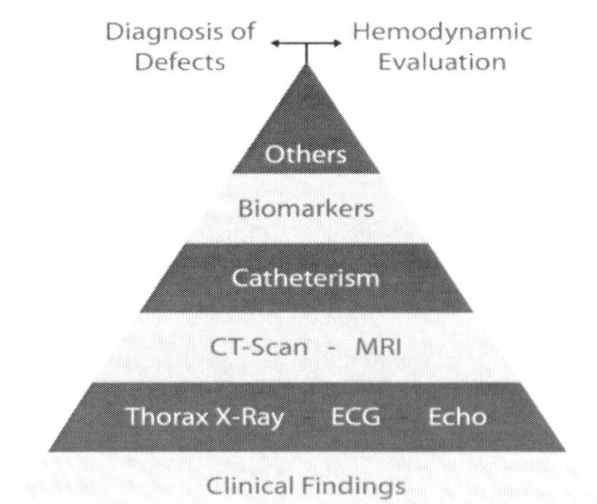

Figure 1. Pyramidal approach proposed for the diagnosis of the patients with pulmonary hypertension: The base of the pyramid represents the clinic findings (currently neglected by technological advances) and the rest of the pyramid includes the entire set of laboratory test results. From the tip of the pyramid emerges the diagnosis of the defect(s) and hemodynamic assessment and from the analysis of these, the therapeutic conduct is defined.

For the study of these patients, a pyramidal approach is suggested; the base of the pyramid consists of the clinical findings and the rest of the pyramid consists of laboratory test results (Figure 1).

In this way, a comprehensive evaluation of the impact of pulmonary hypertension can be made. Moreover, it is essential to make a comprehensive assessment of the child, looking for underlying health conditions that may be influencing pulmonary hypertension, such as upper airway obstruction, sleep apnea, pulmonary parenchymal pathology, etc. In these cases an interdisciplinary approach to treatment is pivotal.

Clinical Findings

Logically in pulmonary hypertension associated with congenital heart defects clinical findings depend largely on the underlying disease; however specific findings are related to the progression of pulmonary hypertension. When there is significant PH, patients begin to feel progressive fatigue with exercise and, in advanced stages, cyanosis appears with exercise, which becomes a permanent cyanosis when Eisenmenger Syndrome is established (discussed later).

Sometimes, the first sign may be a syncopal episode. On palpation, right ventricle hyperactivity intensifies with increasing pulmonary pressure and, in severe cases, even closure of the pulmonary valve is palpable.

Regarding cardiac auscultation, it is important to analyze the 2nd heart sound; initially a permanent split of the second sound is evident, but with increasing pulmonary hypertension, the pulmonary component is intensified and it appears to be a unique and intensive second sound. As pulmonary hypertension progresses, the murmur of VSD or ductus disappears and a mild diastolic decrescendo murmur (Graham Steel murmur) appears at the left upper third of the sternal border, which indicates that there is severe pulmonary hypertension; most likely associated to severe pulmonary vascular disease [17].

In patients with severe pulmonary hypertension, arrhythmias and right ventricular failure may occur, indicating a poor prognosis.

Electrocardiogram

The electrocardiogram findings will also be associated to the underlying heart defect. For example in large VSD´s, when there is hyperkinetic pulmonary hypertension, the characteristic sign of biventricular growth, the Katz Wachtel sign is positive: Wide biphasic RS in three leads (generally V2, V3 and V4 or between V2-V5) with R+S > 45 mm [23, 24] (Figure 2A).

When pulmonary hypertension is severe enough, a significant right ventricular dominance begins to appear with right axis deviation and “R” on the right precordial leads. A peaked “P” in D2 can be found due to right atrial enlargement and diminished reduction of left ventricular forces appear (Figure 2B).

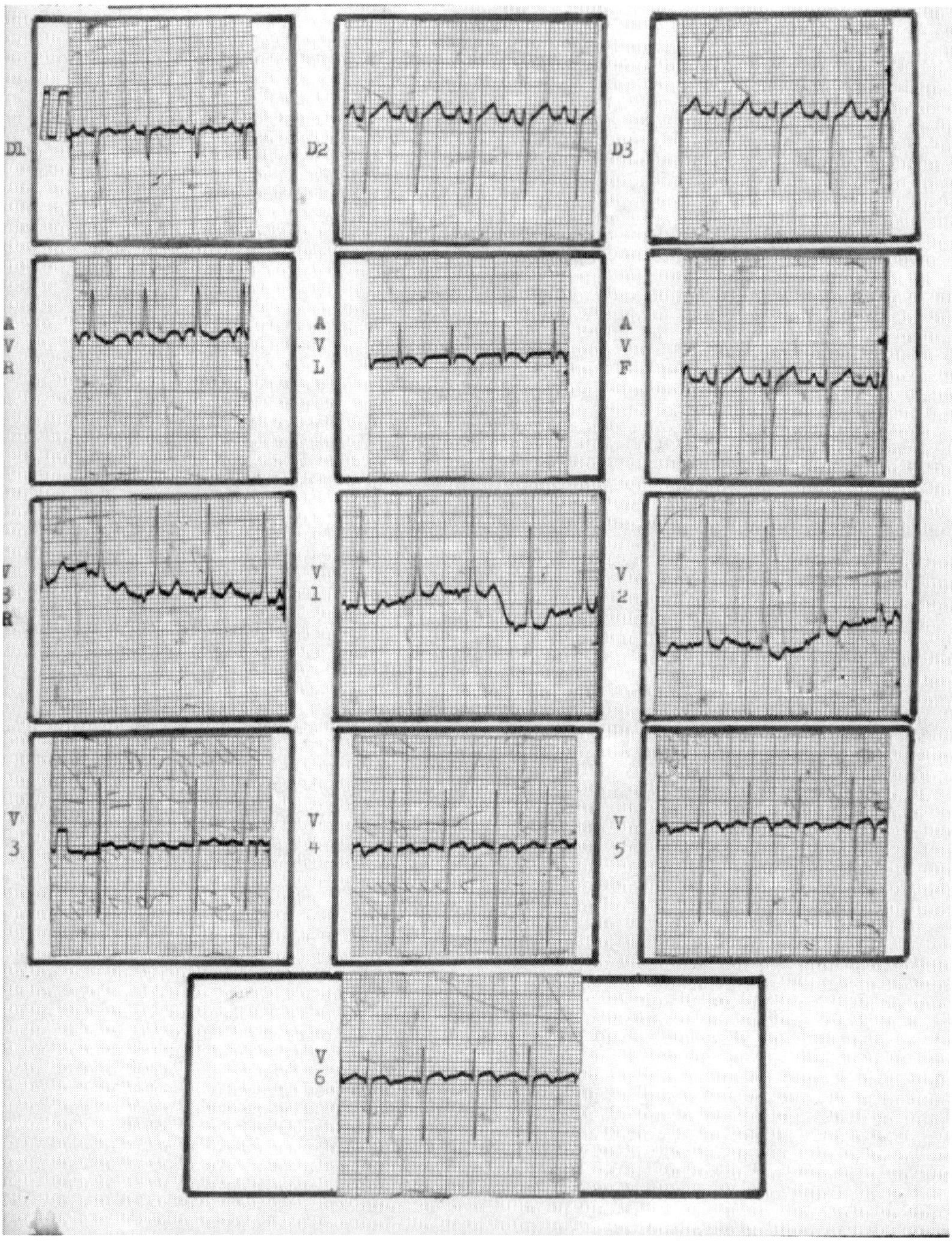

Figure 2A. Electrocardiogram of a five-year-old boy with VSD and hyperkinetic pulmonary hypertension. The EKG shows a positive Katz Wachtel finding (wide biphasic QRS in three precordial leads, with R+S > 45mm) indicating biventricular growth.

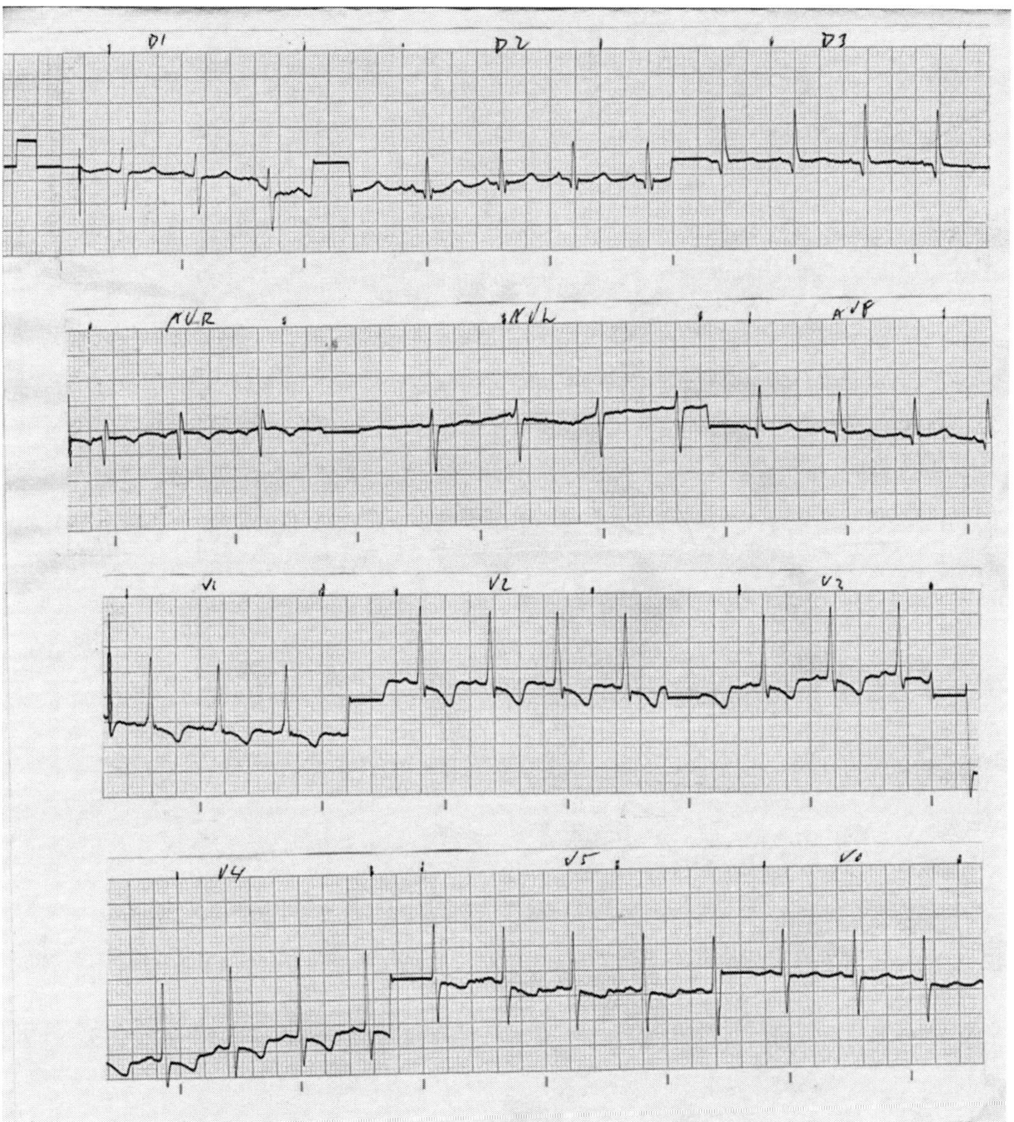

Figure 2B. Electrocardiogram (0.5 V) of a 9-year-old child with Eisenmenger syndrome. Note the R of 26 mm in V1 caused by severe right ventricular hypertrophy.

Chest X- Ray

Usually in large left to right shunts, severe cardiomegaly with biventricular and left atrium enlargement is initially evident, with increased pulmonary flow (Figure. 3A). As pulmonary vascular disease progresses, there is a decrease in the size of the cardiac silhouette and pulmonary flow, and the pulmonary trunk and central pulmonary arteries become prominent. When there is severe pulmonary vascular disease, as in Eisenmenger Syndrome, progressive decrease in the blood flow is observed in the periphery [17] (Figure 3B).

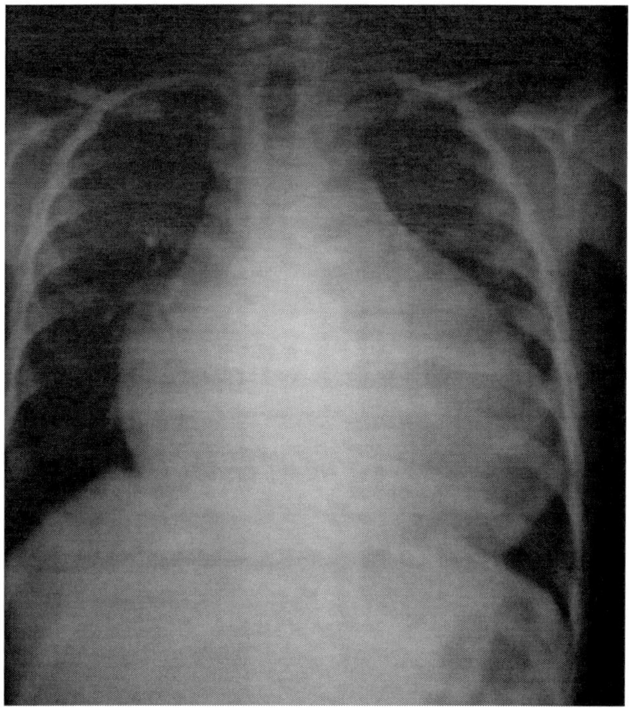

Figure 3A. Chest X-ray of a child with VSD and hyperkinetic pulmonary hypertension showing severe cardiomegaly and increased pulmonary flow. A huge left atrium is shown.

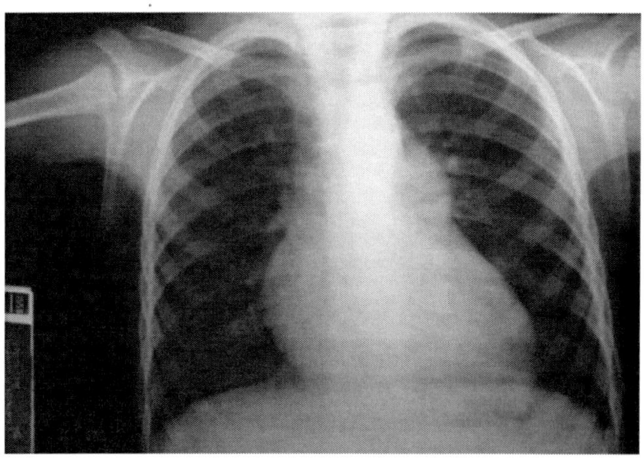

Figure 3B. Chest X ray of a 14-year-old girl with Eisenmenger syndrome. Note that there is no "cardiomegaly", however there is persistent right ventricular growth, significant prominence of the pulmonary trunk and central pulmonary arteries with hypoflow seen in the periphery.

Echocardiography

Echocardiography is essential for the initial diagnosis and monitoring of patients with PH. In this group of patients (congenital heart defects and PH), it allows the identification of the characteristics of the defect, but the main drawback is that this exam is operator-dependent. For this reason, cardiac catheterization is essential for a definitive diagnosis and complete hemodynamic evaluation. Furthermore, for the evaluation of pulmonary pressure by echocardiography, it is important to achieve an ideal registry of the tricuspid insufficiency jet to apply Bernoulli's equation-(gradient = velocity^2 x 4). The pressure of the right atrium must be added to this gradient, a topic of debate. It should be considered that the value that is added should increase with the severity of the pulmonary hypertension. In severe cases, an acceptable value is 10 mm Hg.

Pulmonary pressure in post tricuspid defects can also be evaluated through the interventricular pressure gradient, in the case of VSD, or aortopulmonary pressure gradient, in the case of the aortopulmonary window or ductus arteriosus, by subtracting this pressure gradient from the systemic pressure recorded simultaneously. It is important to emphasize the registration of the optimal curve of the tricuspid regurgitation jet or the defect. Several optimal measurements are recommended (Figure 4). Keep in mind that in young children the curves are often not easy to record if the patient is irritable or constantly moving; in that case the patient must be reassured. When pulmonary insufficiency exists, the pulmonary diastolic pressure can be assessed with reference to the end of the recorded curve and adding the right atrial pressure, while looking for an optimal registration of the curve.

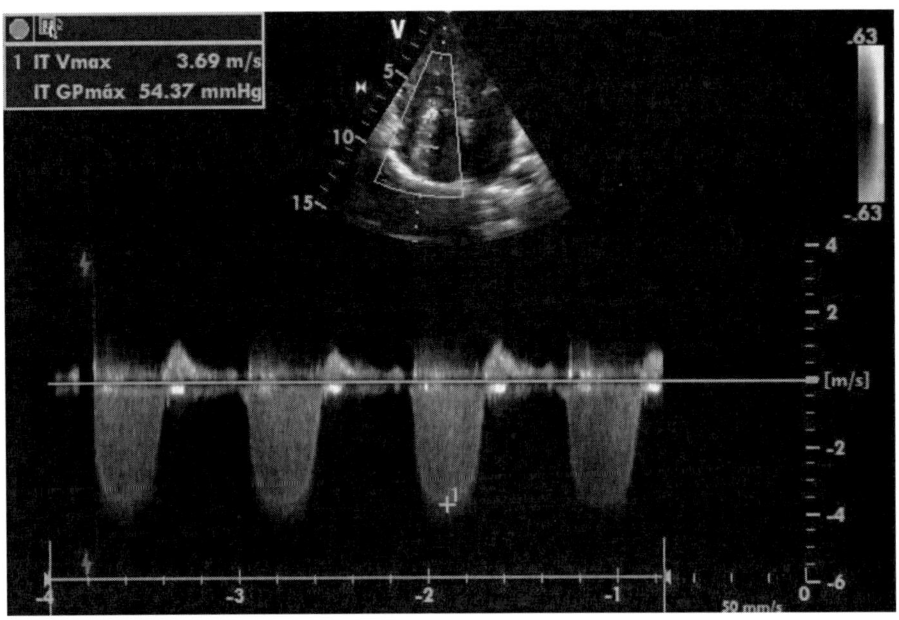

Figure 4. Echocardiogram of a child with severe pulmonary hypertension. An excellent curve of the tricuspid regurgitation is shown.

Besides pulmonary pressure quantification, it is important to assess the right ventricular function, TAPSE, inferior vena cava collapse, morphology of the left ventricle, size of the right atrium, displacement of the atrial septum to the left, and flow through any shunts. The assessment of right ventricular function is very important, but given the geometry of the right ventricle, there is controversy about the reliability regarding the accuracy of the assessment of right ventricular function by echocardiography; assessment by Nuclear Magnetic Resonance is more accurate. An attempt to evaluate different parameters has been made, including right ventricle/left ventricle ratio, tissue Doppler, TEI index and the flattening of the interventricular septum, which is valued very well in short axis. In severe cases, the left ventricular geometry is altered, compromising the filling of the left ventricle and paradoxical movement of the interventricular septum can be found. In the most severe cases, a pericardial effusion can be found which has been associated with poor prognosis. With the analysis of the different parameters, the dysfunction of the right ventricle can be defined. Another even more difficult and less reliable aspect is the evaluation of pulmonary resistance [25-28].

In conclusion the echocardiographic evaluation of patients with pulmonary hypertension is very important, but their study is difficult and requires sufficient time to achieve an ideal assessment of the heart disease, pulmonary pressure, and right ventricular function. These difficulties have led to define the role of echocardiography as essential for the detection, screening, and monitoring of patients, but for an accurate diagnosis, cardiac catheterization is required as previously stated.

Biomarkers

Biomarkers play an important role in the evaluation of pulmonary hypertension [29,30], with brain natriuretic peptide (BNP) considered the principal biomarker in clinical practice [31]. This marker is increased when pulmonary hypertension is significant, especially when patients are clinically decompensated. When the patient is compensated with medical treatment, BNP decreases because BNP does not assess pulmonary pressure but the hemodynamic repercussion of pulmonary hypertension. One drawback of BNP is that an accurate cutoff for sensitivity and specificity has not been established. In 52 patients with persistent pulmonary hypertension of the newborn, a specificity of 87% and sensitivity of 76% was found for a value of 267 pcgr/dl. In the control group of healthy newborns, the value was under 20 pcgr/dl. The presence of circulating endothelial cells is another marker that is under research [32].

Cardiac Catheterization

Undoubtedly, cardiac catheterization is the gold standard for PH evaluation and all patients, suspected of significant pulmonary hypertension, require cardiac catheterization. In this moment, it is important to mention the current trend is the early correction of cardiac defects. If there are no important findings of pulmonary hypertension, with noninvasive diagnosis, surgery can be performed without the need for catheterization [33]. Cardiac catheterization allows us to specify the details of the heart defect and assess not only the features of the malformation and the pulmonary pressure, but also the severity of pulmonary vascular disease. In children, it is very important to analyze the type of sedation for the catheter study since sedation and anesthesia can originate systemic hypotension, and certainly the calculation of resistances and pressures will be distorted. Furthermore, sedation or anesthesia in patients with severe pulmonary hypertension implies a risk factor [34, 35]. It is necessary not only to calculate the pulmonary pressure and pulmonary resistance but also to consider the relationship of pulmonary resistance to systemic resistance and the ratio of pulmonary and systemic pressures. For these calculations, the use of oxygen consumption is ideal but is not available in all catheterization laboratories. The application of the Fick principle is an appropriate method in such cases [33].

As mentioned in the definition, when dealing with large left to right shunt defects, pulmonary pressures may be elevated to systemic or close to systemic levels without necessarily indicating inoperability, as is the case of hyperkinetic pulmonary hypertension. Therefore it is essential to consider pulmonary vascular resistance in the assessment. In patients with significant hypertension and elevated pulmonary resistance, the pulmonary vascular bed reactivity test should be applied to determine the extent of vascular compromise. Nitric oxide, oxygen or both, are often used, but adenosine or prostacyclin might be useful as well. It should be noted that in altitude by hypobaric hypoxia, oxygen plays a pivotal role for the pulmonary vascular reactivity test, (see below). The test is considered positive when there is a 20% decrease in pulmonary vascular resistance compared to baseline.

Magnetic Resonance Image and Computed Tomography

Diagnostic images play an important role in the evaluation of patients with pulmonary hypertension. Magnetic resonance imaging provides more accurate right ventricular function assessment than echocardiography [36-38], which is pivotal before any surgical procedure. Computed tomography is useful in pulmonary vascular bed assessment to rule out intrinsic pulmonary disease as a cause of pulmonary hypertension. In adults with congenital heart defects and pulmonary hypertension, it is essential to evaluate the pulmonary vascular bed since pulmonary thrombosis is a common cause of it [39].

Six-Minute Walk

Although it seems difficult to apply in children, the six-minute walk test is evolving as a cardiovascular performance test, especially in children above 4 years old. There is growing experience in its application in children [40, 41] and there are already reference values available [42].

Lung Biopsy

Previously lung biopsy was used to assess pulmonary vascular disease but its use is decreasing, considering that a lung biopsy sample can be taken from a place with a normal pulmonary vascular bed or one not severely affected. However it continues to have an important role when studied by very experienced professionals or for research studies. Moreover, lung biopsy studies have made large contributions to the study of patients with pulmonary hypertension but there are important limitations [7, 15, 43, 44].

Therapeutic Approach

In patients with pulmonary hypertension associated with congenital heart defects it is important to differentiate between pulmonary hypertension and pulmonary vascular disease. The best therapeutic approach for pulmonary hypertension with CHD is the early detection and treatment of CHD to avoid the remodeling of the pulmonary vascular tree [7] in order to prevent pulmonary vascular disease, as can be seen in Eisenmenger Syndrome. *If CHD are detected and corrected opportunely, the Eisenmenger Syndrome would eventually become a part of pediatric cardiology history.*

In the treatment of patients with severe pulmonary hypertension secondary to congenital heart defects, some aspects related with the operability of patients should be noted [45,46]. According to the 2013 Nice Task Force recommendations (unpublished data), patients are fit for surgical procedures if pulmonary resistance is below 4 WU/m2. On the other hand, when pulmonary resistance is above 8 WU m2, surgery is precluded. There is a grey zone between 4 and 8 WU/m2, a clinical scenario where the decision is not easy. In this type of borderline patients we must resort to other clinical and laboratory procedures, including the prolonged hyperoxia test (especially for patients living at an altitude of more than 2,500 meters above sea level, see below).

Pharmacological Treatment of Pulmonary Hypertension

Mark Humbert described three lines of treatment for patients with pulmonary hypertension, according to the pathophysiology of the disease [47,48]: the use of prostacyclin and its analogues, endothelin inhibitors such as Bosentan, Ambrisentan, and Maticentan (not yet available in the market) [49], and the use of the nitric oxide pathway, which increases cGMP, such as fosfodiasterase 5 inhibitors (Sildenafil) and Riociguat [50].

The major drawback of prostacyclin analogues is the administration route (intravenous), since the catheter is associated with complications that put the patients at risk and is difficult for children to tolerate. This is why its use is not common in pediatric populations, except with inhaled Iloprost [51, 52].

Endothelin antagonists have shown good results in pulmonary hypertension treatment, especially Bosentan, and now represent a good option with dose standardization in children. Based on experience, it is recommended to start with sildenafil, and then evaluate clinical response. If there is no satisfactory response after up to three months of treatment, a combination of Bosentan – Sildenafil is initiated as treatment [53-55].

There is extensive experience with sildenafil for pulmonary hypertension in children, although since 2012, the FDA does not recommend its use in patients below 17 years of age due to the risk of death at high doses [56, 57]. In Europe, conversely, it is approved for use in children. At a dose of 1 mg/kg every six hours, several studies have demonstrated satisfactory results with sildenafil, and with only few complications reported. Hypotension was the adverse effect most commonly presented in patients. Sildenafil has been used in different types of pulmonary hypertension, and the entire spectrum in age presentation in children, including neonates, for the treatment of persistent pulmonary hypertension in newborns with excellent results and safety without long term complications as have been reported by other authors [58-61].

Surgical Treatment

As stated earlier, patients with pulmonary vascular resistance less than 4 Wood units can be taken to surgery to correct this defect and patients with increased pulmonary resistance > 8 units are inoperable. The doubt and difficulty lies in defining the surgical procedure in a borderline patient. Valved patches have been used in patients with VSD [62, 63] and temporarily occluding the ductus during catheterization in order to observe the response and tolerance to the occlusion [64]. If there is more than one defect, for example the presence of a VSD and ductus arteriosus, one possibility that exists is to close the ductus and leave the VSD open to see the patient's evolution and afterward consider its closure.

In "borderline" patients, the inoperable status of the patient must be well established, before definitively rejecting the option of surgery. One example of this is that of a six-year-old girl living at altitude, diagnosed with VSD and severe pulmonary hypertension, and considered nonsurgical after catheterization. She underwent a prolonged hyperoxia test that was positive (see below), so medical treatment with sildenafil began while living at low altitude. Six months later, the patient was catheterized in the same catheterization laboratory; the pulmonary resistance was decreased, permitting the closure of the VSD, and after six years of follow up, the patient is asymptomatic. It must be considered that if a patient with severe pulmonary hypertension and advanced pulmonary vascular disease is taken to surgery, the prognosis is worse than the prognosis of patients with Eisenmenger syndrome and the average lifespan is shorter, similar to patients with idiopathic pulmonary hypertension [65,66].

In patients with severe irreversible pulmonary disease (Eisenmenger syndrome), lung transplantation is a last option for the correction of the defect, or a cardiopulmonary transplantation with acceptable results [67-69]; the drawback is the difficulty in procuring donors.

It is important to keep in mind that in patients with significant pulmonary hypertension undergoing surgery there are three types of patients: a group of patients in which once operated, pulmonary pressures progressively decrease and normalize; another group of patients in whom there are no drops in pulmonary pressure; and a third group of patients in which the pulmonary arterial pressure and pulmonary vascular disease continues to progress after the surgery. This last group of patients is similar to patients with idiopathic pulmonary hypertension and therefore the prognosis is worse than those with Eisenmenger [66] syndrome.

In cases with severe pulmonary vascular disease, there are experimental publications documenting decreased pulmonary vascular disease after performing pulmonary artery banding [70].

Pulmonary Hypertension Associated with Congenital Heart Defects at Altitude. Physiology and physiopathology at Altitude

It is important to note some physiological aspects that occur when the altitude above sea level increases, which are essential to understanding the behavior of the inhabitants of high altitude. Barometric pressure is the pressure exerted by a column of air over any element located on the earth's surface. This pressure is 760 mm Hg at sea level and decreases as altitude rises. This is related to the decreasing of the pressure of alveolar oxygen (PAO2), and pressure of arterial oxygen (PaO2). The oxygen saturation and the partial pressure of oxygen (PO2) also decrease as altitude increase [4]. The oxygen concentration is the same at different altitudes (21%); however, the partial pressure of a gas = barometric pressure, multiplied by its concentration, but barometric pressure is inversely proportional to altitude. So, as the altitude rises, the partial pressure of the gas diminishes. The partial pressure of oxygen (PO2) = barometric pressure, multiplied by the concentration of O2:

At sea level PO2 is 760 X 0.21 = 159.6 mm Hg
Bogota (2.640 mAsl) PO2 is 560 X 0.21 = 117 mm Hg
La Paz (3.600 mAsl) PO2 is 490 X 0.21 = 102 mm Hg

Hypobaric hypoxia refers to the diminished oxygen availability to saturate blood as altitude rises, which in turn markedly influences the hemodynamic parameters of patients living in altitude and alters the characteristics of the pulmonary vascular bed, therefore influencing pulmonary hypertension. For these reasons, the inhabitants of altitudes should not be approached in the same manner as an inhabitant at sea level.

According to the studies by Dante Peñaloza, the effects of altitude are noticeably above 2,500 meters above sea level, following a parabolic curve of rapid ascent [71] (Figure 5).

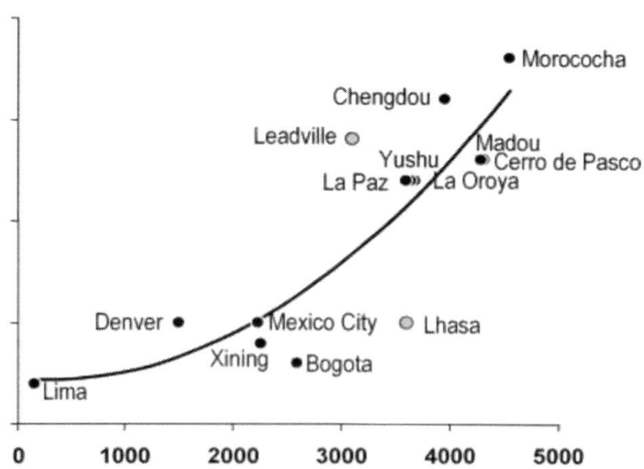

Figure 5. Graph showing the effect of altitude due to hypobaric hypoxia. The effect is significant above 2.500 meters above sea level, following a parabolic curve (with permission from Professor Dante Peñaloza).

Classification of Altitude

For the study of the patient living in altitude and the effects of hypobaric hypoxia, altitude has been classified into several levels. The following classification is used and seems most appropriate:

Low altitude: Up to 1,500 meters above sea level (masl)
Moderate altitude: 1,500 to 3,000 masl
High altitude: 3000 to 5000 masl
Extreme altitude: 5000 to 8000 masl

By the above analysis, it can clearly be seen that altitude is a very important factor in the study of patients with PH due to all the implications of hypobaric hypoxia related to the progressive decrease of barometric pressure and partial pressure of oxygen as altitude increases [71,72].

Usually in patients with PH, regardless of altitude, the recommendations of studies conducted at sea level are followed, including the same values of normality regarding pressure and saturation used at sea level, labeling patients who have normal pulmonary pressure as mild pulmonary hypertensive patients and recommending oxygen in newborns often without need is a mistake.

The decrease in barometric pressure with altitude is related with vasoconstriction of the pulmonary vascular bed secondary to the hypoxia and this is an adaptive mechanism for those who live at altitude. However, this vasoconstriction causes increased pressure and pulmonary vascular resistance, increased cardiac output by increasing the heart rate and may have increased stroke volume to maintain proper release of O2. This sustained vasoconstriction may eventually cause pulmonary vascular disease [73].

The altitude affects both normal patients and patients with different types of PH and therefore patients with congenital heart defects (CHD). In these last patients, the behavior in altitude is different from the behavior at sea level, accelerating PH and pulmonary vascular disease, indicating that at moderate and high altitude CHD must be treated early.

In children, and in general in the inhabitants of high altitudes, hyper-reactivity of the pulmonary vascular bed is an important factor and is more noticeable among younger children [72-74]. This factor must be taken into account in the evaluation of children with pulmonary hypertension associated with congenital heart defects in altitude because it must be differentiated whether pulmonary vascular resistance is elevated by pulmonary vascular disease or by vasoconstriction of the pulmonary vascular bed.

The above factors must be taken into account from the neonatal period and perhaps from the prenatal stage. It is well known that according to studies of the Peruvian group led by Dante Peñaloza [75,76], pulmonary resistance in postnatal life decreases more slowly than at sea level; it is also known that in some infants with left to right shunts, pulmonary vascular resistance cannot fall back to normal in postnatal life. For these reasons, there is a tendency to acquire early vascular disease in these infants compared to people at sea level. This is the case seen in Figure 6, showing advanced pulmonary vascular disease in a 6-month-old infant with large VSD. This is why these patients should have surgery very early.

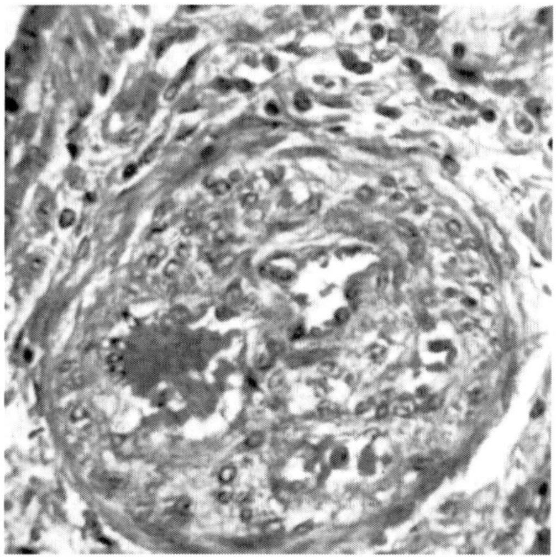

Figure 6. Histological section of a pulmonary arteriole with hematoxylin-eosin staining of a six-month-old infant with large VSD and severe pulmonary vascular disease. Note that there is a light obstruction with recanalization (grade III of Head and Edwards disease classification). (Courtesy of Susana Murcia MD.)

Taking into account hypobaric hypoxia, and that oxygen is very important part in the evaluation of pulmonary vascular bed in the inhabitants of high altitudes, a test has been designed that we named the prolonged hyperoxia test (forthcoming), defined as hyperoxia > 80% oxygen for at least 1 hour and up to 24 hours, performing a baseline echocardiogram and taking a blood sample for BNP prior to the test, and performing another echocardiography after hyperoxia as well as the BNP. With this test we were able to rescue patients defined by catheterization as inoperable or having a poor prognosis, and some have been able to receive surgery or have evolved satisfactorily.

Based on the foregoing, a question arises: In the hemodynamic assessment of pulmonary hypertension in children at altitude, including the child with congenital heart defects associated with pulmonary hypertension, and more specifically in relation to a reactivity test during catheterization, should the same parameters as at sea level be followed or should more importance be given to oxygen levels and therefore to the hyperoxia test? Based on experience, soon to be published, in altitude the parameters to evaluate the reactivity of the pulmonary vascular bed should be reconsidered, including whether the child is an inhabitant of high altitude with congenital heart defects associated with pulmonary hypertension. This is an important research topic and there is still much to learn.

Eisenmenger Syndrome

What is now called Eisenmenger syndrome was first described by Eisenmenger in 1897 in a 32-year-old cyanotic patient who at autopsy was found to have a ventricular septal defect and, histologically, a severe pulmonary vascular disease. These findings were initially called the Eisenmenger complex [12]. In 1958 Paul Wood found eleven pathologies with a similar presentation to that described by Eisenmenger and coined the term Eisenmenger syndrome

[13,77], a term that has persisted since then and is defined as the pathophysiological presentation in which a left to right shunt causes progressive pulmonary vascular damage with increased pulmonary pressures that reach systemic or suprasystemic levels and elevate pulmonary vascular resistance, so that the shunt is reversed, becoming right-to-left or bidirectional shunts, explaining the appearance of cyanosis. In this stage of the disease, an irreversible pulmonary vascular disease has been established with changes greater than grade 3 or more of the Head and Edwards classification [14]. As stated earlier, this state can be avoided if left to right shunts are detected and surgery is early. Eisenmenger syndrome occurs earlier and more frequently in the post tricuspid shunts (VSD, PDA and aortopulmonary window) which occurs in up to 50% of large defects, unlike in pretricupid shunts (ASD) in which ES appears later in about 10% of cases [78]. Logically, in the outcome, other factors are influential, such as the size of the defect, genetic factors and the altitude above sea level where the patient lives.

Clinical Presentation

Patients begin to experience fatigue with exercise, chest pain, and cyanosis can be transient or with exercise, which eventually becomes permanent. With time, the cyanosis is severe with clubbing and conjunctival injection. Initially, a significant number of patients present with syncope. In the clinical examination important hyperactivity of the RV is found and closure of the pulmonary valve is palpable. Upon auscultation there is a significant increase in the intensity of the pulmonary component of the 2nd sound, and an early systolic click is frequently found. The features of the original defect are lost and a small ejection murmur may be found at the upper third of the left sternal border along with a diastolic decrescendo murmur at the same site (Graham Steel murmur) [17]. These signs are indicators that the patient has an irreversible pulmonary vascular disease and should not be sent to surgery.

Treatment

In these patients, the objective is to prolong life and improve the quality of life. Although it is important to note that they live longer than patients with idiopathic pulmonary hypertension; they may live up to 40 or 50 years of age and beyond [78].

To improve quality of life, the current approach of the previously mentioned pharmacological treatment includes combination therapy. Prostacyclin + Bosentan or sildenafil + Bosentan, is used, indicating that the BREATH 5 study has shown improvement in patients with the use of Bosentan as shown in randomized studies [79]. Lately, combined medical and surgical treatments have been encouraged [51-64,80]. If there is right ventricular failure, ACE inhibitors and digoxin can be used but care must be taken with diuretics because they increase polycythemia, which is characteristic in these patients and may promote thrombosis. It is convenient to use antiplatelet medicine but anticoagulation is controversial. If arrhythmias are present, antiarrhythmic medicines are necessary [80, 83]. For the patients that live in high altitudes, it is recommended that they live at a lower altitude above sea level.

As complications of these patients may include thrombosis, bleeding, epistaxis, brain abscesses and arrhythmias. In patients with Eisenmenger syndrome it is important to note that pregnancy is contraindicated because of the high risk of death not only for the mother (about 50%) but also to the fetus (about 40%) [81,82]. A last therapeutic option for patients with ES is lung transplantation with correction of the defect or cardiopulmonary transplantation [67-69].

The Adult with Congenital Heart Defects and Pulmonary Hypertension

This group of patients represents 5-10% of patients with congenital heart defects and increases progressively as the development of pediatric cardiology expands [80-83]. They can be separated into three subgroups of patients: a) patients developing Eisenmenger syndrome (this subgroup should disappear, at least in the cases of simple left to right shunts if they had surgery in a timely manner), mainly in developing countries where there is not an adequate treatment of these pathologies; b) patients with complex congenital heart defects where it was impossible to perform an ideal surgery and finally develop pulmonary vascular disease (for example, patients with pulmonary atresia with VSD and significant collaterals); c) patients developing severe pulmonary hypertension after adequate surgical treatment of the defect.

In the pathophysiology of pulmonary hypertension in these patients, in addition to those factors previously mentioned in the Eisenmenger syndrome, it is necessary to include factors related with chronicity such as polycythemia, coagulation disorders, and intrapulmonary thrombosis, which is found in 30% of patients with Eisenmenger syndrome.

The clinical findings of these patients are basically similar to those found in patients with ES, but modified by the findings of the congenital heart defect, dyspnea and syncope being relatively common.

For diagnosis, the parameters previously indicated for ES are followed, emphasizing the exercise stress test and the 6-minute walk test that helps indicate hemodynamic status, and patient outcome with treatment [83,84]. Also, it is important to study coagulation disorders and consider polyglobulia. In these cases, erythropheresis was often performed but this should be done only if the hematocrit is over 65% and in these cases it is necessary to replace volume, emphasizing that these patients should avoid any risk of dehydration. This means that from the hematologic point of view, these patients require special handling [85]. It should also be remembered that pregnancy carries a high mortality, so in these patients pregnancy should be avoided [81, 82].

This group of patients has benefited greatly from the current treatment of pulmonary hypertension with prostacyclin analogs, endothelin inhibitors and sildenafil. With these new therapies, it has been possible to not only improve the quality of life but to also prolong it.

An important group of patients that must be taken into account are patients undergoing cavopulmonary bypass (Fontan), in which case any increase in pulmonary vascular pressure causes hemodynamic repercussion with heart failure and disorders such as protein-losing enteropathy [83, 84].

B) Cyanotic Congenital Heart Defects with Increased Pulmonary Blood Flow

The prototypes of this group are transposition of the great arteries (TGA) and the common arterial trunk. In patients with TGA, it should be investigated whether there is an intact ventricular septum (IVS) or if it is a TGA with VSD and/or large ductus. In TGA with IVS, pulmonary vascular disease is found between 6 and 40% at the end of the first year of life [86,87].

In TGA with VSD and/or large ductus, irreversible vascular disease is frequent before the first year of life, and this applies to cases of truncus arteriosus as well.

In the 70s, several studies on early pulmonary vascular disease associated with TGA in patients without surgery were carried out, as is documented in the classic study of Neufeld [86].

Hypoxia plays an important role in the origin of vascular disease in these patients since it is a potent vasoconstrictor [73]. Moreover, there is a group of patients with TGA and significant pulmonary hypertension in the neonatal period, which can be considered a persistent pulmonary hypertension of the newborn associated with TGA. This association explains why some patients with TGA with intact ventricular septum do not improve with atrioseptostomy. These patients have been called “bad mixers" [88]. With regard to pulmonary vascular disease in patients not treated surgically; it is fortunately not the current situation because of the tendency of early correction of these patients. It is important to note that some patients, who experienced timely surgery, may still develop pulmonary hypertension later [89-91].

As in TGA, patients with truncus arteriosus have two factors that contribute to the origin of early pulmonary hypertension: hypoxia that leads to vasoconstriction of the pulmonary vascular bed and increased pulmonary blood flow [92]; for this reason, these patients should be corrected early in the first days of life.

C) Heart Defects That Cause Increased Pulmonary Capillary Wedge Pressure

This group includes all heart defects that cause obstruction to pulmonary venous drainage directly by obstruction of the pulmonary veins, or retrogradely by obstruction at the cardiac level or the aorta such as cor triatriatum, congenital mitral stenosis, etc. These pathologies give origin to retrograde pulmonary hypertension, although the main manifestation is heart failure and pulmonary edema [17].

An essential aspect about this group is that once the defect is corrected, pulmonary hypertension regresses very quickly. This group also includes the obstructed of total anomalous pulmonary venous return which causes severe pulmonary hypertension and early heart failure in the neonatal period. These patients require early surgical correction.

D) Heart Defects with Pulmonary Circulation of Systemic Origin or Malformation of the Pulmonary Vascular Bed

In this group, the pulmonary vascular bed receives systemic pressure flow, which causes PH, and may be severe very early on. This group includes the pulmonary artery originating from the aorta and Scimitar syndrome, which is associated with hypoplasia of the right lung [93-95].

E) Complex Congenital Heart Defects

In this group the PH may be secondary to increased pulmonary blood flow, obstruction to systemic or pulmonary venous drainage, etc. This category unites an important medley, although fortunately the defects of this group are not very frequent.

Worth mentioning is the PH secondary to a total atrioventricular septal defect (total AV canal) which causes early severe pulmonary hypertension, especially if associated with Down syndrome. These patients should have surgery before 6 months of age.

Acknowledgment

Thank you to Dr. Carlos E. Diaz for the collaboration in preparation of the chapter.

References

[1] Rabinovitch M. Pulmonary hypertension: updating a mysterious disease. *Cardiovasc Res* 1997; 34:268-72.

[2] Xu W-Q, Jing Z-C. High-altitude pulmonary hypertension. *Eur Respir Rev* 2009; 18: 13–17.

[3] Widlitz A, Barst RJ. Pulmonary arterial hypertension in children. *Eur Respir J* 2003; 21:155-176.

[4] Simonneau G, Robbins IM, Beghetti M et al. Updated clinical classification of pulmonary hypertension. *J Am Coll Cardiol* 2009;54 (1 Suppl):S43-54.

[5] del Cerro MJ, Abman S, Diaz G et al. A consensus approach to the classification of pediatric pulmonary hypertensive vascular disease: Report from the PVRI Pediatric Taskforce, Panama 2011. *Pulmonary Circulation* 2011; 1, 286-298.

[6] Brenner O. Pathology of the vessels of the pulmonary circulation Part 1. *Arch Inter Med* 1935; 56: 211.

[7] Rabinovitch M. Pathophysiology. In *Heart Disease in Infants Children and adolescents* sixth edition. Allen H, Gutgessell HR, Clark E, Driscoll DJ. Lippincot Williams and Wilkins. 2001: 1312-1346.

[8] Rabinovitch M, Andrew M et al. Abnormal endothelial factor VIII associated with pulmonary hypertension and congenital heart defects. Physiology and natural history. Pulmonary hypertension. *Circulation* 1987; 76: 1043-1052.

[9] Schulze-Neick I, Beghetti M. Classifying pulmonary hypertension in the setting of the congenitally malformed heart —cleaning up a dog's dinner. *Cardiol Young* 2008;18: 22-5.

[10] Beghetti M, Tissot C. Pulmonary hypertension in congenital shunts. *Rev Esp Cardiol* 2010; 63:1179–93.

[11] Van Loon R, Roofthooft M, Berger R. Pulmonary arterial hypertension in children with congenital heart disease. *PVRI Review* 2009;1:203-7.

[12] Eisenmenger V. Die Angeborenen Defect der Kammerscheidewand des Harsen. *Z Klin Med* 1897; 32: 1-28.

[13] Brammel H, Vogel J, Pryor R et al. The Eisenmenger syndrome. A clinical and physiologic reappraisal. *Am J Cardiol Reviews.* 1971; 28: 679-92.

[14] Heath D, Edwards JE. The pathology of Hypertensive pulmonary vascular disease. A description of six grades of structural changes in the pulmonary arteries with special reference to congenital cardiac septal defects. *Circulation* 1958 18: 533-547

[15] Rabinovitch M, Haworth S, Castañeda A et al. Lung Biopsy in congenital heart disease: A morphometric approach to pulmonary vascular disease. *Circulation* 1978, 58 (6): 1107-1122

[16] Haworth SG, Reid L. A morphometric study of regional variation in lung structure in infants with pulmonary hypertension and congenital cardiac defect: A justification of lung biopsy. *Br Heart J* 1978; 40: 825-31.

[17] Díaz G, Díaz R. *Hipertensión Pulmonar Secundaria.* En Cardiología Pediátrica. Díaz G, Sandoval N, Vélez JF, Carrillo G eds. McGraw Hill, 2003; 825-837.

[18] Rothman A. Hipertension Pulmonar y Cardiopatia Congenita. En Díaz G.F., Sandoval J., y Sola A. Editores. Hipertensión Pulmonar en Niños. Editorial Distribuna. Bogota, 2011, 207-261.

[19] Haworth SG, Sauer U, Nuhlmeyer K, Read L. The development of pulmonary circulation in ventricular septal defect: a quantitative structural study. *American J Cardiol* 1977; 40: 781-788.

[20] Soudon P, Stijns M, Tremouroux- Walliez M, Vliers A. Precocity of pulmonary vascular obstruction in Down syndrome. *Eur J Cardiol* 1975; 2: 473-476.

[21] Ishikawa S, Miyauchi T, Sakai S et al. Elevated levels of plasma endothelin-1 in young patients with pulmonary hypertension caused by congenital heart disease are decreased after successful surgical repair. *J Thorac Cardiovasc Surg* 1995;110:271-273.

[22] Yoshibayashi M, Nishioka K, Nakao K, et al. Plasma endothelin concentrations in patients with pulmonary hypertension associated with congenital heart defects. Evidence for increased production of endothelin in pulmonary circulation. *Circulation* 1991;84:2280-5.

[23] Dushane JW, Weidman WH, Braundenburg RO et al. The electrocardiogram in children with ventricular septal defect and severe pulmonary hypertension. *Circulation* 1960, 22: 49-54.

[24] Katz LN, Wachtel H. The diphasic QRS type of electrocardiogram in congenital heart disease. *Am Heart J* 1937; 13: 202-206.

[25] Roberts JD, Forfia PR. Diagnosis and assessment of pulmonary vascular disease by Doppler echocardiography. *Pulm Circ* 2011; 1: 160-182.

[26] Pyxaras SA, Pinamonti B, Barbati G. Echocardiographic evaluation of systolic and mean pulmonary artery pressure in the follow-up of patients with pulmonary hypertension. *Eur J Echocardiogr.* 2011; 12: 696-701.

[27] Ivy D. Dunbar. Echocardiographic evaluation of pulmonary hypertension. In: Echocardiographic diagnosis of congenital heart disease. *An embryologic and anatomic approach.* Valdez-Cruz LM, Cayre R eds, Lippincot Raven Publishers, Philadelphia. 1999: 537-547.

[28] Huhta J. Ecocardiografía en Hipertensión Pulmonar. En Díaz G.F., Sandoval J., y Sola A. Editores. *Hipertensión Pulmonar en Niños*. Editorial Distribuna. Bogotá, 2011, 345-359.

[29] Foris V, Kovacs G, Tscherner M, Olschewski A, Olschewski H. Biomarkers in pulmonary hypertension: what do we know? *Chest.* 2013 Jul;144(1):274-83.

[30] Cracowski JL, Leuchte HH. The potential of biomarkers in pulmonary arterial hypertension. *Am J Cardiol.* 2012 Sep 15;110(6 Suppl):32S-38S.

[31] Bernus A, Wagner BD, Accurso F, Doran A, Kaess H, Ivy DD. Brain natriuretic peptide levels in managing pediatric patients with pulmonary arterial hypertension. *Chest* 2009 Mar;135(3):745-51.

[32] Bull TM, Golpon H, Hebbel RP, Solovey A. et al Circulating endothelial cells in pulmonary hypertension. *Thromb Haemost.* 2003 Oct;90(4):698-703.

[33] Lopes AA, O'Leary PW. Measurement, interpretation and use of haemodynamic parameters in pulmonary hypertension associated with congenital cardiac disease. *Cardiol Young.* 2009;19:431-5.

[34] Taylor CJ, Derrick G, McEwan A, Haworth SG, Sury MR.. Risk of cardiac catheterization under anaesthesia in children with pulmonary hypertension. *Br J Anaesth.* 2007 May;98(5):657-61. Epub 2007 Mar 31.

[35] Beghetti M., Berger Rolf M.F., Schulze-Neick I. Diagnostic evaluation of paediatric pulmonary hypertension in current clinical practice. *ERJ September* 1, 2013 vol. 42 no. 3 689-700.

[36] Bradlow WM, Gibbs JS, Mohiaddin RH. Cardiovascular magnetic resonance in pulmonary hypertension. *Journal of Cardiovascular Magnetic Resonance* 2012, 14:6-18.

[37] Montani D., Günther S, Dorfmüller P. Et al. Pulmonary arterial hypertension. Review. *Orphanet Journal of Rare Diseases* 2013, 8:97.

[38] Stevens GR, Fida N, Sanz J. Computed tomography and cardiac magnetic resonance imaging in pulmonary hypertension. *Prog Cardiovasc Dis.* 2012 Sep-Oct;55(2):161-71.

[39] Lang I.M., MD; Plank C, MD and Sadushi-Kolici R, MD; Imaging in Pulmonary Hypertension. *J Am Coll Cardiol Img.* 2010;3(12):1287-1295.

[40] Lammers A.E., Hislop A.A., Flynn Y and Haworth S.G. The six-minute walk test: Normal values for children of 4 -11 years of age. 2008. *Arch. Dis. Child* 93(6), 464-468.

[41] Li AM, Yin J, YU CC, Tsang T, Wong E, Chan D, Hon EK, Sung R. The six-minute walk test in Healthy children: reliability and validity. *Eu Respir J.:* 25 (6): 1057-60.

[42] Priesnitz CV, Rodrigues GH, da Silva Stumpf C, et al. Reference values for the 6-min walk test in children who are healthy aged 6-12 years. *Pediatr Pulmonol.* 2009;44:1174–1179.

[43] Nicod P. and Moser K M. Primary pulmonary hypertension. The risk and benefit of lung biopsy. *Circulation.* 1989;80:1486-1488
[44] Haworth S.G., Radley-Smith R and, Yacoub M. Lung biopsy findings in transposition of the great arteries with ventricular septal defect: Potentially reversible pulmonary vascular disease is not always synonymous with operability. *J. Am Coll Cardiology* 1987; 9: 327–333
[45] Viswanathan S, Kumar RK. Assessment of operability of congenital cardiac shunts with increased pulmonary vascular resistance. *Catheter Cardiovasc Interv.* 2008;71:665-70.
[46] Giglia TM, Humpl T. Preoperative pulmonary hemodynamics and assessment of operability: is there a pulmonary vascular resistance that precludes cardiac operation? *Pediatr Crit Care Med.* 2010;11 Suppl:S57-69.
[47] Humbert M., Sitbon O. and Simonneau G, Treatment of Pulmonary Arterial Hypertension, *New Eng. J. of Med.* 2004 Volume 351 (14):1425-1436.
[48] Galie N., Torbicki A. Barst R. Et al. Guidelines on diagnosis and treatment of Pulmonary Arterial Hypertension. *European Heart J.* 2004; 25: 2243-2298.
[49] Pulido T., M.D., Adzerikho I, M.D.and, Channick R.N. M.D. Macitentan and Morbidity and Mortality in Pulmonary Arterial Hypertension *N Engl J Med* 2013; 369:809-818.
[50] Ghofrani HA., M.D., D'Armini AM., M.D., Grimminger F., M. Det al. Riociguat for the Treatment of Chronic Thromboembolic Pulmonary Hypertension. *N Engl J Med* 2013; 369:319-329.
[51] Mulligan C, Beghetti M. Inhaled iloprost for the control of acute pulmonary hypertension in children: a systematic review. *Pediatr Crit Care Med.* 2012 Jul;13(4):472-80.
[52] Dunbar Ivy D., Doran A, and Smith K J. Short- and Long-Term Effects of Inhaled Iloprost Therapy in Children With Pulmonary Arterial Hypertension Volume 51, Issue 2, 161-169. *JACC* . 2008; 51 ()2:161-169.
[53] Barst R, Ivy D, Widlitz AC, et al Pharmacokinetics, safety, and efficacy of bosentan in pediatric patients with pulmonary arterial hypertension. *Clin Pharmacol Ther* 2003;73(4):372-82.
[54] Rosenzweig EB, Ivy DD, Widlitz A, et al. Effects of Long-Term Bosentan in Children With Pulmonary Arterial Hypertension. *Journal of the American College of Cardiology* 2005 August 16;46(4):697-704.
[55] Beguetti M, Hoeper MM, Kiely DG et al. Safety experience with bosentan in 146 children 2-11 years old with pulmonary hypertension: results from the European Postmarketing Surveillance program. *Pediatr Res.* 2008;64(2)200-4.
[56] Safety Announcement .FDA Drug Safety Communication: FDA recommends against use of Revatio (sildenafil) in children with pulmonary hypertension. *DRUGS.* 8-30-2012.
[57] Abman SH, Kinsella JP, Rosenzweig EB et al. Implications of the U.S. Food and Drug Administration warning against the use of sildenafil for the treatment of pediatric pulmonary hypertension. *Am J Respir Crit Care Med.* 2013Mar 15;187(6):572-5.
[58] Barst RJ, Ivy DD, Gaitan G, et al. A randomized, double-blind, placebo-controlled, dose-ranging study of oral sildenafil citrate in treatment-naïve children with pulmonary arterial hypertension. *Circulation* 2012;125:324-334
[59] Humpl T, Reyes JT, Holtby H, Stephens D, Adatia I. Beneficial Effect of Oral Sildenafil Therapy on Childhood Pulmonary Arterial Hypertension: Twelve-Month

Clinical Trial of a Single-Drug, Open-Label, Pilot Study. *Circulation* 2005 June 21;111(24):3274-80.

[60] Baquero H, Soliz A, Neira F, et al. Oral sildenafil in infants with persistent pulmonary hypertension of the newborn: a pilot randomized blind study. *Pediatrics* 2006;117:1077–83

[61] Keller, R L.; Hamrick, S E.; Kitterman, J A.; et al. Treatment of rebound and chronic pulmonary hypertension with oral sildenafil in an infant with congenital diaphragmatic hernia. *Pediatric Critical Care Medicine*. 2004. March 5 (2):184-187.

[62] Mohan Rao PS, Raju V, and Narayana M. Flap valve closure of ventricular septal defects with increased pulmonary vascular resistance Interactive CardioVascular and *Thoracic Surgery* 11 (2010) 577–580.

[63] Novick WM, Sandoval N, Lazorhysynets VV, Castillo V, Flap valve double patch closure of ventricular septal defects in children with increased pulmonary vascular resistance. *Ann Thorac Surg*. 2005 Jan;79(1):21-8.

[64] JiQ, Feng H and Mei Y. Trans-catheter Closure of Adult Patent Ductus Arteriosus with Severe Pulmonary Hypertension. *Hypertension Research* (2008) 31, 1997–2002.

[65] Van Loon R, Roofthooft M, Berger R. Pulmonary arterial hypertension in children with congenital heart disease. *PVRI Review* 2009;1:203-7.

[66] Hopkins WE, Ochoa LL, Richardson GW, Trulock EP. Comparison of the hemodynamics and survival of adults with severe primary pulmonary hypertension or Eisenmenger syndrome. *J Heart Lung Transplant*. 1996; 15:100–105.

[67] Waddell TK, Bennett L, Kennedy R, Todd TR, Keshavjee SH. Heart-lung or lung transplantation for Eisenmenger syndrome. *J Heart Lung Transplant*. 2002 Jul;21(7):731-7.

[68] George M.P., Champion H.C. and Pilewski J.M. Lung transplantation for pulmonary hypertension. *Pulmonary Circulation*. 1(2): 182-191.

[69] Long J., Russo M.J., Muller C., et al Surgical Treatment of pulmonary Hypertension: Lung Transplantation. *Pulmonary circulation*. 2011, 1 (3): 327-333.

[70] O´Blenes SB, Fisher S, McIntyre B. et al. Hemodynamic unloading leads to regression of pulmonary vascular disease in rats. *J. Thor. Cardiov. Surg*. 2001 121(2): 279-89.

[71] Penaloza D., Sime F. and Ruiz L. Pulmonary Hemodynamic in children living at high altitudes. *High altitude Medicine and Biology*. 2008, 9(3): 199-207.

[72] Díaz G. y Márquez A. Hipertensión Pulmonar a Moderada altura. En Díaz G.F., Sandoval J., y Sola A. Editores. Hipertensión Pulmonar en Niños. Editorial Distribuna. Bogotá, 2011, 295-313.

[73] Stenmark K.R., Fagan K.A. and Frid M.G. Hypoxia-Induced Pulmonary Vascular Remodeling. Cellular and Molecular Mechanisms. *Circ Res*. 2006;99:675-691.

[74] Robbins I.M., Barst R.J. Channick R.N. and Rubin L.J. Pulmonary vasorreactivity in PPH. *J Am. Coll of Cardiol*. 2001; 38:1267.

[75] Sime F, Banchero N, Penaloza D, Gamboa R, Cruz J, Marticorena E. Pulmonary hypertension in children born and living at high altitudes. *Am J Cardiol* 1963; 11: 143-149.

[76] Peñaloza D., Sime F. y Ruiz L. Hemodinámica Cardiopulmonar en Niños nativos de grandes alturas. En Díaz G.F., Sandoval J., y Sola A. Editores. *Hipertensión Pulmonar* en Niños. Editorial Distribuna. Bogotá, 2011, 275-293.

[77] Wood P. The Eisenmenger Syndrome or Pulmonary Hypertension with reversal central shunt brit. *Med. J.* 2: 701-709 and 755-762, 1958.
[78] Berger RM. Pulmonary hypertension associated with congenital cardiac disease. *Cardiol Young.* 2009;19:311-4.
[79] Galie N, Beghetti M, Gatzoulis MA, et al. Bosentan therapy in patients with Eisenmenger syndrome: a multicenter, double-blind, randomized, placebo-controlled study. *Circulation* 2006;114:48–54.
[80] Zuckerman WA., Krishnan U. and Rosenzweig EB. Pulmonary Arterial Hypertension Associated with Congenital Heart Disease. *Curr Pediatr Rep* (2013) 1:92–101.
[81] Swan L, Lupton M, Anthony J. et al. Controversies in pregnancy and congenital heart disease. *Congenit Heart Dis.* 2006;1(1–2):27–34.
[82] Bedard E, Dimopoulos K, Gatzoulis MA. Has there been any progress made on pregnancy outcomes among women with pulmonary arterial hypertension? *Eur Heart J.* 2009;30(3):256–65.
[83] Diller Gp. And Gatzoulis GP. Pulmonary vascular disease in adults with congenital heart disease. *Circulation* 2007, 115: 1039-1050.
[84] Gatzoulis MA., Alonsi Gonzalez R and Beghetti M. Pulmonary arterial hypertension in pediatric and adult patients with congenital heart disease. *Eur. Resp Rev.* 2009 18: 154-161.
[85] Oechslin E. Hematological management of the cyanotic adult with congenital heart disease. *Int J Cardiol.* 2004;97(Suppl 1):109-115.
[86] Newfeld EA, Paul MM, Muster AJ, et al. Pulmonary vascular disease in complete transposition of the great arteries: A study of 200 patients. *Am J Cardiol.* 1974;34:75–82.
[87] Kumar A., Taylor GP., Sandor GG. Et al. Pulmonary vascular disease in neonates with transposition of the great arteries and intact ventricular septum. *Br Heart J* 1993, 69: 442.
[88] Roofthooft MT, Bergman KA, Waterbolk TW, Ebels T, Bartelds B, Berger RM. Persistent pulmonary hypertension of the newborn with transposition of the great arteries. *Ann Thorac Surg.* 2007 Apr;83(4):1446-50.
[89] Torres. M., Coserria J.F. y Gavilán J.L. Desarrollo tardío de hipertensión arterial pulmonar en paciente con transposición de grandes arterias sometido a switch arterial *Rev Esp Cardiol.* 2012;65:1064-5.
[90] Fan H, Hu S, Zheng Z, Li S, Zhang Y, Pan X, Liu Y. Do patients with complete transposition of the great arteries and severe pulmonary hypertension benefit from an arterial switch operation? *Ann Thorac Surg.* 2011 Jan;91(1):181-6.
[91] Nakajima Y, Momma K, Seguchi M, Nakazawa M, Imai Y Pulmonary hypertension in patients with complete transposition of the great arteries: midterm results after surgery. *Pediatr Cardiol.* 1996 Mar-Apr;17(2):104-7.
[92] Williams J.M., De Leeuw M., D Black M, MD; et al. Factors associated with outcomes of persistent truncus arteriosusa. *J Am Coll Cardiol.* 1999;34(2):545-553
[93] Shinora G., Morita K., Uno Y et al. Scimitar syndrome in an infant with right lung hypoplasia, ventricular septal defect, and severe pulmonary hypertension. *Gen Thorac Cardiovasc Surg.* 2010 Oct;58(10):524-7.

[94] Santos M.A. and Pereira Azevedo V.M. Anomalous Origin of One Pulmonary artery from the Ascending Aorta. *Surgical Repair Resolving Pulmonary Arterial Hypertension.* Arquivos Brasileiros de Cardiologia -2004:83, (6), 503-507.

[95] Yamarki S., Suzuki Y, Ishizawa E, et al. Isolated aortic origin of the right pulmonary artery. Report of a case with special reference to pulmonary vascular disease in the left and right lungs. *Chest* 1983; 3: 575-8.

In: Congenital Heart Diseases
Editor: Raúl Cayré and José Milei
ISBN: 978-1-61122-003-2

Chapter 8

The Functionally Univentricular Heart: "40 Years without a Subpulmonary Ventricle"

***Mario Cazzaniga*[1*] *and Renata Revel-Chion*[2,†]**
[1]NISA Hospital-Pardo de Aravaca. Madrid-Spain
[2]Casa di Cura Sta. María Maddalena, Occhiobello (RO) and Mediclinic, Pozzonovo (PD), Italy

Abstract

The term "functionally univentricular heart" embraces heterogeneous categories of complex cardiac malformations that, in the context of congenital heart diseases, exemplify one of the most challenging objectives of the study. The management of patients with an anatomical or functional "single ventricle" represents an unlimited task in the pediatric cardiology and surgical field. The vision of this matter in this "undone chapter" can be summarized in three stages: the prelude, the epic and the future. In the early 1940s, the preface era, an experimental work inspired what is named nowadays as the Fontan/Kreutzer operation – the total right ventricular bypass was first reported in humans in the early 1970s. In the following 40 years several modifications and refinements of the initial surgical design, improved perioperative care and management of algorithms-based protocols produced a drastic increase in perioperative survivors – the heroic epic. However, when patients grew into adulthood, coping with a complete univentricular circulation as a result of the palliative procedures, they faced numerous complications and multi-organ system difficulties that seriously limited their quality of life. Continuous research and multidisciplinary efforts in several directions are needed to answer the future of Fontan failure patients. Perhaps this would include the expected potential clinical application of a mechanical "new neo subpulmonary ventricle" compatible with a normal life span similar to people with a normal biventricular circulation.

* Corresponding author: Email: mario.cazzaniga@gmail.com.
† E-mail: renatarevelchion@yahoo.com.

Introduction

The functionally univentricular heart (UH) is a denomination that encompasses a heterogeneous group of congenital cardiac malformations which, with or without unbalanced ventricular chambers on its myocardial ventricular mass, makes conventional surgical biventricular correction impossible or highly improbable due to their anatomical/functional characteristics or even due to the complex surgical approach [1-5]. The most used therapeutic alternative for patients that fulfil this premise is to create a univentricular hemodynamic model in which at least one dominant ventricular chamber is able to take in series, both the systemic and the pulmonary circulation without any interposition of a subpulmonary pump (Fontan operation) [6]. This strategy is how hearts are currently addressed when a true hypoplasia of one or another ventricle is seen (in univentricular or biventricular atrioventricular arrangement) or perhaps due to the absence or obliteration of ventricular components of its functional anatomical tripartite unit: in any case, the underdeveloped small chamber is not capable of coping with any circulatory system. In a similar manner, some malformed hearts with two well-balanced and completely formed ventricular chambers come up with combined intracardiac lesions that do not allow a surgical approach to restore the optimal biventricular circulation [4,7,8]. As a result of that, the wide morphological expression of structural defects that are not amenable to a 2-ventricle surgical correction can be grouped into the more corrected denomination of functionally UH (Table 1); with no doubt, the management of patients with these anomalies is still an endless challenge in the world of congenital heart diseases (CHD). Seeing the problem in perspective as a whole, three sections can be discerned as involved in its evolution: “the prelude”, “the epic” and “the future”.

Table 1. Heart Malformations with “Single Ventricle Physiology”: Functionally Univentricular Heart

Double inlet ventricle : Left, Right or Indeterminate ventricular type

Two patent atrioventricular valves

Right or left atrioventricular valve atresia -tricuspid or mitral atresia-

Atrioventricular common valve

Unbalanced atrioventricular septal defect

Straddling / overriding atrioventricular valves –unbalanced ventricular mass-

Hypoplastic left heart syndrome

Criss-cross heart

variants of:

Ebstein anomaly

Transposition or double outlet great arteries:

with a combination of non committed ventricular septal defect and/or complex outflow tract obstruction

Pulmonary atresia with intact ventricular septum, hypoplasic right ventricle and coronaries arteries anomalies

The prelude has been built with the efforts of pathologists and clinicians committed to an accurate understanding of the anatomical-clinical substrate; at the same time, active surgical groups have explored, in animal experimentation, the feasibility of a partial or complete right ventricle (RV) bypass using innovative techniques. The epic undoubtedly started from the clinical success of the Fontan procedure described in 1971 and was originally designed to correct the tricuspid atresia, a real adventure that come by to the present day with constant progress in all acting fields such as: variations in the original surgical technique, use of several strategies and renewed therapeutic algorithms, sophisticated -pre, intra and postoperative- care and appropriate clinical follow-up, all that condensed in "the univentricular route". Finally, the future, an exciting stage to be seen in the next decades and that should include several aspects: implementation in the healthcare system of multidisciplinary units specialized in patients that walk into adulthood with fragile hemodynamic conditions that involve clinical difficulties as time goes by; development of innovative projects that consider new strategies of management and/or redesign of current surgical techniques; and the potential clinical application of subpulmonary circulatory assistance with miniaturized devices. Currently, most of the physicians who care about adolescents and adults with Fontan procedure or its modified types have understood that the resulting UH circulation involved in these palliatives surgeries cannot be compared with the biventricular model of the normal population and subsequently a shorter lifespan is expected.

The Prelude

In search of a useful nomenclature of the functionally univentricular heart

The process of nomenclature and classification of the malformations in CHD is a desire that in the last decades has caught the attention of the pathologist, embryologist, cardiologists and surgeons, all of them expert authorities in the matter [9-13]. The efforts to optimize the knowledge and, at the same time, to improve the management of patients with functional univentricular structural anomalies, boost them into a common objective: to formulate a precise method of diagnostic analysis designed with simple rules, objectives and organized with no theoretical or abstract speculations. Not without extended debates, conceptual and semantic, this intent was condensed in two consecutive steps: 1) a lengthy phase of morphologic description of the "univentricular universe" with embryological support and correlation, organized-unified terms and entities, addition of image tools (specifically echocardiography and cardiac magnetic resonance) that are trustworthy to identify connections, morphology and alignment of the different cardiac segments such as an anatomist would do it; and 2) the "anatomical-functional surgical phase" that begins with the revolutionary breakthrough of the Fontan procedure that acts as an unexpected referee reorganizing "the UH playing field" to include other cardiac malformations not initially classified as single ventricle, anticipating in an unquestionable way, that they cannot have as a target the biventricular surgical repair to two ventricles. This background stands for what is currently called segmental and sequential morphologic analysis of the heart and vessels (still with problems to be solved, mainly in the aspects of heterotaxy syndrome), which consist of a methodical model that, not being the only one possible (other experts make use of "different roads to Rome"), evolves in acceptance with accentuated consensus as a method for a precise diagnosis, if not all, for the majority of congenital cardiac malformations [14-17]. The International Pediatric and Congenital Cardiac Code (IPCCC) (www.ipccc.net) and the three specialized Study Committees: Nomenclature Working Group (NWG), Definitions Working Group (DWG) and Congenital Heart Archiving Research Team (CHART) [classifies images and videos] that bring together international experts and integrates – in combination with other methods – the specified model in the encoding process platform and cross-mapping system that is also part of the Congenital Heart Surgery Database [18,19].

Brief historical review on cardiac morphology

From references listed in historical reviews [20-22] it can be assumed that in the XIX century two unique malformed hearts were reported; at the end they came out to be the first paradigms of the UH: double inlet left ventricle (A. Holmes, Canada) and tricuspid atresia (F. Kreysig, Germany) respectively. With evident differences in relation to what we now understand as the atrioventricular connection approach, both lesions shared, among other aspects, two chambers connected in the ventricular mass: a large, dominant chamber and a small, rudimentary one. This starting point attracted the attention of pathologists engaged in defining these structural abnormalities that received in the past different and, in some cases, confusing designations: "cor triloculare biatriatrium", "single ventricle", "univentricular heart", "single ventricle with outlet chamber", "single ventricle with infundibular outlet chamber", "primitive ventricle", "common ventricle", "solitary ventricle" [8,9,23-27]. Participants of avant-garde schools in the field of CHD opened a debate decades ago. It is historical now but no less important to solve controversies and classify these unique anomalies: R. Van Praagh in USA, M.V. de la Cruz in Mexico and R. Anderson in Europe, among other innovators and qualified experts [9,28,29]. This wide-ranging work developed in the theoretical, semantic and informative fields and their influence in the pediatric cardiology and pediatric cardiovascular surgery communities must be acknowledged as it represents the keystone of our current knowledge. Van Praagh [30] taking into account, as criteria, the absence of ventricular sinus ("inflow tract") and ventricular septum (partial or total) proposed the first classification of the "single or common ventricle" defining 4 types:

A) single left ventricle (absence of right ventricle sinus)
B) single right ventricle (absence of left ventricular sinus)
C) common ventricle (rudimentary interventricular septum)
D) undetermined ventricle (absence of inflow tract and interventricular septum)

This analysis was based on specimen collection that, intentionally, did not included cases with mitral or tricuspid atresia. The author pointed out the nature of the "classical single ventricle with rudimentary outlet chamber" that was revealed to be mainly a dominant left ventricle and a right ventricle infundibulum (type A). In addition, he also defined subtypes based on atrial situs and the relationship among the great arteries; in essence, this descriptive scheme anticipated the morphological segmental model of analysis. Later, the same author and other experts in the field, highlighted the connection among atriums and the principal ventricle in these ventricular anomalies can hold two patent atrioventricular valves (double inlet ventricle) or a common atrioventricular valve (common inlet). Finally, and accepting that the single ventricle usually presents two chambers related in the ventricular myocardial mass (the presence of a solitary ventricle is exceptional) means that the dominant ventricular phenotype is recognizable by the morphologic pattern of the apical trabecular component, so it is possible to identify three patterns that, in order of frequency, are left ventricle (LV) type, right ventricle (RV) type and undetermined type (the older type C was re-classified as a large interventricular defect). However, the use of embryologic terms as sinus, conus, outlet chamber, infundibular outlet chamber, foramen bulboventricular (septal defect which communicates both ventricular cavities), as well as the non-inclusion of tricuspid and mitral atresia in the first classification, raised many controversies [2,24,26,30,31].

R. Anderson and cols. [1,7,10,32-34] integrated many scattered criteria and rearranged terms interpreting them in numerous papers with two essential principles that were probably at the base of the debate: 1) the key of the diagnosis of the "single ventricle" is the univentricular type of the atrioventricular (AV) junction (the entire AV junction connects with one ventricle), and in this set two ways of connection are possible: double inlet ventricle [DIV] (two atrium connected with the dominant ventricle) or the absence of one AV connection (one atrium, right or left, does not connect with any ventricular chamber) and in such a way the classic tricuspid (TA) and mitral atresia are, in fact, included in this principle; 2) the ventricle is documented by its anatomical and functional tripartite nature: inlet (identified from the AV junction to the distal insertion of the valve tensor apparatus), apical trabecular portion (typical of trabeculated pattern) and outlet (supports the semilunar valves).

The same group of experts, immersed in an intense debate, supported the concept that with this principle in mind, the so called "outlet infundibular chamber" presented in the double inlet LV is, actually, an incomplete RV (absence of inlet), rudimentary (underdeveloped), which apical trabecular portion is separated from its homonymous of the dominant LV by an interventricular septum well recognizable by the distribution of the conductive tissue and the perforate branches of the coronary vessels. They also point out that the intrinsic morphological characteristics of the rudimentary RV are similar in both types of univentricular AV connections: double-inlet ventricle and absent right sided AV connection (classic TA). With morphological and topographic description, Van Praagh and de la Cruz [15,35) proposed the first classification for complex heart malformations and Anderson and the European group [13,14] developed and extended the sequential-segmental analysis that not only integrates all the data but focuses attention onto the implication of recognizing, amid other aspects, the nature of the inter-segmental connection of the 3 segments or cardiac blocks [atrial chambers, ventricular mass and great vessels] with systematic rules to obtain the most complete and adjusted diagnosis. The method of morphologic sequential and segmental analysis includes the following steps:

- Definition of the atrial arrangement
- Type of atrioventricular connection
- Morphology of the atrioventricular valves
- Ventricular morphology, size, topology and inter-chamber relationship
- Infundibular morphology
- Great arteries relationship
- Position of the heart in the chest with base-apex orientation
- Abdominal-thoracic arrangement (visceral situs)
- Associated cardiovascular malformations
- Non-cardiac anomalies – syndrome or genetic context will be analysed

The sequence to obtain this systematic information is variable according to the observational method employed, the clinicians' expertise and the available diagnostic tools. Echocardiography would be the initial diagnostic approach [36] but magnetic resonance image (MRI) will overcome many of the limitations for the extra cardiac features. Both techniques will be the non-invasive diagnostic images for a complete view of the cardiac and extra-cardiac components. To develop the sequential and systemic methodology is essential to recognize the diverse and persistent anatomical elements that belong to each segment of the heart or cardiac block and, what is more important, to keep in mind that these explicit constant morphological references are present in normal hearts as well as in malformed ones; these are:

1. Morphology of the atrial appendage to be able to recognize each atrium [right: triangular, broad base, ploughed by pectinate muscles extended up to the orifice of the coronary sinus; left: narrow opening, hook shaped and spare pectinate forms]
2. Pattern of the apical trabeculated portion to identify ventricular chambers [LV: thin trabecular arrangement; RV: thick bands configuration]
3. Define the origin of the coronary arteries and the superior distribution of the arterial tree [aorta: arterial branches run toward the superior half of the body and, at least, the presence of one coronary ostium at the Valvalsa sinus level; pulmonary artery: the remaining vessel that does not accomplish the previous description]

Epidemiological data

Epidemiological studies, either previous or most recent, point out that the incidence of CHD is located in a range between 4-10% of live newborns. TA and DILV are represented in 0.05-0.08% of live newborns, and between 1.3-2.7% of the entire CHD. DILV is prevalent (70%) with respect to DIRV (< 20%); the type of undetermined ventricular morphology is uncommon (<10-15%) and often is part of the heterotaxy syndrome. In the DILV the ventricular-arterial discordance (L-transposition) prevails, hardly present with normally related great vessels ("Holmes heart"); the double outlet or malposition of the great vessels is more frequent in the DIRV and in the undetermined ventricle. In the double inlet ventricle with right atrioventricular valve atresia (classic TA) the relationship of the great vessels is mainly concordant (70%), in the smaller percentage of the discordant subtype. From Hoffman's study [37] the estimated prevalence of "major forms" of CHD per 1000 live newborns can be assumed: single ventricle (SV) 0.83, hypoplasic left heart syndrome (HLHS) 0.22, atrioventricular septal defect (AVSD) 0.34, tricuspid atresia (TA) 0.9, double-outlet RV 0.12, transposition of the great arteries (TGA) 0.30, many of them categorized as functional UH.

The surgical history of partial / total right heart bypass

For centuries physiologists considered the dual concept of the pulmonary circulation, vital for life: the RV behaves as a subpulmonary pump propelling blood through the pulmonary vessels toward the left chambers, a task that contributes with the same purpose with another mechanism, the respiratory cycle with the couple inspiration/expiration. Animal experiments carried out in the 40s in which the right myocardium was damaged questioned that argument as it was found that, in the acute period and under certain circumstances, the pulmonary blood flow was kept even with absent or altered RV function [38,39]. Years later there was the onset of what was intended as the Fontan procedure [40], a period of several experimental attempts with different surgical approaches intended to demonstrate that the total or partial exclusion of the RV was possible. As reflected in historical review papers [40-42] numerous surgical attempts with various technical details proposed the current operating scenery that we know nowadays. Hurwitt in 1955, unsuccessfully attempted the atriopulmonary anastomosis (total RV bypass) in a dying child with TA employing the concept of "pump action of the right atrium" as an anticipation of the yet to come Fontan procedure [43]. From all the clinical and experimental attempts, the partial exclusion of the RV by means of the cavopulmonary shunt (end to side superior vena cava to right pulmonary artery) turned out to be extremely useful and soon its clinical application spread widely to palliate different cyanotic congenital heart diseases. Although the first clinical successes were reported in the 1950s, in an almost simultaneous manner in Italy, Russia and France, it was W. W. Glenn in USA who confirmed its clinical usefulness in numerous patients and alleged that around 30-40% of the superior systemic venous flow is distributed in the right pulmonary field; this technique became commonly called the classic unidirectional Glenn shunt [44,45]. Due to the late morbidity (occurrence of pulmonary arteriovenous malformations) this technique was side lined in the 70s. By that time the first clinical attempts with the bidirectional cavopulmonary shunt were reported – successfully by the way – [46-48] and gradually joined the surgical arsenal of the UH with the name of bidirectional Glenn shunt (BDGS) *["the rescue of the Glenn's !"].*

The EPIC

Another subject that arouses so much attention in the international biomedical community and some other connected disciplines is univentricular circulation, a particular circulatory model in human subjects. We are now getting into the 4th decade for palliative reconstruction in CHD with no amenable biventricular surgical correction, however… "the odyssey continues" [49]. Proof of that is the large amount of quotations provided by several biomedical webs [Medline, PubMed, journals and books on line]: more than 3,000 reports come out when you search for a bibliographic review with the key word "Fontan procedure", "Fontan operation", "Fontan-Kreutzer operation" or "cavopulmonary anastomosis".

No doubt the epic started with the complete bypass of the RV and the early surgical successes reported by Fontan in 1971 and Kreutzer in 1973 [6,50] with a technique initially intended for patients with TA and reduced pulmonary flow: the atriopulmonary anastomosis (APa). The original technique was set up with: 1) classic Glenn anastomosis, 2) APa that provided blood flow to the left pulmonary branch and 3) closure of the interatrial defect that ended the right to left mixing blood.

Rather soon, different technical details were corrected improving the initial procedure, to mention some**:** the use of valved grafts positioned at the entry of the inferior vena cava into right atrium and/or at level of the pulmonary artery anastomosis (position in which also was briefly used as the native pulmonary valve) that was later abandoned**;** the anterior anastomosis prone to have a sternal compression was replaced by a wider posterior with no chance of extrinsic compression and, pretty important, the anastomosis encompassed both pulmonary artery branches with no need of previous classic Glenn or related procedures (another additional native or surgical source of pulmonary flow were abolished); the potential pump function of the right atrium was taken into consideration [it was well known to pathologists that the myocardial wall of the atrium was thicker in TA [51] totalling a combined support of adequate diastolic ventricular function and an optimal mechanism of pulmonary ventilation that supports the hemodynamic concept of the surgical technique. All these aspects together set for the first time a successful survival with a remarkable hemodynamic in human being, commonly known as "Fontan circulation" or univentricular circulatory model. With some more advantageous modifications it became popular worldwide and also extended the anatomical substrate to which was intended for other malformations different to DILV or TA in which the morphological type of the main ventricle was right or undetermined [52-56]. Other old techniques are already considered to be past history [57-59].

Almost at the same time the classic Glenn was modified to the present BDGS with benefit [47,48] being both stated as a "versatile complement" to the Fontan operation and adjusted upon clinical demand [60-63]. Likewise, the BDGS was used in 1984 (Kawashima operation) in patients with heterotaxy syndrome and left isomerism who had absence of the intrahepatic segment of the inferior vena cava with azygos vein system continuation. This peculiar anatomy involves the entire systemic venous flow distributed in both lungs by the superior vena cava except the hepatic veins that remain connected to the atrium; with the BDGS the patient improves oxygenation but the so called "hepatic angiogenesis factor" eludes the vascular pulmonary field with the resultant advent of pulmonary arteriovenous malformations [64].

Little more than a decade after the Fontan-Kreutzer operation, other problems must be noted, the occurrence of a severe progressive right atrial enlargement that promotes arrhythmias with a poor intrinsic kinetic energy to lead the systemic venous flow to the lungs. In 1988 Marc de Leval developed and applied, both in animal experiments as well as in clinical trials, the so-called total cavopulmonary connection (TCPC) which, in its original concept, involved two concomitant procedures: BDGS and a tubular intra-atrial tunnel with a baffle that goes from the inferior vena cava to the proximal right pulmonary artery (with extended atrial line sutures). This last part of the procedure was named and is expressed in the literature as a lateral tunnel (LT) [65-69]. This new approach obtained: lower power losses of the venous pathway that reach the pulmonary vascular bed without systolic impulse, better circulatory efficiency and, over time, less incidence of arrhythmias since only a part of the atrial myocardium would be affected by the high pressure of the venous circuit. In the 1990s new progress appeared: 1) the BDGS became used as an interim before Fontan and its modifications (two stage strategy); 2) some groups modified the BDGS that becomes the hemi-Fontan with an easier surgical approach and with anticipation of eventual Fontan completion with a LT, and 3) the implant of a prosthetic extra cardiac conduit (ECC in the literature) that leads the flow on the outside of the heart from the inferior vena cava to the pulmonary artery (it does not require difficult atrial sutures, so a lower incidence of arrhythmias is expected) [70-75] (Figure 1). An important improvement, no less important, was the baffle fenestration of the LT (easy to do) or in the ECC (more complicated to perform) deliberately created by the surgeon (it was applied to children with possibly reversible or treatable risk factors). Rapidly, its indication was enlarged for patients with pre-Fontan standard-risks). It is a single communication at the level of the LT or the ECC with the "pulmonary venous atrium" that allows a "right to left shunt", which guarantees a consistent contribution to the cardiac output for better circulatory adaptation in the immediate postoperative: low mortality, significantly less pleural effusion and significantly shorter hospitalization even if it induces a mild degree of cyanosis [76-78].

The feasibility of performing such techniques without extracorporeal circulation, or with minimal circulatory support was successfully explored [79]. William Norwood took a big step forward with the procedure that bears his name on the way to palliate neonates with HLHS and gave an impulse toward other recommendations: the algorithms of the two-staged procedure, as a sequence of planned actions not due to clinical requirements, performed at a young age to reach the complete Fontan; this strategy attempted to reach a more effective and early unloading of the systemic ventricle that positively impacted morbidity and mortality [80-83]. Other advances in the perioperative field – clinical management, anesthesia or intraoperative procedures – are already well established in the everyday routine. One of the them, the modified ultrafiltration after weaning off cardiopulmonary bypass, significantly reduced the systemic inflammatory response (suppression of cytokines and harmful factors for the myocardial function and the pulmonary vascular resistance) confirmed as independent variables associated with a decreased incidence and duration of the pleural effusions, improved pulmonary and ventricular function and decreased postoperative bleeding following Fontan [assured a "more comfortable" immediate postoperative period] [84,85].

In some selected patients (for example in a small RV or Ebstein malformation), palliative surgery can be used, named the one and one half ventricle repair (BDGS plus closure of the interatrial communication) dividing the two circuits, pulmonary and systemic, keeping intact the normal connection of the inferior vena cava with the right sided heart and their normal pulmonary artery at the same time [86,87].

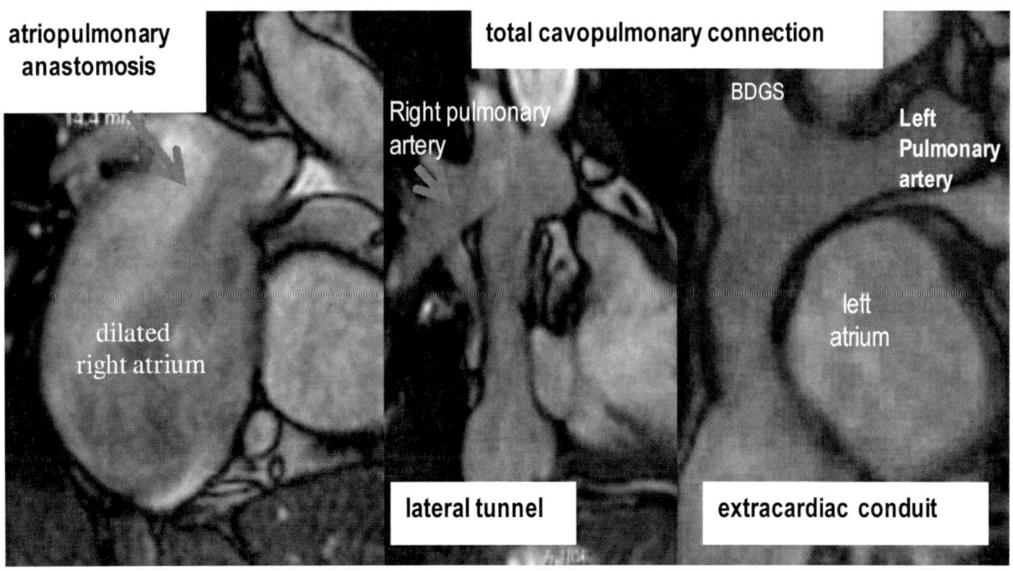

Figure 1. The three types of Fontan procedure – MRI.

Single ventricle physiology

Since the fetal stage and already in the postnatal period, patients with a single ventricle present a model of circulation in parallel: a "super ventricle" ejects simultaneously to the pulmonary and to the systemic arterial system (via ductus or through a native outlet) depending upon the resistance of each circuit. This ventricle is dilated, with some degree of hypertrophy in accordance (it is estimated that it works with more than 200% of the expected volume with respect to a normal LV in biventricular fashion); both conditions are more obvious when a consequence of the normal decrease of pulmonary vascular resistance is blood flow increase, through an unobstructed outflow tract, after palliation by an aortopulmonary shunt or "untightened" pulmonary band. In the past, this period of parallel circulation protracted in time with a detrimental impact on ventricle and pulmonary vascular bed. Immediately after single non-staged Fontan there is a sudden reduction of ventricular size (< 50-70% of the normal value indexed with the body surface area) with myocardial mass prevalence (mismatch mass/size and abnormal diastolic function) that affects the postoperative progress [88]. The BDGS as 1st stage lessens this mechanism so that it contributes to a slow-paced unloading without an uneven overgrowth. Some authors avoid any simultaneous pulsatile additional flow (more cyanosis, effective ventricular "unloading"), others prefer to maintain an additional source of pulsatile flow appropriately regulated ("a little additional flow") to induce the normal development of arteries and distal pulmonary bed without a disproportionate increase of the ventricular preload, at the same time there is less hypoxemia. Gewillig points out: "not too much for the ventricle, not too little for the lungs" [89]. This difficult balance is not always easy to obtain in practice but it is essential for the patient. When the Fontan circulation is completed as 2nd stage, the single ventricle preload depends almost exclusively (the so called suction effect has not been fully understood) of the pulmonary vascular resistance (transpulmonary flow/gradient). Without doubt, it is the intrinsic condition of the total univentricular model in series in a way that the single ventricle suffers a chronic preload deprivation with little or poor functional reserve on exercise (there is no prepulmonar systolic impulse). All that, contrary to what happens in normal subjects, explains the chronic low output – more evident on effort – that is not sufficiently compensated, neither with the afterload nor with the contractility, only with a modest increase of the heart rate. The "chronotropic auto regulation" theory in the univentricular circulation is interesting: a very high heart rate on effort (usually the rule in normal people) would reduce in excess the diastolic time with the consequent severe impairment of the cardiac output. The slow-paced ventricular unloading earlier imposed and the protection of the pulmonary vascularity has created a reduction of hospital morbi-mortality and at midterm, as well, an effect of "recruitment of new candidates for Fontan" (reduction or disappearance of AV valve insufficiency, low pulmonary resistances, lessening of the hypertrophy, among others). Redington, Gewillig, and other experts reviewed in detail the univentricular physiology and its palliations [90-95]: the final model subsists with 3 well known conditions: 1) chronic low systemic output [in essence regulated by the non-pulsatile resistance of pulmonary vascular bed], 2) chronic increase of the systemic venous pressure [paradox physiology: > venous pressure and < pulmonary pressure] and 3) normalization of hypoxemia (in absence of fenestration). A remarkable aspect is, being the arteriolar pulmonary resistance is a determinant factor for early and late success in univentricular circulation, the hemodynamic determination of the pre Fontan operation has less reliable data (different source of flows, stenosis or distortions in the pulmonary arteries, mathematics assumptions, etc.). Also obtaining a low transpulmonary gradient preFontan does not guarantee the desired value (between 5-8 mmHg) in the early and late postoperative period. Choussat described in 1978 as many as 10 requisites to select the most favorable patients with acceptable conditions for palliation with the Fontan technique and not following them would become a therapeutic failure. Since 1986 the criteria have been reviewed or reformulated (for example Fontan circulation can be completed at an earlier age, the pulmonary arteriolar resistance has to be ≤ 2 units/m^2), some were excluded, some others not reflected before were added (systemic obstruction with ventricular hypertrophy, significant AV valve regurgitation). In addition, different independent variables associated with the immediate mortality were reported (Down's syndrome, geographic altitude, lack of fenestration, among others) [96-100].

Current Phases of the Univentricular Route

Currently, for optimal diagnosis and medical-surgical management of the heterogeneous varieties of functionally UH, diverse algorithms have emerged, all of them attempting to complete the Fontan circulation. To achieve this goal it is necessary to have an adequate level of development and complexity of the perioperative neonatal and cardiovascular surgery program of the center. A great deal of the current approach in innovative teams is due to the impulse and relevant impact that was introduced by the Norwood operation. Nevertheless, there are differences in management among institutions, some conceptual, other operative or related to the preferences of the surgical team. In any case, several fields of controversy exist for example, in the application of early procedure strategy. Some experts propose the early univentricular route as a scheme of a more updated management in the different phases, medical, interventional and surgical with the expectancy of obtaining a reduction of the early and late morbi-mortality, extend the Fontan circulation longevity and decrease the incidence of complications [27, 101-106].

The suggested phases of the univentricular route are (see Table 2):

Table 2. Current Management: "The Univentricular Route" "... phases, stages, strategies ...."

A ⟹ ***Fetal and Postnatal diagnosis*** .... *parents information, counseling, in-útero and / or postnatal cath-interventions, individualized care*

B ⟹ **1° stage-surgery ...** *[univentricular circulation "in parallel"] aorto-pulmonary shunt – pulmonary banding - Norwood op. - DKS procedure "interstage care " - cath-interventions*

C ⟹ **2° stage-surgery ...** *[partial univentricular circulación] Cath or MRI before: bidireccional Glenn shunt / hemiFontan / concomitants procedures*

D ⟹ **3° stage-surgery ...** *[total univentricular circulación "in serie"] Cath or MRI before: total cavopulmonary anastomosis: lateral tunnel vs. extracardiac conduit*

E ⟹ ***Late follow-up*** ... *multidisciplinary care: univentricular follow-up units functional status, quality of life, specialized studies*

Phase A

Fetal diagnosis and management. A fetal diagnosis of a great deal of the anomalies of the functionally UH by echocardiography is possible in skillful hands between weeks 18-20 of gestation paying attention to a 4 chambers view that visualizes the type of the atrioventricular junction and the presence of one small ventricle. The study is completed with other echocardiographic views addressed to complete the sequential-segmental analysis indicating in the first echo scan: 1) the degree of under developed ventricle, 2) characteristic of the foramen ovale and its Doppler flow pattern, 3) relationship of the great arteries and the asymmetry among them (anticipate potential development/progression of systemic or pulmonary obstruction), and 4) extra cardiac associated malformations. However, it is well known that anomalies that form the subgroup of the HLHS undergo changes during the pregnancy, in part due to flow disturbances; that's the reason why some prenatal care units propose serial tests for any variety of UH for a longitudinal screening of the fetal hemodynamic and verification of progress/changes in the structures. This fetus follow-up strategy not only adds to the knowledge and interpretation of the mechanisms that influence the development of heart disease in utero but allows for planning interventions, if applicable in selected cases (pulmonary or aortic valvuloplasty, atrial septostomy), and even anticipates an approximation of the postnatal prognosis which assists the selection of a specialized center for the delivery in agreement with the ongoing programs of neonatal cardiovascular surgery. From reports that analyse the outcome of a fetus with UH, some information has emerged: 1) the detection rate in tertiary perinatal centers is 80-95% and anticipates quite rightly the neonatal therapeutic actions in more than > 60%, 2) 20-25% of the total number of fetuses with extracardiac malformations or syndromes, 3) the "in-utero" demise is infrequent < 3-5%, 4) termination-abortion after parents-counselling fluctuates between 15-50%, 5) fetal loss for complications in "intention to-treat" or secondary to fetal intervention is observed in < 10-20%. No less important are two other aspects that are highlighted in the literature: a) the postnatal mortality is not affected by in-uterus diagnosis, and b) the positive impact of the prenatal diagnosis is significant for morbidity and patient clinical status in the neonatal period [early application of treatment before the onset of circulatory failure or shock secondary to ductus closure]. The prenatal diagnosis of CHD allows the parents to know in detail the characteristic and nature of the malformation, the intervention and/or surgical repair needed for survival, the immediate postnatal prognosis and the long-term therapeutic strategies to be applied. Simultaneously, the prenatal unit team offers genetic counselling to the couple whose importance is remarkable: the risk of having CHD in siblings of patients with HLHS may reach 35% while in some other categories of UH, the risk for siblings and offspring doesn't seem to exceed 5%. In any case, this multidisciplinary management of information and early counselling to parents get them ready to face the care of a child with life-threatening CHD who will require multiple attentions throughout his life and, at the time, gives them the opportunity to reflect on the choice of termination of pregnancy. It should be pointed out that, even with a precise fetal diagnosis, in some varieties and subtypes of the functional UH it is not possible to anticipate if they will be suitable or not to univentricular palliation [107-115].

Phase B

Postnatal period, diagnosis reassessment, treatment strategy, 1st stage palliation, inter-stage evaluation. The importance and expression of clinical impact in the newborn or neonate with single ventricle physiology will depend upon well-defined anatomical features: obstruction to the systemic or pulmonary flow, obstruction to the "ventricular inflow" (obstruction or intact atrial septum in right or left AV valve atresia), systemic or pulmonary venous return abnormalities (heterotaxy syndrome) and presence/grade of AV valve regurgitation (more frequent in hearts with common AV valve). The basic axes of procedures and management in this phase depend to a large extent on whether the diagnosis is previously known (prenatal), if "de novo" is suspected as a consequence of routine application of neonatal screening strategies during the usual newborn hospital stay or it is recognized weeks later after the appearance of clinical signs and symptoms (mainly cyanosis for insufficient pulmonary blood flow, heart failure due to overload or circulatory collapse/shock when the systemic circuit is ductus-dependant). The significant neonatal action includes: 1) fast and detailed confirmation of the anatomical diagnosis (echocardiography is vital in this process, it is especially necessary to appeal to more sophisticated imaging techniques such as MRI) and 2) prompt medical management in the Neonatal Intensive Care Unit (NICU) in order to reach the clinical stability (Prostaglandin E is mandatory to preserve the ductal permeability), optimize the total cardiac output and the systemic oxygen delivery. Once defined and the scenarios described, and according to the anatomical malformation category, four types of 1st stage palliation can be required:

1) *Total aortic reconstruction*: Norwood operation or hybrid process for neonates with HLHS or single ventricle variants with severe aortic obstruction. The reported hospital survival with this approach fluctuates between 70-93%; 10-15% of neonates require ECMO or cardiopulmonary resuscitation in the post-operative period; at 12 months transplant-free survival is around 75%. Currently the primary heart transplant is unusual in patients with HLHS or its variants; only exceptionally will it be indicated as an alternative in the presence of RV dysfunction and/or severe tricuspid AV valve [101,116,117].
2) *Aortic arch repair in association with unrestricted pulmonary blood flow*: coarctation repair associated with the Damus-Kaye-Stansel (DKS) operation in neonates with evident or potential subaortic obstruction (due to restricted ventricular septal defect). To adapt the pulmonary flow a systemic-pulmonary anastomosis is simultaneously performed through a prosthetic graft (modified Blalock-Taussig shunt-BT). The association between the pulmonary banding and the appearance/progression of subaortic stenosis in the setting of DILV or TA with transposed great arteries is well known. It is possible to substitute the DKS operation with a pulmonary banding if the two requisites are satisfied: the banding is left in place for a short period of time and a scheduled close echocardiographic surveillance (early planning for 2nd stage palliation in 2-3 months). This last action plan does not permanently rule out the DKS operation, which may be performed concomitantly with the 2nd stage palliation if the subaortic stenosis progresses to an obstructive degree. In some centers the palliative arterial switch has been proposed as an alternative to sort out the systemic obstruction and with well-selected cases the results are encouraging. The hospital survival with this varied approach of surgical palliation ranges between 85-90% [118-121].
3) *Excessive pulmonary blood flow*: in the absence of subpulmonary stenosis the initial approach to reduce the pulmonary over circulation is the pulmonary banding. Disadvantages of this "simple" procedure are: migration of the banding with obstructive consequence in one or both pulmonary branches, uncontrolled flow and pulmonary pressure ("little tightening) so it will perpetuate the signs and symptoms of heart failure, or too tight with severe reduction of the pulmonary flow that

clinically expresses itself by severe cyanosis; any of these symptoms must be solved. With these problems in mind, some groups propose dividing the pulmonary trunk and regulating the pulmonary flow with a BT shunt. With any of these actions hospital mortality fluctuates between 5 and 13% [122,123].

4) *Insufficient pulmonary blood flow*: the modified BT shunt (small graft of 3 or 3,5 mm) is the therapeutic choice for increasing/adjusting the inappropriate pulmonary flow in neonates with atresia or severe pulmonary stenosis. The reported mortality with this strategy stands for 5 and 15%, so it is not surprising that interventional cardiologists perform ductal stenting in neonates to avoid the initial surgical palliation and go straight for a BDGS. The postoperative therapy with antithrombotic agents is essential as the main cause of graft occlusion is related to thrombosis; in some selected cases it may turn to interventional catheterization (thrombolysis plus stent implant into the shunt) [124,125]

The exception to all this perioperative medical and surgical management in the neonatal age is reduced to a small proportion of patients (<10%) with UH variants because of their "very good balanced circulation": Qp/Qs 0,9-1:2 and arterial oxygen saturation around 80-85%.

Phase C

2nd stage palliation ("the unloading ventricle process"). It is intended to perform, between 3-6 months, the cavopulmonary shunt with two technical options depending on the preference of the surgical group and largely anticipating the next step or path towards the complete Fontan: BDGS or HemiFontan (wide side to side superior vena cava-right atrium junction and right pulmonary branch plus closing the created communication between the atrium and pulmonary artery with a patch). From the hemodynamic viewpoint they are equivalent; the first one is used more frequently, is easier and preferred for surgeons that will complete Fontan with an ECC. The second one is more complex, requires working closely to the sinus node (with potential injury to the tributary vessel or their innervation) and is preferred by teams that go for LT. The associated anomalies, if it is necessary should be corrected in a concomitant approach (severe AV insufficiency, distortions or stenosis of the pulmonary branches, subaortic stenosis, among others). Some groups prefer to abolish any kind of additional pulsatile pulmonary flow at the moment of the BDGS (less post-operative incidence of pleural effusion at the expense of more cyanosis) while others prefer to maintain pervious pulsatile flow – systemic-pulmonary shunt, pulmonary banding, and native subpulmonary stenosis – relying on better oxygenation in the postop and a favorable effect on the pulmonary vascular tree development growth. The immediate postoperative risk factors are**:** bilateral Glenn, preoperative mean pulmonary artery pressure >15-17 mmHg, arrhythmia and ventricular dysfunction. The operative mortality of this phase tends to be < 5% [126,127]. Again, it has to be highlighted that around 10% of neonates and infants with functionally UH, due to a good systemic /pulmonary blood flow balance, will not need any previous intervention to the BDGS.

Phase D

3rd stage palliation. Total cavopulmonary anastomosis, the last step to complete the Fontan circulation. Around 2-4 years of age the univentricular circulatory model in series is completed with the deviation of the infra-diaphragmatic systemic venous return conveying the inferior vena cava to the pulmonary artery by two technical options: 1) the LT or 2) the ECC. Both techniques have advantages and disadvantages although currently the majority of the centers prefer the ECC, even if there is a controversy about it; some surgical groups prefer a routine fenestration. The operative mortality of this phase is < 5% [128-132]. It must be considered that some patients with acute or subacute failed Fontan completion require early surgical management: 1) Fontan takedown to a BDGS and/or arterial shunt in order to stabilize the univentricular circulation or 2) heart transplantation. Almond reported the outcome of 53 patients in whom a takedown was performed at the time of the Fontan operation itself (22%), or before a year after Fontan completion (78%), among survivors (29/53, 55%), 65% were submitted to redo-Fontan (> 2 years later), 10% underwent cardiac transplantation and 24% with BDGS as definitive palliation [132]. The Fontan completion performed by interventional catheterization was reported [133].

During the transition between phases B, C and D the child passes a relatively short period of cyanosis with little clinical significance, therefore they require a close clinical surveillance. In summary, the combination of a prompt operative strategy and strict selection of the candidate improves the immediate outcome, although it remains to be endorsed whether this protocol increases longevity and quality of life of survivors. Cardiac catheterization is necessary before the BDGS and the modified Fontan completion to define the hemodynamic condition and add the possibility of performing interventional procedures.

Phase E

Adolescents and adults. Late scheduled program of personalized assessment of survivors (specialized Fontan circulation clinic team with interdisciplinary distinctive in a collaborative working group that discusses each patient with other subspecialists) to monitor progression and solve the clinical and hemodynamic problems secondary to low chronic output and the endothelial dysfunction that this condition promotes [protein-losing enteropathy, demineralized bone, somatic growth, neurological disorders, hepatic disease, thromboembolic phenomena, among others]. Also to monitor extra cardiac procedures, pregnancy counseling, antibacterial prophylaxis, social support and other kinds of support the patient requires. [134].

Late Complications – Failing Fontan

A substantial variety of complications happen in the mid- and long-term follow-up of patients palliated with the Fontan procedure and/or its modifications [135-141]. There is agreement that these are largely time-dependent and many of them secondary to the "intrinsic hemodynamic properties" in Fontan circulation. At the same time, the technical modifications and the different algorithms used for patient management that were, and are, applied over the years embraces a set of complications that, at first glance, includes survivors of the initial surgical techniques. So, in order to have a realistic and truthful scrutiny, we have to wait a couple of decades to validate if the present process of precocity adopted in the current univentricular route involves lengthier longevity, less incidence of complications, interventions, redo and/or less "late gradual attrition" than the one observed in "older patients". In any case, these remarks do not invalidate active approaches to palliate, ameliorate or anticipate the complications already recognized in the literature or even unexpected (Figure 2). Furthermore, there is an agreement about the aggressive study of these patients and the periodical assessment of the Fontan circuit by means of catheterization or MRI (eventually cardiac CT angiography to specific issues) to anticipate residual lesions or sequels that can be amended with interventional cardiology or surgery before they have a florid clinical expression [142].

Complications have been gathered under the name of "failing Fontan" [143-147]. A second late gradual rising hazard function for death 5-10 years after the APa is well known; the survival estimated curve was predicted to be 70-75% al 15 years of follow-up, among others, one of the identified risk factors was older age at operation [98,148-152]. Currently the overall late survival predicted and well documented, is around 80-85% at 15-20 years follow up [153-155], yet, there is no evidence whether this rate could be improved with the techniques and current algorithms in follow up longer than 25-30 years. The actuarial freedom according to mode of death at 25 years follow-up was: event-free survival related to heart failure 95.6% (increasing hazard risk after 10 years follow-up), related to sudden death 96.3% (annual incidence of 0.15%), and related to thromboembolism 91% [151]. The recognized risk factors associated with late mortality have been summarized in: 1) the type of ventricular morphology (the right seems to induce worst late results in respect to LV type although there is a debate about this specific issue), 2) the heterotaxy syndrome (common AV with significant insufficiency), 3) protein-losing enteropathy, 4) elevated right atrium pressure after Fontan, 5) arrhythmia, 6) thromboembolism (due to lack of aspirin prescription or any other anticoagulant therapy) and 7) reoperations (pacemaker, Fontan revision and conversion, heart transplant).

Functional capacity, quality of life and some other complications.- When the functional class is estimated with the NYHA classification it is remarkable that around 70-80% of patients are allocated in class I and II, however over time such percentage seems to decline for many reasons of sudden, unexpected and insidious onset. This fact emphasizes the need for a multidisciplinary and programmed screening to study and anticipate, if possible, the different late clinical problems that happen in this particular population during the follow up. Another aspect of interest in this field is the discordance between the perception in the assessment of health reflected by the patient and close relatives and the objective measurements that assess the clinical status. Different reports from the Pediatric Heart Network Investigators - Fontan Cross-Sectional Study - National Heart, Lung, and Blood Institute [www.pediatricheartnetwork.com] suggest that not only is there a functional limitation in survivors but that, at the time, this affects their quality of life (Child Health Questionnaire CHQ and ADH adult model: www.pedsql.org). One of the most investigated parameters has been the functional exercise performance; in 546 patients Paridon detected, at 8 years post Fontan, an average for maximum oxygen consumption of 65% with respect to the expected normal, this percentage value is less in the older Fontan population in Diller´s report; and finally there is an increased risk of hospitalization [156,157]. Van den Bosch reports a reduction of physical functioning; mental health and general health perception in 36 adult survivors with an average of 15 years follow up [158]. The evaluation of the cardiopulmonary response to exercise reflect levels of interaction between the reduction of the functional capacity and the concomitant ventilatory disorders; the factors associated with these observations are: inappropriate chronotropic response, atrioventricular asynchrony, ventricular-arterial uncoupling, presence or not of hypoxemia (due to fenestration or non-filiation right to left shunt), restrictive phenomena of the pulmonary function (for example thoracic distortion secondary to previous palliation or scoliosis) and increased post pubertal body mass. In any case, the most important limiting factor of the functional capacity is an inadequate cardiac output to meet the metabolic demands to the maximum effort (inability to meet the demand of high transpulmonary flow due to limited preload rather than of abnormal single ventricle systolic function). A functional score was recently developed coupling ventricular ejection fraction (by echo), predicted maximal oxygen consumption (%), child health questionnaire and brain natriuretic peptides. Risk factors for poor functional scores were found to be: RV morphology, elevated preoperative end diastolic pressure, pre Fontan oxygen saturation and parental incomes. Other traditional non-dependent variables were also analysed and interestingly enough the functional score only detected around 18% of the risk factors. This means that there are still many areas to know and understand [159-161]. McCrindle [162] obtained information from 537 families (Parents Report Questionnaire) and pointed out the problems with pattern disturbances for attention and learning (around 46%) as well as behavior problems (23%). The issue of neurodevelopment is controversial; recent information links it with fetal hemodynamic disorders and/or related with neonatal surgical procedures (circulatory bypass, aortic clamping and others). It is, anyway, a serious matter to be concerned with [163,164].

Arrhythmia

The lost or absence of the normal sinoatrial-ventricular synchrony is an undesirable complication for Fontan circulation. The development of atrial arrhythmias at mid- and long-term is a well-known factor for morbi-mortality; they are more prevalent in atrio-pulmonary anastomosis (up to 60%) in regard to cavo-pulmonary techniques (between 10-30%), with an annual incidence between 4 to 15%. They can be at slow rate (sinus node dysfunction, junctional rhythm and complete AV block) or at a fast rate (intra-atrial re-entrant tachycardia, focal atrial tachycardia, atrial flutter and atrial fibrillation). The variable associated to these atrial arrhythmia are: severe dilatation of the right atrium, length of follow up, older age at operation, heterotaxy syndrome, severe AV regurgitation and previous bradi-arrhythmias. Altogether they induce a marked hemodynamic instability of the fragile univentricular circulation, ventricular dysfunction, thromboembolism, reduction of the quality of life, several hospitalizations and, are particularly well-known causes of sudden death. As a result it is mandatory for prompt therapeutic actions and hemodynamic investigation and/or exhaustive diagnosis by imaging to detect disorders that could be potentially repairable by interventional cardiology (obstructions along the Fontan pathways) or by surgery [165-169]. The sinus node dysfunction can be observed in the preoperative period (7%) but there is an increment in the staged Fontan (between 10-15% in the postoperative Hemi Fontan or BDGS) due to potential lesion of the sinus node [170,171]. Some authors claim major incidences with the lateral tunnel (22%), others, on the contrary, do not detect significant differences; also, the intra/extra techniques with less atrial sutures seems to be a better approach. Even if some patients recover the sinus rhythm inter-stage or post Fontan, in the vast majority the problem persists and even 10-13% of patients require a definitive pacemaker. The junctional rhythm – absence of sinus rhythm – is considered to be a risk factor for tachyarrhythmia and fibrotic hepatic lesion. The tachyarrhythmias are prevalent and the most common (75%) is the intra-atrial tachycardia due to macro re-entrant circuits, usually complex and/or numerous. It is followed in frequency by tachycardia caused by ectopic focus in 15%; atrial flutter and atrial fibrillation are reported mainly in adult patients and is a kind of arrhythmia often present in patients sent for surgical conversion. There are no significant differences in the incidence of intra-atrial tachycardia between the lateral tunnel and external conduit. Recently, a multicenter trial analysed the occurrence of arrhythmia (defined as the need of treatment at the time of onset) in 1271 patients divided into two groups: A) intracardiac Fontan (602 pts) and B) extracardiac Fontan (669 pts). The incidence of bradyarrhythmias were: early postoperative 4% in group A and 11% in group B, late outcome 18% in group A and 9% in group B. In regards to tachyarrhythmia: early postoperative 5% in group A and 11% in group B, late outcome 10% in group A and 3% in group B. The follow up was longer in group A (average 9.2 years) in respect to group B (average 4.7 years) [172,173].

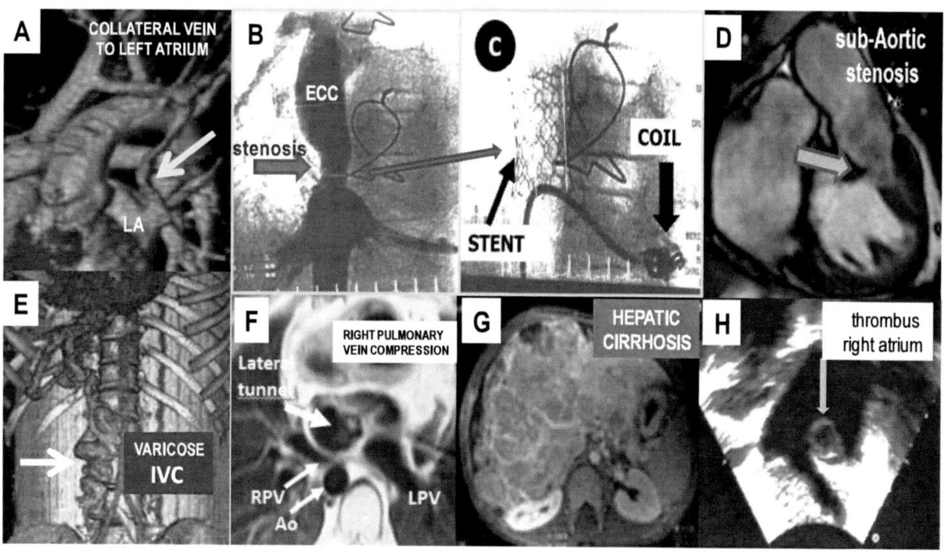

Figure 2. Different types of complications.

The usually protocol to safely perform an electrical cardioversion is a useful form of acute therapy to immediately improve the hemodynamic instability; on the other hand, anti-arrhythmic drugs such as sotalol, propafenone, and beta blockers can appropriately control the heart rate but only between 20-30% of patients resolve the problem. The immediate success with the ablation by catheterization reaches 70-80% but new arrhythmias reappear early in more than half of the patients in spite of performing procedures with new techniques of 3D mapping. Another treatment reported for arrhythmia control in Fontan patients is the different and sophisticated pacing modalities. In this sense, and considering that the viability of the venous access to atriums is limited in the external conduit, preventive epicardial atrioventricular leads are routinely implanted in Fontan second stage to avoid new mini thoracotomy. The APa or LT conversion to ECC with surgery for the concomitant arrhythmia (right atrial maze for intra-atrial tachycardia and left mode for patients with fibrillation) drastically reduces the incidence of arrhythmia even if there is a recurrence of 15% reported in the last type. This therapeutic approach is a good alternative that, in specialized centers, offers satisfactory results with low mortality even if around 6-8% will require heart transplant [174-176]

Protein-Losing Enteropathy

This is a serious, limiting and "active" clinical condition which etiopathogenesis, although not fully elucidated, is assumed to be multifactorial, interacting hemodynamic and inflammatory factors. It is hypothesized that chronic low cardiac output induces an increase of the splanchnic arterial resistance (determined by the Doppler technique at the superior mesenteric artery and celiac artery), regional phenomena that, together with the increased infra-diaphragmatic systemic venous pressure, place in action as a cascade; inflammatory factors that slowly, silently and gradually will injury the integrity of the intestinal mucosae. This condition may be present in patients with any type of Fontan design and can be either in the early as well as the late follow up. The average interval between the Fontan procedure and the clinical onset of this syndrome is between 3.7 years and 8.6 years (with a range of 0.3 and 19 years post Fontan), with a cumulative risk at 10 years of 13.4% [177-180]

The variables associated with this syndrome are non-LV ventricular morphology, immediate post-operative renal failure, long cardiopulmonary bypass time and hospital stay and high end-diastolic ventricular pressure. It is characterized by a significant enteral loss of plasmatic protein with a long half-life and the diagnosis (in the absence of hepatic or renal failure) is done with the finding of hypoalbuminemia (< 3 gr) and a high quantity of alfa-1-Antitrypsin in a 24-hour stool clearance test. Other remarkable laboratory findings (by the way similar to other causes of PLE) are: reduction of immunoglobulin – IgG, IgM and IgA-, lymphocytopenia (reduction of lymphocytes CD4 and B), elevated proinflammatory cytokines (tumor necrosis factor-alpha, PCR and interferon-y), hypocalcaemia and altered prothrombotic factors such as anti-thrombin III, proteins C and S. Intestinal mucosae lymphangiectasis confirmed by biopsy and histological examinations were observed in gastric endoscopies [181].

Clinically there is edema, abdominal distension and ascites, pleural and/or pericardial effusion, occasional or chronic diarrhea and finally malnutrition if the syndrome persists. Different pharmacological stratagems have been attempted with partial success: angiotensing-converting-enzyme inhibitors, steroids, high molecular weight heparin (to alleviate the cellular injury of the intestinal membrane), parenteral albumin, pulmonary vasodilators and specific diet (medium-chain triglycerides). If there is a source amenable to be repaired it is desirable to do it by catheter intervention: to enlarge obstructions present in Fontan circuit or create a fenestration, occlusion of aortopulmonary collaterals or overlooked and pervious systemic-pulmonary shunts, atrioventricular pacing and resynchrony (in bradyarrhythmias). Of course it will be better off to convert the APa to cavopulmonary or heart transplant. The multicenter trial done by Mertens [178] proved that half of the patients will be dead in 5 years and will survive, only 20%, at 10 years if the syndrome is not solved. Any kind of lesion subject that can be fixed must be repaired either by cardiac catheterization (desirable) or by surgery. An important issue is the bone demineralization, a condition that happens in children and adolescents secondary to steroid therapy or related to the underlying abnormal Fontan hemodynamic (abnormal osteoblasts function). A bone densitometry scan is a study to be performed periodically and measurement of osteoblast function biomarkers is mandatory [182].

Plastic Bronchitis

An infrequent but extremely serious complication is the appearance of pulmonary distress due to an obstructed airway by fibrinomucoid and cellular casts considered to be a consequence of abnormal lymphatic fluid drainage even if some other factors are also incriminated in this problem. Plastic bronchitis is a potentially fatal condition that begins with cough, dyspnea and expectoration (the material mimic the bronchial shape), sometimes recurrent, with regional atelectasis and it may progress to severe respiratory distress, even leading to death. An incidence of < 3% is reported, present in any form of surgical Fontan circuit design and at mid or long term follow up. Its pathogenesis and physiopathology are considered to be multifactorial and in some aspects similar to those that originate the protein-losing enteropathy: pro-inflammatory phenomena, defined immune phenotype, increase of the systemic venous pressure, and low cardiac output, a possible role of genetic factors still to be determined. Different therapeutic strategies have been applied in relation to the clinical severity of the problem; therapy must be focused on solving the pulmonary obstruction and to immediately determine the anatomy and physiology of the Fontan circuit. Having been tried, with variable rates of success at midterm: bronchoalveolar lavage, high frequency ventilation, steroids, aerosolized urokinase or tissue plasminogen activator, pulmonary vasodilators, Fontan fenestration, atrial pacing and heart transplant. Neutrophils, eosinophil, macrophages, and B lymphocytes were identified in cast samples; there were only fewer T lymphocytes. Fibrin was an abundant protein in the cast proteome. Histone H4 was also abundant and by immunofluorescence microscopy was demonstrated to be mostly extracellular. The cytokine profile of plastic bronchitis casts was proinflammatory. The cast formation cannot be explained simply by lymph leak into the airways as they are composed of fibrin and are cellular and inflammatory in nature. Consequences of cellular necrosis including extracellular histones and, the apparent low number of T cells, indicates that a derangement in inflammation resolution likely contributes to cast [183-188].

Thromboembolism

Both, thrombus formation and embolism, present either in the early or late follow up, are not infrequent and could be present in 20-30% of survivors. Even if this percentage is not sufficiently convincing it is estimated that between 13-17% of patients can have a silent thrombus in some part of the Fontan pathway or even pulmonary embolism without any clinical manifestation. The stasis and systemic venous hypertension, the slow circulatory velocity, arrhythmias, prosthetic material in the venous circuit, presence of cul-de-sac, older age at Fontan, procoagulant hematological disorders (antithrombin III, protein S and protein C reduction, platelet reactivity), and non-antiplatelet treatment, are some of the well-known risk factors. The silent pulmonary thromboembolism impacts in a negative way on the pulmonary arteriolar resistance (increased resistance and emphasizing the chronic Fontan low output), if it is especially massive should potentially be, the cause of sudden death. It has been pointed out in the literature that systemic embolism can affect the neurological area (stroke), coronary system or some other areas; the origin can be founded at the APa level (arrhythmia), ventricular myocardium (significant systolic dysfunction), ligated pulmonary trunk (thrombus seated between the cul-de-sac and the pulmonary valve close to the systemic circuit), also the systemic embolic phenomena was described in patients with a patent fenestration. Anyhow, the coagulation algorithms are currently under debate as there are many arguments for and against preventive anticoagulation; nevertheless the common tendency, particularly in adult patients, is to keep a prophylactic antithrombotic therapy and to replace it with warfarin or acenocumarol in a thromboembolic episode. An issue to be of concern is the presence of varicose syndrome in adolescents or adults probably due to the combination of venous obstruction due to previous cardiac catheterization and the increase of systemic venous pressure [190-195].

Liver Dysfunction

Usually upon physical examination, there is hepatomegaly secondary to venous congestion in any type of Fontan circuit. Hepatic dysfunction, increased enzymes and coagulation conditions are not infrequent, in fact more than 50% of patients have disorders of this kind yet it has been indicated that, in some cases, there is a fluctuation in serial lab tests; the length of follow up is a risk factor for this condition. More recently attention has been focused on the slow and progressive evolution toward fibrosis, cirrhosis and/or hepatoma, with different degrees of clinical manifestation. This progression to severe and limiting hepatic disease has not been fully understood. Among the identified mechanisms are not only chronic hepatic congestion but also regional alterations of the hepato-splachnic system resistance or insult, or hepatic injuries in pre Fontan stage. In any case, these observations reinforce the necessity of a multidisciplinary team for follow up. Close and frequent surveillance of the liver, using different diagnostic tools (Doppler flow pattern of portal and hepatic veins and arteries, magnetic resonance imaging, multi-sliced TAC) in some selected cases the possibility of liver biopsy could be considered. The relevance of "hepatic problem" can be noted in the need – exceptional but already indicated – for a particular patient having an indication for heart and liver transplantation [196-199].

Cyanosis and Collateral Venous Circulation

The vast majority of patients have an oxygen arterial saturation not less than 92-95%; values below that level must be investigated as to the aetiology of the desaturation. Generally they are due to: intended surgical fenestration, residual interatrial communication (leaks), collateral systemic veins from infra/supra diaphragmatic origin that connect with the left atrium or pulmonary vein, arteriovenous pulmonary malformations or intrinsic pulmonary pathology (restrictive physiology due to thoracic deformities, diaphragmatic palsy, pneumonia, pulmonary embolism). In the pathogenesis of the arteriovenous pulmonary malformations, the absence of hepatic flow ("hepatic factor") in the pulmonary circuit play a role, so this disease is more prevalent in patients with classic Glenn, in heterotaxy syndrome with intra/extrahepatic porto-systemic shunt, or operated on with the Kawashima technique, and also in a suboptimal Fontan circuit design (unbalanced pulmonary flow distribution). In selected cases (with detailed hemodynamic evaluation to pondering pros and cons – benefit/risk), a good deal of these permeable vascular anomalies or residual localized shunts can be occluded with interventional catheterization as long as collaterals are not due to a "needed leakage" mechanism for elevated venous pressure. The catheter occlusion of the surgical fenestration is still controversial; some groups advocate the closure in their management protocol, on the other hand it is considered that the open fenestration "for lifelong" is for the patient's safety [76,200-202]

Aortopulmonary Collaterals

After BDGS or Fontan completion, the presence of aortopulmonary collaterals is considered a risk factor to influence the perioperative outcome. It is not known if this condition appears to compensate for the low systemic cardiac output; in any case controversy persists about the clinical or hemodynamic impact. The benefit of coil embolization is advocated for different investigators, but a practice variation exists between centers. The left-to-right shunt that the aortopulmonary collaterals produce can be measured accurately by non-invasive phase-contrast MRI, and then the indication of coiling intervention can be adjusted [203,204].

Heart Failure

As the time of follow up passes by, some patients develop heart failure recognizable by peripheral edema, ventricular, renal or hepatic dysfunction. Around 30% of the patients have reduced systolic function measured by echocardiography or magnetic resonance: myocardial regional asynchrony, abnormal ventriculo-arterial coupling, atrioventricular electrical disturbances, incoordinate relaxation and diminished beta-adrenergic reserves related to limited preload, are some of the observations reported. Even a generalized approach with inter-centers variation, the conventional therapy (afterload inhibitors, beta blockers) is inconsistent. Diuretics and aldosterone antagonists are required and frequently used with success for the treatment of Fontan failure. In selected cases, anecdotally, resynchronization has been used with beneficial results. The RV, in the setting of the HLHS, acts as a single chamber and its ability to pump after Fontan completion will be prevalent in the next years; therefore, it will be very interesting to watch their function in the long-term follow-up [93, 205-207].

Mechanical Assisted Devices – Heart Transplant

Some patients with failing/failed Fontan require advanced cardiac support due to unsuccessful conventional therapeutic attempts. In the last few years ventricular assist devices (VADs) as a bridge to heart transplant have been used with increasing frequency not only in adults but also in children. Orthotopic heart transplant is the latest opportunity of effective treatment or solution for these patients even though the indication and timing are under debate. Most studies report a perioperative transplant mortality of 30% and a 50% survival estimated at 10 years [208, 209].

Fontan Procedure in Adults

The Fontan operation is possible in adult patients (>18 years old). The analysed reports include the 3 types of surgical technique applied to children. The vast majority of patients have a previous palliation with aorto-pulmonary or cavopulmonary shunts. The hemodynamic study before the Fontan operation is mandatory and patient selection is very strict to avoid including patients with risk factors. The creation of fenestration is variable, even minority. Hospital mortality is reported below 10%. Two aspects are relevant: 1) arrhythmias are frequent pre and post-operatively and 2) albeit the functional state measured by NYHA scale in survivors is better than preoperative, an early decline of the ventricular function has been noticed. The life survival is 65% at 15 years with free-from-operations of 80% at 15 years [210-212].

Long-Term Complications

- Arrhythmias – Sudden death
- Plastic bronchitis
- Protein-Losing Enteropathy
- Thromboembolism – sudden death, silent pulmonary embolism
- Bone demineralization-abnormal osteoblast function
- Liver disease, cirrhosis, hepatoma
- Impairment Ventricular Function-Heart Failure
- Worsening cyanosis
- Somatic Growth – Anthropometric abnormalities
- Pathway obstructions
- AV Valve – Aortic valve regurgitation
- Neurodevelopment Disturbances
- Increase Pulmonary Vascular Resistance
- Decline Functional Status – Exercise Capacity
- Atriomegaly, dilated coronary sinus, compression of pulmonary veins

The Future

Numerous researchers realize the adversities and doubts that lurk in the long-term longevity of the univentricular model with any technique used. The failure of traditional medical care leads us to promote the heart transplant – in addition with liver transplantation in some cases - as the only one effective and definitive treatment of the failing or failed Fontan. Some clues can be derived from the following information: 1) the incidence of complications increase when the univentricular circulation is completed if compared to the partial model (BDGS) [213,214] 2) the permeable fenestration "at least at mid-term" (increase the cardiac output and reduce the systemic venous pressure) offers better functional expectations even at the cost of maintaining some degree of hypoxemia [200], 3) the progressive endothelial dysfunction with unfavorable multi-organ impact is a reality [215], at the pulmonary level where the non-pulsatile flow promotes a slow and insidious rise of the vascular resistance - evidence of vascular disease after cardiac transplant in Fontan patients [216] and disorder in the modulation and release of endothelin-1 and nitric oxide among other factors, or, at the level of other systemic pulsatile subsystems (splanchnic bed) where the regional arteriolar resistance increases secondary to chronic low cardiac output, 4) the promising chronic therapy with 5-phosphodiesterse inhibitors – sildenafil – with well-known benefits associated with improved exercise performance [217], 5) computation models performed in the experimental field demonstrated flow abnormalities in the TCPC surgical pathways at rest or at computer-generated stimulus; an optimization of the system design (Y-shaped form or direct connection inferior vena cava-pulmonary artery to obtain a more equivalent pulmonary flow distribution) by means of the bio-engineers based on imaging patient-specific simulations is needed [218], and 6) innovative experts have designed new devices for potential implant in the extra cardiac conduit with the view to actively promote the systemic venous circulation to the pulmonary circuit with the purpose of increasing the cardiac output (mimics a "subpulmonary ventricle") yet without clinical application [219-221].

There are several unsolved challenges in the next decades that will require the contribution of some other scientific disciplines for a better understanding of the nature of the different clinical disorders as well as the potential adjusted-treatment. These are only some of the problems to be solved: a) to elucidate if the clinical pictures depend on compensatory adjustments of the univentricular physiology or if they are only pathological consequences of the procedures, b) to identify the molecular starting point responsible of the pulmonary arteriovenous malformations (the so-called circulating "hepatic factors") as liable to induce potential misbalance between pro and antiangiogenic signals and/or find the link between those vascular malformations and bone morphogenetic protein-9 (222-225), c) to define the link between exogenous growth hormone given to Fontan patients with short stature and the increase in arteriovenous malformations or worst PLE syndrome (226), and d) a possible approach with new molecular therapy and cell replacement to repair or replace abnormal tissues during morphogenesis (227,228). Perhaps only few questions but they merge the need of a multidisciplinary approach to this new generation of survivors. Are we doing correctly or are we just leading a complex pathway with an intricate end?. Many difficult questions to be answered yet and they are on the air.

The concept of multidisciplinary team units expert in the knowledge and management of patients with UH physiology whom survive longer is imperative, not only to face the related cardiovascular problems but also to give support and care in fields like non-cardiac surgery, pregnancy, insurances, employment, psychological support and social activities (135,137,200,229-234). Therefore, what it has been reported here just support our adherence to what forward-looking physiologists advised already centuries ago: the subpulmonary right ventricle is essential for the human life.

References

[1] Anderson, RH; Cook, AC. Morphology of the functionally univentricular heart. *Cardiol Young*, 2004, 14 (Suppl. 1), 3-12.

[2] Wilkinson, JL; Anderson, RH. Anatomy of functionally single ventricle. *World J Pediatr Congenit Heart Surg*, 2012, 3, 159-64.

[3] Jacobs, ML; Anderson, RH. Nomenclature of the functionally univentricular heart. *Cardiol Young*, 2006, 16, 3-8.

[4] Freedom, R; Van, Arsdell, GS. Biventricular hearts not amenable to biventricular repair. *Ann Thorac Surg*, 1998, 66, 641-3.

[5] Delius, RE; Rademecker, MA; de, Leval, MR; et al. Is a high-risk biventricular repair always preferable to a single ventricle repair?. *J Thorac Cardiovasc Surg*, 1996,112, 1561-9.

[6] Fontan, F; Baudet, E. Surgical repair of tricuspid atresia. *Thorax,* 1971, 26, 240-8.

[7] Cook, AC, Anderson, RH. The anatomy of hearts with double inlet ventricle. *Cardiol Young*, 2006, 16 (Suppl. 1), 22–26.

[8] Weinberg, PM. Morphology of single ventricle. *Progr Pediatr Cardiol*, 2002, 16, 1-9.

[9] Van Praagh, R; Plett, JA; Van Praagh, S. Single ventricle: pathology, embryology, terminology, and classification. *Herz*, 1979, 4, 113-50.

[10] Wilkinson, JL; Becker, AE; Tynan, M; et al. Nomenclature of the univentricular heart. *Herz*, 1979, 4, 107-12.

[11] Tynan, MJ; Becker, AE; Macartney, F; et al. Nomenclature and classification for congenital heart disease. *Br Heart J*, 1979,41, 544-53.

[12] Anderson, RH. How should we optimally describe complex congenitally malformed hearts?. *Ann Thorac Surg*, 1996, 62, 710-716.

[13] Ho, SY. Cardiac Morphology and Nomenclature. Chapter 2, pp. 7-18. In: Gatzoulis MA, Webb GD, Daubeney PEF, eds. Diagnosis and Management of Adult Congenital Heart Disease. Churchill Livingstone, 2003.

[14] Anderson, RH; Shirali, G. Sequential segmental analysis. *Ann Pediatr Cardiol*, 2009, 2, 24-35.

[15] Van Praagh, R. The segmental approach to diagnosis in congenital heart disease. In: Bergsma D, ed. Birth defects original article series, VIII nº5. The fourth conference on the clinical delineation of births defects. The National Foundations-March of Dimes. Baltimore: Williams and Wilkins, 1972, pp.4-23.

[16] Jacobs, JP; Anderson, RH; Weinberg, PM; et al. The nomenclature, definition and classification of cardiac structures in the setting of heterotaxy. *Cardiol Young*, 2007, 17 (Suppl. 2), 1-28.

[17] Strickland, MJ; Riehle-Colarusso, T; Jacobs, JP; et al. The importance of nomenclature for congenital cardiac disease: implications for research and evaluation. *Cardiol Young*, 2008, 18 (Suppl. 2), 92–100.

[18] Jacobs, JP; Franklin, RC; Colan, S; et al. Classification of the functionally univentricular hearts: unity form mapped codes. *Cardiol Young*, 2006, 16, 9-21.

[19] Jacobs, JP; Jacobs, ML; Maruszewskic, B; et al. Initial application in the EACTS and STS Congenital Heart Surgery Databases of an empirically derived methodology of complexity adjustment to evaluate surgical case mix and results. *Eur J Cardiothorac Surg*, 2012, 42, 775–80.

[20] Dobell, ARC; Van Praagh, R. The Holmes heart: historic associations a pathologic anatomy. *Am Heart J*, 1996, 132, 437-45.

[21] Rashkind, WJ. Tricuspid atresia: a historical review. *Pediatr Cardiol*, 1981, 2, 85-8.

[22] Evans, WN; Acherman, RJ, Anderson, RH. One hundred years of texts describing congenitally malformed hearts from 1814 to 1914. *Cardiol Young*, 2009, 19, 12-9.

[23] Lev, M; Libertson, RR; Kirkpatrick, JR; et al. Single (primitive) ventricle. Circulation, 1969, 39, 577-86.

[24] de la Cruz, MV. Different concepts of univentricular heart. Experimental embryological approach. *Herz*, 1979, 4, 67-73.

[25] Quero Jimenez, M; Cameron, AH; Acerete, F; et al. Univentricular hearts: pathology of the atrioventricular valves. *Herz*, 1979, 4, 161-5.

[26] Anderson, RH; Becker, AE; Freedom, RM; et al. Problems in the nomenclature of the univentricular heart. *Herz*, 4, 97-106.

[27] Khairy, P; Poirier, N; Mercier, LA. Univentricular heart. *Circulation*, 2007,115, 800-12

[28] de la Cruz, MV; Miller, BL. Double inlet left ventricle. Two pathological specimens with comments the embriology and or its relation to single ventricle. *Circulation*, 1968, 37, 240-60.

[29] Anderson, RH; Becker, AE; Tynan, MJ; et al. The univentricular atrioventricular connection: getting to the root of a thorny problem. *Am J Cardiol*, 1984, 5, 281-8.

[30] Van Praagh, R; Ongley, PA; Swan, HJ. Anatomic types of single or common ventricle in man: morphologic, geometric aspects of 60 necropsied cases. *Am J Cardiol*, 1964,13, 367-86.

[31] Muñoz Castellanos, L; Ramirez, S; Kuri Nivon, M; Salinas, Sanchez, HC. Doble entrada ventricular izquierda. Morfopatología quirúrgica. *Arch Inst Cardiol Mex*, 2000, 70, 136-47.

[32] Anderson, RH; Wilkinson, JL; Gerlis, LM; et al. Atresia of the right atrioventricular orifice. *Br Heart J*, 1977, 39, 414-28.

[33] Deanfield, JE; Tommasini, G; Anderson, RH; Macartney, FJ. Tricuspide atresia: analysis of coronary artery distribution and ventricular morphology. *Br Heart J*, 1982, 48, 485-92.

[34] Anderson, RH; Becker, A; Wilkinson, JL; et al. Morphogenesis of univentricular hearts. *Br Heart J*, 1976, 38, 558-72.

[35] de la Cruz, MV; Nadal-Guinard, B. Rules for the diagnosis of visceral situs, truncoconal morphologies, and ventricular inversions. *Am Heart J*, 1972, 84, 19-32.

[36] Valdés Cruz, LM; Cayré, RO. Anomalies of the ventricles. Chapter 17, pp. 297-313. In: Valdés Cruz LM, Cayré RO, eds. Echocardiographic diagnosis of congenital heart disease. *An embryologic and anatomic approach*. Lippincott-Raven Publishers 1999.

[37] Hoffman, JIE; Kaplan, S. The Incidence of Congenital Heart Disease. *J Am Coll Cardiol*, 2002, 39, 1890 –900.
[38] Starr, I; Jeffers, WA; Meade, RH. The absence of conspicuous increments of venous pressure after severe damage to the right ventricle of the dog, with a discussion of the relation between clinical congestive failure and heart disease. *Am Heart J*, 1943, 26, 291-301.
[39] Bakos, ACP. The question of the function of the right ventricular myocardium: an experimental study. *Circulation*, 1950, 1, 724-32.
[40] Robicsek, F; Watts, LT. A prelude to Fontan. *Pediatr Cardiol*, 2007, 28, 422–425.
[41] Sanger, PW; Robicsek, F; Taylor, FH; et al. Observations on partial and complete circulatory exclusion of the right heart. *J Cardiovasc Surg (Torino),* 1965, 6, 30-48.
[42] Cowgill, LD. The Fontan Procedure: A Historical review. *Ann Thorac Surg*, 1991, 51, 1026-30.
[43] Hurwitt, ES; Young, D; Escher, DJW. The rationale of anastomosis of the right atrial appendage to the pulmonary artery in the treatment of tricuspid atresia. *J Thorac Surg*, 1955, 30, 503-12.
[44] Glenn, WWL. Circulatory bypass of the right side of the heart. IV. Shunt between superior vena cava and distal right pulmonary artery-report of clinical application. *N Engl J Med*, 1958, 259, 117-20.
[45] Bickford, BJ; Edwards, FR. Cavo-pulmonary anastomosis. *Thorax*, 1960, 15, 165-8.
[46] Dogliotti, AM; Venere, G; Tarquini, A; et al. L'intervento di anastomosi vena cava-arteria polmonare nella tetrade di Fallot e in altre cardiopatie. *Minerva Cardioangiol*, 1961, 9, 577–93.
[47] Haller, JA; Adkins, JC; Rauenhorst, J. Total bypass of the superior vena cava into both lungs. *Surg Forum*, 1964, 15, 264–265.
[48] Azzolina, G; Eufrate, S; Pensa, P. Tricuspid atresia: experience in surgical management with a modified cavopulmonary anastomosis. *Thorax*, 27, 111-115, 1972.
[49] Backer, CL. The Fontan procedure: our odyssey continues. *J Am Coll Cardiol*, 2008, 52, 114-16.
[50] Kreutzer, G; Galindez, E; Bono, H; et al. An operation for the correction of tricuspid atresia. *J Thorac Cardiovasc Surg*, 1973, 66, 613-21.
[51] Sanchez-Quintana, D; Climent, V; Ho, SY; et al. Myoarchitecture and connective tissue in hearts with tricuspid atresia. *Heart*, 1999, 81, 182–191.
[52] Doty, DB; Marvin, WJ; Lauer, RM. Modified Fontan procedure: methods to achieve direct anastomosis of the right atrium to pulmonary artery. *J Thorac Cardiovasc Surg*, 1981, 81, 470-5.
[53] Kreutzer, GO; Vargas, FJ; Schlichter, A; et al. Atriopulmonary anastomosis. *J Thorac Cardiovasc Surg*, 1982, 83, 427-36.
[54] Puga, FJ; Chavareli, M; Hagler, DJ. Modification of the Fontan operation applicable to patients with left atrioventricular valve atresia or single atrioventricular valve. *Circulation*, 1987,76, III-53-60.
[55] Jonas, RA; Castaneda, AR. Modified Fontan procedure: Atrial baffle and systemic venous to pulmonary artery anastomosis techniques. *J Cardiac Surg*, 1988, 3, 91-96.
[56] Mayer, J; Helgason, H; Jonas, R; et al. Extending the limits for modified Fontan procedures. *J Thorac Cardiovasc Surg*, 1986, 92, 1021-8.

[57] Björk, VO; Olin, CL; Bjarke, BB; et al. Right atrial–right ventricular anastomosis for correction of tricuspid atresia. *J Thorac Cardiovasc Surg*, 1979,77, 452.
[58] Bowman, FO; Malm, JR; Hayes, CJ; et al. Physiologic approach to surgery for tricuspid atresia. *Circulation*, 1978, 58, 83-6.
[59] Brock, R. Tricuspid atresia. A step toward corrective treatment. *J Thorac Cardiovasc Surg*, 1964,47, 17-25.
[60] Pennington, DG; Nouri, S; Ho, J; Secker-Walker, R; et al. Glenn shunt: long-term results and current role in congenital heart operations. *Ann Thorac Surg*, 1981, 31, 532—9.
[61] DeLeon, SY; Idriss, FS; Ilbawi, MN; et al. The role of the Glenn shunt in patients undergoing the Fontan operation. *J Thorac Cardiovasc Surg*, 1983, 85, 669–677.
[62] Hopkins, RA; Armstrong, BE; Serwer, GA; et al. Physiological rationale for a bidirectional cavopulmonary shunt: a versatile complement to the Fontan principle. *J Thorac Cardiovasc Surg*, 1985, 90, 391–8.
[63] Mazzera, E; Corno, A; Picardo, S; et al. Bidirectional cavopulmonary shunts: clinical application as staged or definitive palliation. *Ann Thorac Surg*, 1989, 47, 415–20.
[64] Kawashima, Y; Kitamura, S; Matsuda, H; Shimazaki, Y; Nakano, S; Hirose, H. Total cavopulmonary shunt operation in complex cardiac anomalies: a new operation. *J Thorac Cardiovasc Surg*, 1984, 87, 74-81.
[65] de Leval, M; Kilner, Ph; Gewillig, M; et al. Total cavopulmonary connection: a logical alternative to atriopulmonary connection for complex Fontan operations. *J Thorac Cardiovasc Surg*, 1988, 96, 682-95.
[66] Lamberti, JJ; Spicer, RL; Waldman, JD; et al. The bidirectional cavopulmonary shunt. *J Thorac Cardiovasc Surg*, 1990, 100, 22–9.
[67] Bridges, ND; Jonas, RA; Mayer, JE; et al. Bidirectional cavopulmonary anastomosis as interim palliation for high-risk Fontan candidates: early results. *Circulation*, 1990, 82 (Suppl. 5), 170–76.
[68] Kopf, GS; Laks, H; Stansel, HC; et al. Thirty-year follow-up of superior vena cava-pulmonary artery (Glenn) shunts. *J Thorac Cardiovasc Surg*, 1990, 100, 662-71.
[69] Castaneda, AR. From Glenn to Fontan: a continuing evolution. *Circulation*, 1992, 86 (Suppl. II), 80-4.
[70] Pridjian, AK; Mendelsohn, AM; Lupinetti, FM; et al. Usefulness of the bidirectional Glenn procedure as staged reconstruction for the functional single ventricle. *Am J Cardiol*, 1993,71, 959-62.
[71] Quero Jimenez, M; Maitre Azcárate, MJ; Brito, JM; et al. Anastomosis cavo-atriopulmonar. *Rev Esp Cardiol*, 1993, 46 (Supl. 2), 101-18
[72] Mainwaring, RD; Lamberti, JJ; Moore, JW. The bidirectional Glenn and Fontan procedures-integrated management of the patient with a functionally single ventricle. *Cardiol Young*, 1996, 6, 198-207.
[73] Fernandez Pineda, L; Cazzaniga, M; Villagrá, F; et al. La operación de Glenn bidireccional en 100 casos con cardiopatías congénitas complejas. Factores determinantes del resultado quirúrgico. *Rev Esp Cardiol*, 2001, 54, 1061-74.
[74] Douville, EC; Sade, RM; Fyfe, DA. Hemi-Fontan operation in surgery for single ventricle: a preliminary report. *Ann Thorac Surg*, 1991, 51, 893-900.
[75] Marcelletti, C; Corno, A; Giannico, S; et al. Inferior vena cava-pulmonary extracardiac conduit: a new right ventricular by-pass. *J Thorac Cardiovasc Surg*, 1990, 100, 228-32.

[76] Bridges, N; Lock, JE; Castaneda, A. Baffle fenestration with subsequent transcatheter closure: modification for the Fontan operation for patients at increased risk. *Circulation*, 1990, 82, 1681-9.
[77] Bridges, ND; Mayer, JE Jr.; Lock, JE; et al. Effect of baffle fenestration on outcome of the modified Fontan operation. *Circulation*, 1992, 86, 1762–69.
[78] Lemler, MS; Scott, WA; Leonard, SR; Stromberg, D; Ramaciotti, C. Fenestration improves clinical outcome of the fontan procedure: a prospective, randomized study. *Circulation*, 2002, 105, 207–12.
[79] Burke, R; Jacobs, J; Ashraf, M; et al. Extracardiac Fontan operation without cardiopulmonary bypass. *Ann Thorac Surg*, 1997, 63, 1175-7.
[80] Norwood, WI Jr. Hypoplastic left heart syndrome. *Ann Thorac Surg*, 1991, 52, 688-95.
[81] Norwood, WI Jr. Jacobs, ML; Murphy, JD. Fontan procedure for hypoplastic left heart syndrome. *Ann Thorac Surg*, 1992, 54, 1025-30.
[82] Norwood, WI Jr.; Jacobs, ML. Fontan´s procedure in two stages. *Am J Surg*, 1993,166, 548-51.
[83] Jacobs, ML; Norwood, WI Jr. Fontan operation: influence of modifications on morbidity and mortality. *Ann Thorac Surg*, 1994, 58, 945-52.
[84] Koutlas, TC; Gaynor, JW; Nicolson, SC; et al. Modified Ultrafiltration reduces postoperative morbidity after cavopulmonary connection. *Ann Thorac Surg*, 1997, 64, 37–43.
[85] Hiramatsu, T; Imai, Y; Kurosawa, H; et al. Effects of dilutional and modified ultrafiltration in plasma endothelin-1 and pulmonary vascular resistance after the Fontan procedure. *Ann Thorac Surg*, 2002, 73, 862–85.
[86] Billingsley, AM; Laks, H; Boyce, SW. Definitive repair in patients with pulmonary atresia and intact ventricular septum. *J Thorac Cardiovasc Surg*, 1989, 97, 46-54.
[87] Van Arsdell, G; Williams, W; Maser, C; et al. Superior vena cava to pulmonary artery anastomosis: an adjunct to biventricular repair. *J Thorac Cardiovasc Surg*, 1996, 112, 1143-9.
[88] Gewillig, M. The Fontan circulation. *Heart*, 2005, 91, 839–46.-
[89] Gewillig, M; Brown, SC; Heying, H; et al. Congenital volume load paradox while preparing for the Fontan: not too much for the ventricle, not too little for the lungs. *Interact Cardiovasc Thorac Surg,* 2010, 10, 262–5.
[90] Redington, A. The physiology of the Fontan circulation. *Progr Pediatr Cardiol*, 2006, 22, 179-86.
[91] Bull, K. The Fontan procedure: lessons from the past. *Heart*, 1998, 79, 213-4.
[92] La Gerche, A; Gewillig, M. What limits cardiac performance during exercise in normal subjects and in healthy Fontan patients?. *Inter J Pediatr*, 2010, 791291, 1-8.
[93] Gewillig, M. Ventricular dysfunction of the functionally univentricular heart: management and outcomes. *Cardiol Young*, 2005, 15, 31–34.
[94] Gewillig, M; Brown, S; Eyskensa, B. The Fontan circulation: who controls cardiac output?. *Interact Cardiovasc Thorac Surg*, 2010, 10, 428-33.
[95] Scwartz, SM; Dent, LC; Musa, ML; et al. Single ventricle physiology. *Crit Care Clin*, 2003, 19, 393-41.
[96] Choussat, A; Fontan, F; Besse, P; et al. Selection criteria for Fontan's procedure. In: Anderson RH, Shinebourne EA, eds. Pediatric Cardiology. Edinburgh: Churchill Livingstone, NY 1978, pp 559-66.

[97] Graham, TP; Jr. Johns, JA. Preoperative assessment of ventricular in patients considered for Fontan procedure. *Herz*, 1992, 17, 213-9.

[98] Kirklin, J; Blackstone, E; Pacifico, A. The Fontan operation: ventricular hypertrophy, age and date of operation as a risk factor. *J Thorac Cardiovasc Surg*, 1986, 92, 1049-64.

[99] Driscoll, D; Offord, K; Feldt, R; et al. Five- to fifteen-year follow-up after Fontan operation. *Circulation*, 1992, 85, 469-96.

[100] Stern, HJ. Fontan "ten commandments". Revisited and revised. *Pediatr Cardiol*, 2010, 31, 1131-4.

[101] Feinstein, JA; Benson, DW; Dubin, AM; et al. Hypoplastic left heart syndrome. Current considerations and expectations. *J Am Coll Cardiol*, 2012, 59 (Suppl. S), S1-S42.

[102] Said, SM; Burkhart, HM; Dearani, JA. The Fontan connections: past, present and future. *World J Pediatr Cong Heart Surg*, 2012, 3, 171-82.

[103] Maroto Monedero, C; Camino Lopez, M; Girona, JM; et al. Guías de práctica clínica de la Sociedad Española de Cardiología en las cardiopatías congénitas del recién nacido. *Rev Esp Cardiol*, 2001, 54, 49-66.

[104] Caffarena, JM; Jr. Gómez Ullate, JM. Corazón univentricular con estenosis subaórtica. Paliación en el recién nacido. *Cir Cardiov*, 1997, 4, 48-55.

[105] Jaquiss, RDB; Imamura, M. Single ventricle physiology, surgical options, indications and outcomes. *Curr Opin Cardiol*, 2009, 24, 113-8.

[106] Cazzaniga, M; Vazquez Martinez, JL. Protocols SECPCC. Cap. 28, pp 377-415. Atresia tricúspide y corazón univentricular, 2010, www.secardioped.org.

[107] Berg, C; Lachmann, R; Kaiser, C; et al. Prenatal diagnosis of tricuspid atresia, intrauterine course and outcome. *Ultrasound Obstet Gynecol*, 2010, 35, 183–190.

[108] Wald, RM; Tham, EB; McCrindle Outcome after prenatal diagnosis of tricuspid atresia, a multicenter experience. *Am Heart J*, 2007, 153, 772–778.

[109] Donofrio, MT; Bremer, YA; Moskowitz, WB. Diagnosis and management of restricted or closed foramen ovale in fetuses with congenital heart disease. *Am J Cardiol*, 2004, 94, 1348–1351.

[110] Cazzaniga, M; Sabadell, C; Castellanos, P; et al. Diagnóstico prenatal del corazón univentricular. *Prog Obstet Ginecol*, 2001, 44, 132-7.

[111] Tham, EBC; Wald, R; McElhinney, DB; et al. Outcome of fetuses and infants with double inlet single ventricle. *Am J Cardiol*, 2008, 101, 1652-6.

[112] Roman, KS; Fouron, JC; Nii, M; et al. Determinants of outcome in fetal pulmonary valve stenosis or atresia with intact ventricular septum. *Am J Cardiol*, 2007, 99, 699-703.

[113] Gill, HK; Splitt, M; Sharland, GK; et al. Patterns of recurrence congenital heart disease: an analysis of 6,640 consecutive pregnancies evaluated by detailed fetal echocardiography. *J Am Coll Cardiol*, 2003, 42, 923-9.

[114] Weigel, TJ; Driscoll, DJ; Michels, VV. Occurrence of congenital heart defects in siblings of patients with univentricular heart and tricuspid atresia. *Am J Cardiol*, 1989, 64, 768-71.

[115] Nelle, M; Raio, L; Pavlovic, M; et al. Prenatal diagnosis and treatment planning of congenital heart defects - possibilities and limits. *World J Pediatr Congenit Heart Surg*, 2009, 5, 18-22.

[116] Stasik, CN; Goldberg, CS; Bove, EL; et al. Current outcomes and risk factors for the Norwood procedure. *J Thorac Cardiovasc Surg*, 2006, 131, 412-7.

[117] Ohye, RG; Sleeper, LA; Mahony, L; et al. Comparison of shunt types in the Norwood procedure for single-ventricle lesions. *N Eng J Med*, 2010,19, 648-56.

[118] Shimada, M; Hoashi, T; Kagisaki, K; et al. Clinical outcomes of prophylactic Damus-Kaye-Stansel anastomosis concomitant with bidirectional Glenn procedure. *J Thorac Cardiovasc Surg*, 2012,143, 137-43.

[119] Fiore, AC; Rodefeld, M; Vijay, P; et al. Subaortic obstruction in univentricular heart, results using the double barrel Damus-Kaye-Stansel operation. *Eur J Cardiothorac Surg*, 2009, 35, 141-148.

[120] McElhinney, DB; Reddy, VM; Silverman, NH; Hanley, FL. Modified Damus-Kaye-Stansel procedure for single ventricle, subaortic stenosis, and arch obstruction in neonates and infants: midterm results and techniques for avoiding circulatory arrest. *J Thorac Cardiovasc Surg*, 1997,114, 718-26.

[121] Heinle, JS; Carberry, KE; McKenzie, ED; et al. Outcomes after the palliative arterial switch operation in neonates with single-ventricle anatomy. *Ann Thorac Surg*, 2013, 95, 212-9.

[122] Takayama, H; Sekiguchi, A; Chikada, M; e al. Mortality of pulmonary artery banding in the current era, recent mortality of PA banding. *Ann Thorac Surg*, 2002, 74, 1219-24.

[123] Bradley, SM; Simsic, JM; Atz, AM; et al. The infant with single ventricle and excessive pulmonary blood flow: results of strategy of pulmonary artery division and shunt. *Ann Thorac Surg*, 2002, 74, 805-10.

[124] McKenzie, ED; Khan, MS; Samayoa, AX; et al. The Blalock-Taussig shunt revisited: a contemporary experience. *J Am Coll Surg*, 2013,216, 699-06.

[125] Gewillig, M; Boshoff, DE; Dens, J; et al. Stenting the neonatal arterial duct in duct-dependent pulmonary circulation: new techniques, better results. *J Am Coll Cardiol*, 2004, 43, 107-12.

[126] Gérelli, S; Boulitrop, C; Van Steenberghe, M; et al. Bidirectional cavopulmonary shunt with additional pulmonary blood flow: a failed or successful strategy?. *Eur J Cardiothorac Surg*, 2012,42, 513-9.

[127] Ferns, SJ; El Zein, C; Multani, K; et al. Is additional pulsatile pulmonary blood flow beneficial to patients with bidirectional Glenn?. *J Thorac Cardiovasc Surg*, 2013, 145, 451-4.

[128] Petrossian, E; Reddy; V; McElhinney, D; et al. Early results of the extracardiac conduit Fontan operation. *J Thorac Cardiovasc Surg*, 1999, 117, 688-96.

[129] Stewart, RD; Pasquali, SK; Jacobs, JP; et al. Contemporary Fontan operation: association between early outcome and type of cavopulmonary connection. *Ann Thorac Surg*, 2012, 93, 1254-61.

[130] Backer, CL; Deal, BJ; Kaushal, S; et al. Extracardiac vs. intra-atrial lateral tunnel Fontan: extracardiac is better. *Semin Thorac Cardiovasc Surg Pediatr Card Surg Annu*, 2001, 14, 4-10.

[131] Petrossian, E, Reddy, VM; Collins, KK; et al. The extracardiac conduit Fontan operation using minimal approach extracorporeal circulation: early and midterm outcomes. *J Thorac Cardiovasc Surg*, 2006, 132, 1054-63.

[132] Almond, ChSD; Mayer, JE Jr.; Thiagarajan, RR; et al. Outcome after Fontan failure and takedown to an intermédiate palliative circulation. *Ann Thorac Surg*, 2007, 84, 880-7.

[133] Hausdorf, G; Schneider, M; Konertz, W. Surgical preconditioning and completion of total cavopulmonary connection by interventional cardiac catheterisation: a new concept. *Heart*, 1996, 75, 403-9.

[134] Goldberg, DJ; Dodds, K; Rychik, J. New concepts: development of a survivorship programme for patients with a functionally univentricular heart. *Cardiol Young*, 2011, 21 (Suppl. 2), 77-9.

[135] Jacobs, ML. Late complications associated with the Fontan circulation. *Cardiol Young*, 2006, 16 (Suppl. 1), 80-4.

[136] Rychik, J. Forty years of the Fontan operation: a failed strategy. *Sem Thorac Cardiovasc Surg Pediatr Card Surg Annu*, 2010,13, 96-100.

[137] Mondèsert, B; Marcotte, F; Mongeon, FP; et al. Fontan circulation: success or failure?. *Can J Cardiol*, 2013, 29, 811-20.

[138] Lastinger, L; Zaidi, AN. The adult with a Fontan: a panacea without a cure?. *Circ J*, 2013, 77, 2672-81.

[139] Kaulitz, R; Ziemer, G; Paul, Th; et al. Fontan-type procedures: residual lesions and late interventions. *Ann Thorac Surg*, 2002, 74, 778-85.

[140] Atik E. Fontan operation: reflections on its current evolution and perspectives. *Arq Bras Cardiol*, 2006, 87, e72-e74.

[141] Freedom, RM; Hamilton, R; Yoo, S-J; et al. The Fontan procedure: analysis of cohorts and late complications. *Cardiol Young*, 2000, 10, 307-31.

[142] Chung, T. Assessment of cardiovascular anatomy in patients with congenital heart disease by magnetic resonance imaging. *Pediatr Cardiol*, 2000, 21, 18-26.

[143] Deal, B; Jacobs, M. Management of the failing Fontan circulation. *Heart*, 2012, 98, 1098-04.

[144] O´Donnell, CP; Landzberg, MJ. The "failing" Fontan circulation. *Progr Pediatr Cardiol*, 2002, 16, 105-14.

[145] Huddleston, CB. The failing Fontan: options for surgical therapy. *Pediatr Cardiol*, 2007, 28, 472-76.

[146] Martin, LD; Joffe, DC; Richards, M. An update on the Fontan operation: morbidity, mortality and late complications. *Congenit Cardiac Anesth Soc,* 2011, www.ccasociety.org.

[147] McRae, ME. Long-term issues after Fontan procedure. *Adv Crit Care*, 2013, 24, 264-82.

[148] Gentles, T; Mayer, JE Jr. Gauvreau, K; et al. Fontan operation in five hundred consecutive patients: early and late outcome. *J Thorac Cardiovasc Surg*, 1997, 30, 1032-8.

[149] Lan, Y; Chang, R; Laks, H. Outcome of patients with double-inlet left ventricle or tricuspid atresia with transposed great arteries. *J Am Coll Cardiol*, 2004, 43, 113-9.

[150] Cazzaniga, M; Fernandez Pineda, L; Villagrá, F; et al. Single-stage Fontan procedure: early and late outcome in 124 patients. *Rev Esp Cardiol*, 2002, 55, 391-412.

[151] Khairy, P; Fernandes, SM; Mayer, JE; Jr. et al. Long-term survival, modes of death, and predictors of mortality in patients with Fontan surgery. *Circulation*, 2008, 117, 85-92.

[152] Earing, MG; Cetta, F; Driscoll, DJ; et al. Long-term results of the Fontan for double inlet left ventricle. *Am J Cardiol*, 2005, 96, 291-98.

[153] Mair, D; Puga, F; Danielson, G. The Fontan procedure for tricuspid atresia: early and late results of a 25-year experience with 216 patients. *J Am Coll Cardiol*, 2001, 37, 933-9.

[154] Stamm, C; Friehs, I; Mayer, JE; et al. Long-term results of the lateral tunnel operation. *J Thorac Cardiovasc Surg*, 2001, 121, 28-41.

[155] Schreiber, C; Horere, J; Vogt, M; et al. Nonfenestrated extracardiac total cavopulmonary connection in 132 consecutive patients. *Ann Thorac Surg*, 2007, 84, 894-99.

[156] Paridon, SM; Mitchell, PD; Colan, SD; et al. A cross-sectional study of exercise performance during the first 2 decades of life after the Fontan operation. *J Am Coll Cardiol*, 2008, 52, 99-107.

[157] Diller, GP; Giardini, A; Dimopoulos, K; et al. Predictors of morbidity and mortality in contemporary Fontan patients: results from a multicenter study including cardiopulmonary exercise testing in 321 patients. *Eur Heart J*, 2010, 31, 3073–83.

[158] van den Bosch, AE; Roos-Hesselink, JW; van Domburg, R; et al. Long-term outcome and quality of life in adult patients after the Fontan operation. *Am J Cardiol*, 2004, 93, 1141-5.

[159] Anderson, PA; Sleeper, LA; Mahony, L; et al. Contemporary outcomes after de Fontan procedure: a Pediatric Heart Network multicenter study. *J Am Coll Cardiol*, 2008, 52, 85-98.

[160] Williams, IA; Sleeper, LA; Colan, S; et al. Functional state following the Fontan procedure. *Cardiol Young*, 2009, 19, 320-30.

[161] Gersony, WM. Fontan operation after 3 decades. What we have learned. *Circulation*, 2008, 117, 13-15.

[162] McCrindle, BW; Williams, RV; Mitchell, PD; et al. Pediatric Heart Network Investigators: Relationship of patient and medical characteristics to health status in children and adolescents after Fontan procedure. *Circulation*, 2006, 113, 1123-29.

[163] Wernovsky, G. Current insights regarding neurological and development abnormalities in children and young adults with complex congenital heart disease. *Cardiol Young*, 2006, 16 (Suppl. 1), 92-104.

[164] Forbess, J; Visconti, K; Bellinger, D; Jonas, R. Neurodevelopmental outcomes in children after Fontan operation. *Circulation*, 2001, 104, I-127-32.

[165] Knott-Craig, C; Danielson, G; Schaff, H; et al. The modified Fontan operation: an analysis of risk factors for early postoperative death or takedown in 702 consecutive patients from one institution. *J Thorac Cardiovasc Surg*, 1995,109, 1237-43.

[166] Balaji, S; Gewillig, M; Bull, C; et al. Arrhythmias after the Fontan procedure: comparison of total cavopulmonary connection and atriopulmonary anastomosis. *Circulation*, 1991, 84 (Suppl. 2), 162-7.

[167] Giannakoulas, G; Dimopoulos, K; Yuksel, S; et al. Atrial tachyarrhythmias late after Fontan operation are related to increase in mortality and hospitalization. *Int J Cardiol, 2012*,157, 221-6.

[168] Fishberger, S; Wernovsky, G; Gentles, TH; et al. Factors that influence the development of atrial flutter after the Fontan operation. *J Thorac Cardiovasc Surg*, 1997, 113, 80-6.

[169] Gardiner, H; Dhillon, R; Bull, C; et al. Prospective study of the incidence and determinant of arrhythmia after total cavopulmonary connection. *Circulation*, 1996, 94 (Suppl. 2), 17-21.
[170] Cohen, MS; Wernovsky, G; Vetter, V; et al. Sinus node function after systematically staged Fontan procedure. *Circulation*, 1998, 98, II352-8.
[171] Lee, JR; Keak, J; Kim, KC; et al. Comparison of lateral tunnel and extracardiac conduit Fontan procedure. *Interact Cardiovasc Thorac Surg*, 2007, 6, 328-30.
[172] Balaji, S; Daga, A; Bradley, DJ; et al. An international multicenter study comparing arrhythmia prevalence between the intracardiac lateral tunnel and the extracardiac conduit type of Fontan operations. *J Thorac Cardiovasc Surg*, 2013 S0022-5223(13)01067.
[173] Brown, JW; Ruzmetov, M; Deschner, BW; Rodefeld, MD; Turrentine; MW. Lateral tunnel Fontan in the current era: is it still a good option?. *Ann Thorac Surg*, 2010 Feb; 89,556-63.
[174] Backer, CL; Deal, BJ; Mavroudis, C; et al. Conversion of the failed Fontan circulation. *Cardiol Young*, 2006, 16 (Suppl. 1), 85-91
[175] Mavroudis, C; Backer, CL; Deal, BJ. Late reoperations for Fontan patients: state of the art invited review. *Eur J Cardiothorac Surg*, 2008, 34, 1034-40.
[176] Marcelletti, C; Hanley, F; Mavroudis, C; et al. Revision of previous Fontan connections to total extracardiac cavopulmonary anastomosis: a multicenter experience. *J Thorac Cardiovasc Surg*, 2000, 199, 340-6.
[177] Feldt, RH; Driscoll, DJ; Offord, KP; et al. Protein-losing enteropathy after the Fontan operation. *J Thorac Cardiovasc Surg*, 1996, 112, 672-80.
[178] Mertens, L; Hagler, DJ; Sauer, U; et al. Protein-losing enteropathy after the Fontan operation: an international multicenter study. PLE study group. *J Thorac Cardiovasc Surg*; 1998; 115; 1063-73.
[179] Johnson, JN; Driscoll, DJ; O'Leary, PW. Protein-Losing Enteropathy and the Fontan operation. *Nutr Clin Pract*, 2012, 27, 375-84.
[180] Rueda, J; Zoiro; E; Arnau; MA; et al. Resolución de enteropatía pierde proteínas tras el trasplante cardiaco en pacientes jóvenes. *Rev Esp Cardiol*, 2009, 62, 937-940.
[181] Camarero, C; Tamariz, R; García Trujillo, JA; et al. Enteropatía pierde-proteínas tras operación de Fontan. *An Pediatr (Barc)*; 2001; 54; (Supl. 3); 39-42.
[182] Chin, AJ; Stephens, P; Goldmuntz, E; et al. Serum alkaline phosphatase reflects post-Fontan hemodynamics in children. *Pediatr Cardiol*, 2009, 30, 138-45.
[183] Seear, M; Hui, H; Magee, F; et al. Bronchial casts in children: a proposed classification based on nine cases and review of the literature. *Am J Respir Crit Care Med*, 1997,155, 364-70.
[184] Wilson, J; Russel, J; Williams, W; Benson; L. Fenestration of the Fontan circuit as treatment for plastic bronchitis. *Pediatr Cardiol*, 2005, 26, 717-9.
[185] Larue, M; Gossett, JG; Stewart, RD; et al. Plastic bronchitis in patients with fontan physiology: review of the literature and preliminary experience with fontan conversion and cardiac transplantation. *World J Pediatr Congenit Heart Surg*, 2012, 3, 364-72.
[186] Grutter, G; Di Carlo, D. Plastic bronchitis after extracardiac Fontan operation: further evidence *Ann Thorac Surg*, 2013, 95, 2214-5.
[187] Racz, J; Mane, G; Ford, M; et al. Immunophenotyping and protein profiling of Fontan-associated plastic bronchitis airway casts. *Ann Am Thorac Soc*, 2013,10, 98-107.

[188] Mendoza Soto, A; Galletti, P; Gomez de Quero, MV; et al. Bronquitis plástica. A propósito de un caso y revisión de los casos asociados a cirugía de Fontan. *An Pediatr (Barc)*, 2005, 62, 72-5.
[189] Van Nieuwenhuizen, R; Peteres, M; Lubbers, L; et al. Abnormalities in liver function and coagulation profile following the Fontan procedure. *Heart*, 1999, 82, 40-6.
[190] Odegard, K; McGowan, F; Zurakowski, D; et al. Procoagulant and anticoagulant factor abnormalities following the Fontan procedure: increased factor VIII may predispose to thrombosis. *J Thorac Cardiovasc Surg*, 2003, 125, 1260-7.
[191] Kaulitz, R; Ziemer, G; Bergmann, F; et al. Atrial thrombus after the Fontan-operation. Predisposing factors, treatment and prophylaxis. *Cardiol Young*, 1997, 7, 37-43.
[192] Grewal, J; Al Hussein, M; Feldstein; J. et al. Evaluation of silent thrombus after the Fontan operation. *Congenit Heart Dis*, 2013, 8, 40-7.
[193] Varma, C; Warr, MR; Hendler, AL; et al. Prevalence of "silent" pulmonary emboli in adults after the Fontan operation. *J Am Coll Cardiol*, 2003, 41, 2252-8.
[194] Marrone, C; Galasso, G; Piccolo, R; et al. Antiplatelet versus anticoagulation therapy after extracardiac conduit Fontan: a systematic review and meta-analysis. *Pediatr Cardiol*, 2011, 32, 32-9.
[195] Jacobs, ML; Pourmoghadam, KK. Thromboembolism and the role of anticoagulation in the Fontan patient. *Pediatr Cardiol*, 2007, 28, 457-64.
[196] Kiesewetter, CH; Sheron, N; Vettukattill, JJ; et al. Hepatic changes in the failing Fontan circulation. *Heart*, 2007, 93, 579-84.
[197] Rychik, J; Veldtman, G; Rand, E; et al. The precarious state of the liver after a Fontan operation: summary of a multidisciplinary symposium. *Pediatr Cardiol*, 2012, 33, 1001-12.
[198] Schwartz, MC; Sullivan, LM; Glatz, AC; et al. Portal and sinusoidal fibrosis are common on liver biopsy after Fontan surgery. *Pediatr Cardiol*, 2013, 34, 135-42.
[199] Mahle, WT; Border, WL. Fifty years of surgery for single ventricle: now what ?. *J Pediatr*, 2012, 16, 186-90.
[200] Ono, M; Boethig, D; Goerler, H; et al. Clinical outcome of patients 20 years after Fontan operation – effect of fenestration on late morbidity. *Eur J Cardiothorac Surg*, 2006, 30, 923-9.
[201] McElhinney, DB; Marx, GR; Newburger, JW. Congenital portosystemic venous connections and other abdominal venous abnormalities in patients with polysplenia and functionally univentricular heart disease: a case series and literature review. *Congenit Heart Dis*, 2011, 6, 28-40.
[202] Garrido-Lestache, E; Cazzaniga, M; Perez de León, J. Hepato-left atrial vein causing cyanosis after bicavopulmonary shunt. *Rev Fed Arg Cardiol*, 2012, 41, 121-3.
[203] Grosse-Wortmann, L; Al-Otay, A; Yoo, S-J. Aortopulmonary collaterals after bidirectional cavopulmonary connection or Fontan completion: quantification with MRI. *Cir Cardiovasc Imaging*, 2009, 2, 219-25.
[204] Banka, P; Sleeper, LA; Atz, AM; et al. Practice variability and outcomes of coil embolization of aortopulmonary collaterals prior to Fontan completion: a report from the Pediatric Heart Network Fontan Cross-Sectional Study. *Am Heart J*, 2011,162, 125-30.

[205] Anderson, PA; Breitbart, RE; McCrindle, BW; et al. The Fontan patient: inconsistencies in medication therapy across seven Pediatric Heart Network centers. *Pediatr Cardiol*, 2010, 31, 1219-28.
[206] Senzaki, H; Masutani, S; Kobayashi, J; et al. Ventricular afterload and ventricular work in Fontan circulation: comparison with two-ventricle circulation and single ventricle circulation with Blalock-Taussig shunt. *Circulation*, 2002,105, 2885-92.
[207] Nakamura, Y; Yagihara, T; Kagisaki, K; et al. Ventricular performance in long-term survivors after Fontan operation. *Ann Thorac Surg*, 2011, 91, 172-80.
[208] Davies, RR; Chen, JM; Mosca, RS. The Fontan procedure: evolution in technique, attendant imperfections and transplantation for "failure". *Semin Thorac Cardiovasc Surg Pediatr Card Surg Annu*, 2011,14, 55-66.
[209] Davies, RR; Sorabella, RA; Yang, J; et al. Outcomes after transplantation for "failed" Fontan, a single-institution experience. *J Thorac Cardiovasc Surg*, 2012 ,143, 1183-92.
[210] Burkhart, HM; Dearani, JA; Mair, DD; et al. The modified Fontan procedure: early and late results in 132 adult patients. *J Thorac Cardiovasc Surg*, 2003,125, 1252-9.
[211] Ovroutski, S; Alexi-Meskishvili, V; Ewerta, P; et al. Early and medium-term results after modified Fontan operation in adults. *Eur J Cardiothorac Surg*, 2003, 23 311–6.
[212] Veldtman, GR; Nishimoto, A; Siu, S; et al. The Fontan procedure in adults. *Heart*, 2001, 86, 330–5.
[213] Day, RW; Etheridge, SP; Veasy, GL; et al. Single ventricle palliation, greater risk of complications with the Fontan procedure than with the bidirectional Glenn procedure alone. *Int J Cardiol*, 2006, 106, 201-10.
[214] Heh, Th; Williams, W; McCrindle, B; et al. Equivalent survival following cavopulmonary anastomosis shunt: with or without procedure. *Eur J Cardiothorac Surg*, 1999, 16, 111-6.
[215] Mahle, WT; Todd, K; Fyfe, DA. Endothelial function following the Fontan operation. *Am J Cardiol*, 2003, 91, 1286-88.
[216] Mitchell, MB; Campbell, DN; Ivy, D; et al. Evidence of pulmonary vascular disease after heart transplantation for Fontan circulation failure. *J Thorac Cardiovasc Surg*, 2004,128, 693-72.
[217] Giardini, A; Balducci, A; Specchia, S; et al. Effect of sildenafil on hemodynamic response to exercise and exercise capacity in Fontan patients. *Eur Heart J*, 2008, 29, 1681-7.
[218] de Zèlicourt, DA; Marsden, A; Fogel, MA; et al. Imaging and patient-specific simulations for the Fontan surgery: current methodologies and clinical applications. *Progr Pediatr Cardiol*, 2010, 30, 31-44.
[219] Lacour-Gayet, FG; Lanning, CJ; Stoica, S; et al. An artificial right ventricle for failing Fontan: in vitro and computational study. *Ann Thorac Surg*, 2009, 88, 170-6.
[220] Rodefeld, MD; Boyd, JH; Myers, CD; et al. Cavopulmonary assist, circulatory support for the univentricular circulation. *Ann Thorac Surg*, 2003, 76, 1911-6.
[221] Throckmorton, Al; Ballman, KK; Myers, CD; et al. Mechanical cavopulmonary assist for univentricular fontan circulation using a novel propeller blood pump. *ASAIO J*, 2007,53, 734-41.
[222] David, L; Mallet, C; Keramidas, M. Bone morphogenetic protein-9 is a circulating vascular quiescence factor. *Cir Res*, 2008, 102, 914-22.

[223] Chin, AJ; Whitehead, KK; Watrous, RL. Insights after 40 years of the Fontan operation. *World J Pediatr Congenit Heart Surg*, 2010, 1, 328-43.

[224] Kodo, K; Yamagishi, H. A decade of advances in the molecular embryology and genetics underlyng congenital heart defects. *Circ J*, 2011, 75, 2296-04.

[225] Kim, GB; Kwon, BS; Bae, EJ; et al. Significance of circulating hepatocyte growth factor in protein-losing enteropathy after Fontan operation. *Pediatr Cardiol*, 2011, 32, 917-23.

[226] Grattan, MJ; McCrindle, BW. Recurrent exacerbations of protein-losing enteropathy after initiation of growth hormone therapy in a Fontan patient controlled with spironolactone. *Congenit Heart Dis*, 2010, 5, 165-7.

[227] Olson, EN. Gene regulatory networks in the evolution of the heart. *Science*, 2006, 313, 1922-7.

[228] Srivastava, D; Olson, NE. Gene regulatory networks in the evolution of the heart. *Nature,* 2000, 407, 221-6.

[229] Opotowsky, AR; Siddiqi, OK; Webb, GD. Trends in hospitalization for adults with congenital heart disease in the U.S. *J Am Coll Cardiol*, 2009,54, 460-7

[230] Cannobio, MM; Mair, D; van der Velde, M; Koos, B. Pregnancy outcomes after Fontan repair. *J Am Coll Cardiol*, 1996, 28, 1126-32.

[231] Cohen, M; Bush, D; Ferry, RJ; et al. Somatic growth failure after the Fontan operation. *Cardiol Young*, 2000, 10, 438-9.

[232] Pike, NA; Evangelista, LS; Doering, LV; et al. Clinical profile of the adolescent and adult Fontan survivor. *Congenit Heart Dis*, 2011, 6, 9-17.

[233] Baumgartner, H; Bonhoeffer, P; de Groot, NM; et al. ESC Guidelines for the management of grown-up congenital heart disease (new version 2010). *Eur Heart J*, 2010, 31, 2915-57.

[234] Ladouceur, M; Dugardin, B; Gourdin, S; et al. Loan applications in adult patients with congenital heart disease: a French study. *Arch Cardiovasc Dis*, 2011, 104, 375-80.

In: Congenital Heart Diseases
Editor: Raúl Cayré and José Milei
ISBN: 978-1-61122-003-2

Chapter 9

Restrictive Cardiomyopathy in Children

***Alejandra Villa*[1*] *and Marisa Di Santo*[2,†]**
[1]Head of Echocardiography.Cardiology Department.Hospital de Pediatria J.P. Garrahan, Buenos Aires, Argentina
[2]Head Pediatric Cardiology. Hospital Universitario FundacionFavaloro, Buenos Aires, Argentina

Abstract

Restrictive cardiomyopathy is a rare disease in childhood characterized by ventricular diastolic dysfunction usually with preserved systolic function, with a progressive clinical course and poor outcome. This chapter reviews the definition, epidemiology, genetics, natural history, clinical presentation, role of diagnostic tools, outcome, and current management of pediatric populations with this uncommon disease based on our clinical experience and literature studies. Restrictive cardiomyopathy in childhood is a rare entity with high mortality rates that still arises controversy around its definition and treatment. The stratification of risk factors for sudden death, cardiac failure, thromboembolic events and increase in pulmonary vascular resistance requires prospective longitudinal studies with large pediatric populations in order to acquire better knowledge of the course and outcome of this disease. The identification of specific genetic mutations is paving the way for a better understanding of the molecular pathology of restrictive disorders. This line of research will most probably lead to the design of new therapies that can delay or reduce the need for heart transplant.

Introduction

Cardiomyopathies (CM) are a heterogeneous group of diseases. There are many classifications in the literature and sometimes they are contradictory. One of the classifications that is important to mention is the one outlined by The European Society of

* E-mail: avilla@arnet.com.ar.
† E-mail: mdisanto@ffavaloro.org.

Cardiology. They proposed a clinically oriented classification system in which heart muscle disorders are grouped according to ventricular morphology and function. This classification has become the most useful method for diagnosing and describing a cardiomyopathy. Thus, a cardiomyopathy is defined as a myocardial disorder in which the heart muscle is structurally and functionally abnormal, in the absence of coronary artery disease, hypertension, valvular disease and congenital heart disease, sufficient to cause the observed myocardial abnormality.

In this chapter we will focus on the restrictive cardiomyopathy (RCM), which is a disease of the myocardium with diastolic dysfunction as the principal abnormality specifically, restricted ventricular filling [1].

Definition and Epidemiology

The World Health Organization (WHO) defines RCM as a myocardial disease characterized by restrictive filling and reduced diastolic volume of either or both ventricles with normal or near-normal systolic function and wall thickness. But why is still difficult in daily practice to classify patients with RCM?

1. Probably because of the use by the American Heart Association (AHA) and the WHO of such terms of poor specificity as ‘mild hypertrophy’ and ‘near normal diastolic volume’, which seem to be left to individual medical judgment as to what exactly is ‘mild’ or ‘near normal’.
2. Because the term restrictive cardiomyopathy is based on the description of the ventricular physiology and there are various conditions that can affect the filling of the heart, such as amyloidosis, sarcoidosis, carcinoid heart disease, scleroderma, anthracycline toxicity or other morphologic entities like hypertrophic cardiomyopathy (HCM), dilated (DCM) or left ventricular non-compaction [2].
3. Because although histology helps identifying primary and secondary forms of the disease, it is normally non-distinctive and can show normal findings or non-specific degenerative changes, including myocyte hypertrophy, disarray, a degree of interstitial fibrosis, and as much as 40% of cases look like hypertrophic cardiomyopathies (HCM).

RCM is a rare form of cardiomyopathy accounting for 2.5–5% of all idiopathic cardiomyopathies in childhood. [1-3]Although the exact prevalence is unknown.

A few series with limited number of patients have been published documenting the clinical course after the diagnosis of RCM in childhood. Due to the small size of patient population in these studies, its pathogenesis, natural history, and treatment are still object of research. Some investigators have divided RCM into the following subtypes: (1) pure restrictive cardiomyopathy; (2) hypertrophic-restrictive cardiomyopathy, and (3) mildly dilated restrictive cardiomyopathy. [4] This classification arises because even though restrictive cardiomyopathy (RCM) has been subclassified individually, evidence exists for considerable overlap between this entity and hypertrophic cardiomyopathy (HCM). Moreover, in the familial type of RCM, some family members present with mutations expressed as classic hypertrophic cardiomyopathy. [5] The prevalence of pure familial versus sporadic RCM is not known.The first sarcomeric protein for which mutations have been associated with restrictive cardiomyopathy is human cardiac troponin I (TNNI). The location of the mutation within different functional domains of TNNI results in different clinical phenotypes. RCM has also been associated with the intermediate filament protein Desmin abnormalities. The mechanism(s) by which these mutations affect muscle contraction are still being investigated [6].

Genetic

The last consensus of 2006 by the American Heart Association (AHA) [7] developed Contemporary Definitions and a Classification of the Cardiomyopathies. They list the known causes of RCM, however, in the pediatric population in most no specific cause has been identified with increasing reports of specific gene mutations in this age group.

In the past two decades, advances in molecular analysis have pointed out the important role of mutations in genes encoding sarcomeric proteins associated with RCM [8] and, although less frequent, with non-sarcomeric proteins such as desmin.

Sarcomeric Protein Disease and RCM

In the current era genetic investigations have revealed that RCM forms part of the hereditary sarcomeric contractile protein disease spectrum [5-8].

The most common mutations in the sarcomeric protein encoding gene were identified in *TNNI3* Beta-myosin heavy chain *(MYH7)*, *Troponin 2(TNNT2)*, and α-Cardiac actin (*ACTC)*.

It is necessary to briefly consider the normal regulation of muscle contraction [9].

The troponin complex, which is composed of three subunits, troponin C (TNNC), troponin I, and troponin T (TNNT), is located within the thin muscle filament, and its function is to control the interaction between the thick and thin filament during muscle contraction and relaxation, dependent on the intracellular concentration of Ca2+.

Troponin I binds to actin-tropomyosin and prevents muscle contraction by inhibiting actomyosin activity. This inhibitory effect is reversed by troponin C following binding of Ca2+, which introduces changes in the entire troponin complex. The myosin head is binding to actin and ATP to myosin, causing displacement of the myosin head along the thin filament and ATP hydrolysis, leading to muscle contraction. The mutations in sarcomeric proteins have the potential to cause alterations in thin muscle filament with an increase in Ca2+ concentration triggering disturbances in contraction, cardiomyopathy, arrhythmias, and sudden cardiac death (SCD) [10].

Specially mutations in troponin have been identified causing RCM. The subunit TNNT acts modulating actomyosin ATPase activity, Ca2 sensitivity of contraction, and maximal forcein muscle contraction, one of the main factors necessary for normal contraction. Sarcomeric protein gene mutations in the cardiac troponin I gene (TNNI3), in the troponin T (TNNT2), and α-Cardiac actin were the first mutations identified associated with RCM. [11] No mutation in the gene encoding for TNNC has been detected yet. [11] Histopathology from explanted hearts with a TNNT2 mutation shows interstitial fibrosis and myocyte disarray with loss of sarcomeric architecture.

The TNNT gene can express four different isoforms: isoform 1 is predominant in fetal hearts and isoform 3 in adult hearts, being the main difference between them the absence of exon 5 from the N-terminal domain of the adult isoform 3 present in the fetal heart [12].

In this aspect fetal troponin isoforms in the developing heart revealed a protective role in maintenance of normal physiological parameters during stress situations, such as acidosis. [12] The switch of TNNI can be seen on the fourth day after birth and goes on until day fourteen. Mutations in gene encoding for troponin I may produce serious effects just after birth explaining the symptoms and aggressive course.

Pinto et al. describe the protective role of fetal troponin (TN) isoforms and the way they rescue increased Ca2 sensitivity produced by a TNNT gene mutation in RCM, preventing lethality of the fetus during gestation [12].

During the development of the heart, TNNT is expressed continuously and thus, it is expected that RCM may manifest at the end of gestation or produce spontaneous abortions, which may explain why the conditions have not been completely identified yet. More than 20 mutations linked to RCM [10] have been reported in the genes of cardiac desmin, actin, myosin heavy chain, T troponin (TNNT), and troponin I (TNNI) compared to more than 900 mutations reported for HCM. [6] Nevertheless, several gene mutations in sarcomeric proteins have been reported in association with RCM, but they may cause the hypertrophic and dilated cardiomyopathy phenotype in some family members, showing a phenotypic overlap caused by the same underlying gene alteration [13].

Mogensen et al. identified a novel mutation in troponin I in a large family in which several individuals were affected by either hypertrophic or restrictive cardiomyopathy. The index case was an 11-year-old boy with IC. [8] The members of the family had HCM with only mild to moderate hypertrophy and the majority presented with enlarged atria and evidence of restrictive ventricular filling, suggesting phenotypic variability of the same mutation [8].

In a follow-up study by Mogensen et al. [8] and Kubo et al. [14] reported a group of adults with HCM and a restrictive phenotype. Eight of 15 patients had identifiable mutations of the sarcomeric genes, four in β- myosin heavy chain gene and four in troponin I. All eight patients had a bad prognosis.

Kaski et al. published a series of 12 pediatric patients with RCM, four of whom had a positive family history for cardiomyopathy, but with variable phenotypes including non-compaction cardiomyopathy and RCM. [11] The mutations identified were located in the troponin I (TNNI3), troponin T (TNNT2), and cardiac alpha-actin (ACTC) genes.

The diversity in phenotypic features of troponin expression in family members suggests that both genetic and environmental factors may play a role in the disease expression [15].

Alterations in other contractile proteins, such as β myosin, present a genotypic-phenotypic overlap as well. This has been shown in a report by Olson et al. [16] who described a mutation in myosin light chain causing cardiomyopathy with mild hypertrophy with a restrictive physiology which was inherited in an autosomal recessive manner. The index case was a boy with two older brothers who had cardiomyopathies with dilated atria and died due to thromboembolic complications. Clinically non-affected family members were heterozygotes or lacked the mutant allele.

Ware et al. described a β-myosin heavy chain mutation in an infant with RCM who received a heart transplant. [10] These β-myosin heavy chain mutations account for approximately 40 % of the mutations found in adults with HCM, but are infrequent in children. Phenotypicoverlap of RCM and non-compaction cardiomyopathy has also been observed and thus, this type of cardiomyopathy should also be looked for in children from families with RCM [17-19].

Non-Sarcomeric Protein Disease and RCM

Additionally to those of the sarcomeric proteins, cell structures of other proteins may be altered. Some examples are titin (TTN) and desmin mutations. [20, 21] Peled et al. first showed that TTN mutations may cause RCM. [20] The giant filament TTN is a determinant of a resting tension of the sarcomere and the study provides genetic evidence for its crucial role in diastolic function based on a family with six affected individuals between 12 and 35 years of age. Eighteen candidate genes for the alteration were studied. Sequence analysis identified a novel mutation in exon 266 of the TTN gene, resulting in a tyrosine by cysteine substitution p.Y7621C affects a highly preserved region of the protein within the fibronectin-3 domain, belonging to the A/I junction region of TTN [20].

Desmin mutations have been described associated with RCM and conduction anomalies, including AV block, as well as skeletal myopathy. [22] Inheritance may be autosomal dominant, or the mutations may be sporadic [22, 23] however, no large cohort studies have been conducted in pediatric patients with RMC and thus, the role of the disease in childhood remains to be determined [23, 24].

Genetic alterations in the plasmatic proteins of transthyretin causing amyloidosis associated with RMC have been found, but none of them in children. Coffin-Lowry syndrome is a disorder due to mutations of the *RSK2* gene located on the X chromosome, Xp22.2.29, causing facial dysmorphism, low stature, progressive skeletal deformities, and RMC. [25] Emery-Dreifuss dystrophy is an emerin disorder of autosomal dominant inheritance caused by mutations in the gene encoding for lamin A and C on chromosome 1 q21.2 – q21.3.31 and has also been linked to chromosome Xq28.31. Both variants may produce cardiomyopathy, atrial and ventricular arrhythmias, conduction disturbances, and sudden death, however, the restrictive phenotype has not been reported [25].

Pathophysiology

In order to understand the pathophysiology of RCM we must briefly recall the mechanism by which cardiomyocyte contraction is generated.

The sarcomere is surrounded by a membrane system (sarcoplasmic reticulum). It is formed by myosin bands in the center separated on each side by actin filaments. At rest, myosin filaments are neatly surrounded by actin in a way both filaments coincide, though they remain separate. That is so thanks to troponin and tropomyosin that form a complex around the actin filaments preventing them from getting stuck to the myosin ones. Troponin is a complex. Each troponin is formed by 3 subunits:

- troponin C, has affinity for Ca2+.
- troponin T, binds to tropomyosin.
- troponin I, inhibits formation of myosin-actin bridges.

When calcium concentration increases in sarcoplasm, it binds to troponin, causing inhibition of the block caused by tropomyosin. Actin-tropomyiosin complex is hence formed, acting as a bridge. We must remember that Troponin is a complex formed by three subunits: troponin C, with affinity for calcium; troponin T, united to tropomyosin and troponin I, which inhibits the formation of bridges between myosin and actin.

When the bridge is formed the ATPase function on the myosin head is activated and ATP is dissociated in ADP+Pi (inorganic phosphorus), this process requires Mg2+. When phosphate leaves the myosin head it generates a rotation or movement of it causing the actin filament to move along the myosin filament towards the center of the sarcomere, generating a shortening of the fiber [11].

Alternatively, during diastole, Ca2+ levels decrease, troponin C dissociates allowing Mg2+ to binds to C-terminals. This generates relaxation of the fiber, allowing the ventricular filling to take place.

Restrictive physiology is characterized by an abrupt cessation of ventricular filling in early diastole, with minimal mid and late diastolic flow causing a dip-plateau pattern on the ventricular pressure tracing. [26, 27] This typical pattern is the haemodynamic hallmark of restrictive cardiomyopathy. Why does this process occur? Any functional and structural defects in any of these troponin subunits may cause alterations in the Ca2 regulation of muscle contraction.

The fibers containing RCM mutations show incapacity to fully relax, and this improper relaxation is believed to be related to the high Ca2 sensitivity and the altered relaxation properties of the fibers themselves. As Gomes et al. have demonstrated in an *in vitro* study, the mutations in TNNI3 associated with RCM show similar *in vitro* physiological characteristics as TNNI HCM mutations but with a greater increase in Ca2 sensitivity, higher levels of basal force and higher levels of basal ATPase activity. Furthermore, mutations in TNNT2 have also been reported in association with infantile RCM. [9] and familial dilated cardiomyopathy (DCM) [11].

What determines the different expression of the same mutation is under study; environmental factors or other genetic factors could probably be involved. This ultimately results in decreased compliance of the ventricle with development of atrial dilation with the typical characteristics of normal systolic function, although with the progression of the disease, this can be deteriorated, and increase pulmonary pressure and resistance.

Natural History

When we think of the natural history of RCM, we must bear in mind that it is an infrequent disease, that the series published have a small sample size and that the number of patients that have subclinical RCM is unknown. Once the symptoms develop, morbidity and mortality are high.

Denfield and coworkers stated that little is known about the causes and outcome of RCM in childhood. They described twelve cases of RCM and they concluded that the prognosis of RCM is poor, since 33% of patients presented with embolic events, 75% of patients died within 6.3 years, and within 1 to 4 years of diagnosis, patients developed a markedly elevated pulmonary vascular resistance index. Therefore, they recommended that transplantation should be considered early [28].

Also, Cetta et al. [29] found that children with RCM who had symptoms of dyspnea and pulmonary venous congestion had the highest risk of death, and they suggested early consideration of cardiac transplant.

In our series of 36 patients, the survival rate was 86 months (IC 95%; 59–113), and 43 months in the case of children under 5 years of age (CI 95%; 35–57). In a multivariate analysis, the risk factors for poor prognosis were shortening fraction (SF)<28% and a relationship left atrium /aortic root (LA/AO) greater than 2.3. Only 2 patients presented thrombosis and another 2 patients, signs of ischemia on Holter monitoring.

If we compare RCM with other types of cardiomyopathies analyzed in the literature, we can see that children with restrictive CM were younger at diagnosis and had a significantly higher pulmonary vascular resistance index (PVRI) [30].

All studies in the literature agree that patients should be considered for orthotopic cardiac transplantation before the development of severe pulmonary hypertension, but patient selection criteria can be difficult to define. An elevated pre-transplant PVRI greater than 6 U.m2, and transpulmonary gradient (TPG) >15 have historically been a contraindication for cardiac transplantation, since they are associated with an increased risk of posttransplant mortality and right heart failure [30].

The development of new mechanical support options pre and post transplant plus the new set of drugs available for the treatment of pulmonary hypertension seem to have expanded the therapy options. Hughes et al. [30] published a successful orthotopic cardiac transplantation with a PVRI > 6 U.m2 in the presence of pulmonary reactivity, and they concluded that pulmonary vascular reactivity may be a more important prognostic factor than the absolute resistance index.

Thus, we can conclude that RCM is a severe, progressive disease with a mortality rate of up to 50% during the first 2 years after diagnosis. Children with a more chronic course show progressive heart failure, risk for acute onset events such as dysrhythmias, stroke, and sudden death. [31] Concerning this, Rivenes et al. reported a series of 18 patients; the patients at risk for sudden death showed at presentation chest pain, syncope or both in the absence of congestive heart failure. Holter monitor evidence of ischemia predicted death within months. The authors proposed the use of b blockade, implantable cardioverter defibrillator (ICD) therapy, and listing for cardiac transplant [32].

The natural history of RCM in childhood shows that it is a rare disorder with poor outcome. The early detection and current development of new drugs and tools for the treatment of cardiac failure and arrhythmias can probably contribute to changing the poor results in the long term.

Clinical Profile

Physical Examination

Physical examination findings can be variable and indistinct; in patients who are only mildly affected, standard studies may be normal. These studies usually evaluate the degree of congestion from the diastolic dysfunction of the affected ventricle. When the left ventricle is affected, pulmonary edema, pulmonary hypertension and decreased myocardial reserve result in reactive airway disease, recurrent lower respiratory tract infections, dyspnea on exertion, palpitations, syncope, sudden death or/and thromboembolic events [31-33].

Mitral regurgitation and tricuspid insufficiency commonly develop over time. The presence of murmurs and S3 or S4 gallop rhythms are common, as well. With the development of pulmonary hypertension, S2 becomes louder. Right-side congestion is expressed as hepatomegaly, jugular venous distention, and Kussmaul sign, either because of right-side RCM or pulmonary hypertension secondary to left-side RCM. When the disease progresses, patients present with peripheral edema, ascites and frank congestive heart failure.

In our series, at diagnosis 27/36 patients (75%) were symptomatic: 13 presented clinical signs of left heart failure; 3 patients, right heart failure, and 11 had signs of global heart failure.

Electrocardiogram

The electrocardiogram is abnormal in about 100% of cases, with frequent biatrial enlargement and nonspecific ST-T wave abnormalities (Figure 1). Right or left ventricular hypertrophy and also conduction abnormalities can be present, such as second degree atrioventricular block (AV B) and complete heart block.

The use of Holter monitoring as complementary study for the detection of arrhythmias and ischemias is mandatory. Arrhythmias are not uncommon in RCM (approximately 15%), including atrial fibrillation, flutter, ectopic tachycardia and ventricular tachycardia [31].

In our cohort, all 36 patients (100%) presented sinus rhythm and auricular hypertrophy, and 64.3% had alterations in repolarization. No ST-T wave abnormalities, signs of AVB, or conduction abnormalities were observed. Holter monitoring evidenced no arrhythmias or conduction abnormalities at the time of admission.

Chest X-Ray

The chest x-ray is usually abnormal, and with this simple test it is possible to suspect diagnosis of the disease. Cardiomegaly secondary to atrial enlargement and venous congestion are typical features of this pathology.

In our study, the cardiothoracic ratio was >65% at the expense of atrial enlargement in all patients; 42.7% presented alterations of the pulmonary flow due to passive congestion (Figure 2).

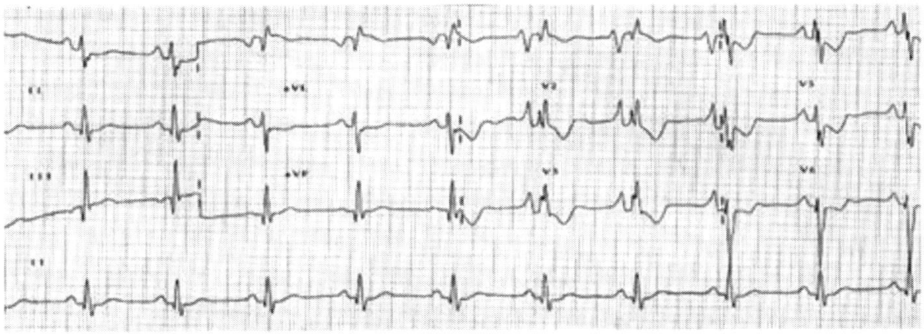

Figure 1. Characteristic ECGs in restrictive cardiomyopathy. Prominent tall and biphasic P waves in the precordial chest leads are seen, with obliquely elevated ST-T segments and notched or biphasic T waves in the precordial leads.

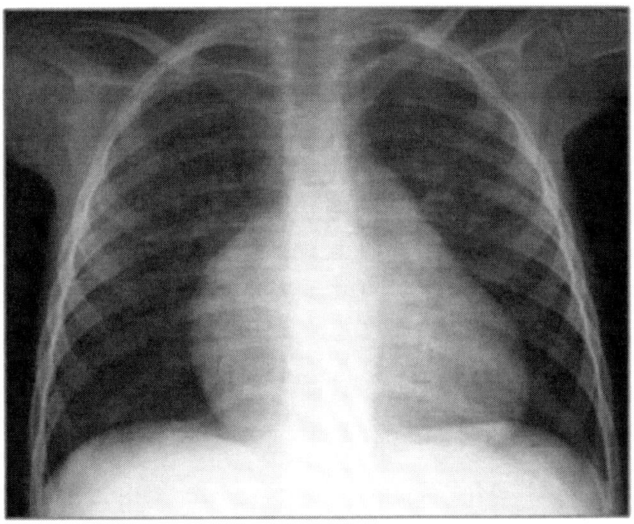

Figure 2. Chest x ray showing marked enlargement of the cardiac silhouette, predominantly due to biatrialdilatation and pulmonary venous congestion.

Cardiac Catheterization

The elevated left or right ventricular end diastolic pressures and the classic pattern in pressure tracings, typical square root or dip-plateau pattern, help to confirm left or right diastolic dysfunction (Figure 3).

Since noninvasive techniques have evolved and proved to be useful for hemodynamic assessment, the modern role of cardiac catheterization in restrictive cardiomyopathy is the direct assessment of pulmonary hypertension and calculation of pulmonary vascular resistance. When resistance is high, pulmonary reactivity tests are fundamental to preclude from orthotopic heart transplant. Endomyocardial biopsy can be helpful although it is not risk-free [30].

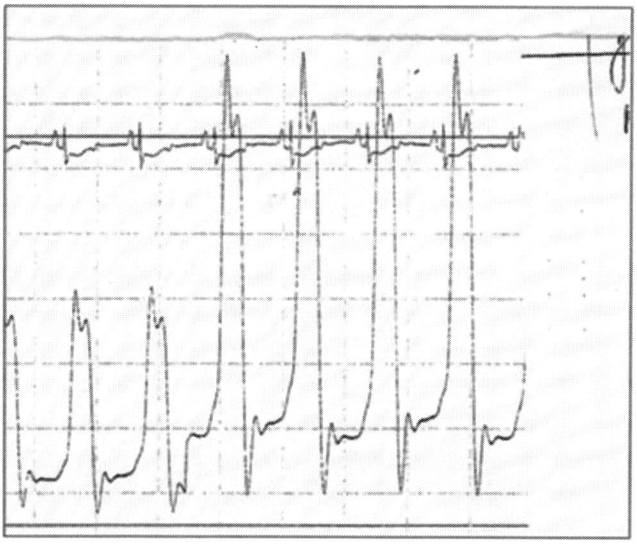

Figure 3. Left ventricular pressure tracing with dip-and-plateau (square-root sing).

In our cohort, 18 patients underwent hemodynamic studies. The left atrial (LA) and pulmonary capillary pressure was 17 ± 6 mmHg (range, 12-30 mmHg). Left atrial enlargement was observed in all patients. The mean pulmonary pressure was 34 ± 6 mm Hg (range, 28-40 mm Hg). The left ventricular end diastolic pressure (LV) was 19 ± 6 mm Hg (range, 12-30 mm Hg). Only 50% of patients showed the square root or dip-plateau pattern on the left ventricular pressure. Angiography evidenced signs of diminished ventricular distensibility.

Echocardiography

RCM can be diagnosed with an echocardiogram based on the markedly dilated atria in the absence of significant atrioventricular valve regurgitation.

Systolic function is typically preserved, although some degree of systolic dysfunction has been seen in some patients at presentation, and deterioration of systolic function over time has also been reported in children [34].

Diastolic patterns present according to LV distensibility and it has been reported in the adult population that very symptomatic patients have restrictive mitral flow, the E wave predominating over the A with a diastolic isovolumetric period of < 70 ms and E wave deceleration time of generally< 100 ms.

The left restrictive flow correlates with a pulmonary vein inflow [15] characterized by an increase in the velocity of the pulmonary reversed A flow > 35cm/s and a duration of > 30ms than that of the mitral A flow when the LV end diastolic pressure is over 20-25 mmHg.

A predominant antegrade diastolic flow without changes during the different phases of the respiratory cycle is seen as the left-sided filling is permanently increased [31].

In the tricuspid valve restricted flow is observed which increases the E wave with inspiration, not more than 10% basal flow during apnea (unlike in constrictive pericarditis in which it is typically more than 15%), with a clearly shorter tricuspid flow deceleration time compared to patients with constrictive pericarditis. Maximum velocity of tricuspid regurgitation is used for the estimation of pulmonary systolic pressure, which is generally high. Pulmonary pressure is often higher than 40mmHg while the pressure is lower in constrictive pericarditis [34].

In children, findings consistent with restrictive filling and increased left ventricular end diastolic pressure include elevated mitral valve Doppler E/A ratios, short mitral deceleration times, increased pulmonary vein atrial reversal velocity, and duration and pulmonary vein atrial reversal duration greater than mitral A wave duration.

Doppler echocardiography allows differentiation from constrictive pericarditis which, unlike restrictive cardiomyopathy, respiratory-phase changes in mitral, pulmonary vein, and systemic vein inflow [35].

In RCM, an inflow with a predominant antegrade diastolic flow throughout the respiratory cycle is found in the suprahepatic veins and in the superior vena cava.

In the pulmonary and hepatic veins, the systolic is much higher than the diastolic flow velocity. An increase in diastolic low inversion is seen in the hepatic veins during inspiration as well as an increase in the velocity and duration of atrial flow inversion in the pulmonary veins.

Tissue Doppler echocardiography has also proved to be useful for the differentiation of RCM from constrictive pericarditis based on telediastolic mitral ring velocity or measuring the gradient of posterior wall velocity [36, 37].

The combined use of an averaged S' cutoff value <8 cm/s as well as an E' cutoff value <8 at the lateral and septal MA demonstrated 93% sensitivity and 88% specificity for the diagnosis of RCM.

Tissue E velocity of less than 0.8 cm/s has been described and a tissue E wave/mitral E wave ratio of less than 0.11 strongly suggests restriction.

The recently developed technique of the M color mode [38] is also useful for the differentiation of RCM from constrictive pericarditis. In the inflow an E and A wave similar to those on Doppler echocardiography are observed. In the restriction, baseline and total propagation velocity to the apex are markedly decreased (typically less than 0.45 cm/s) the basal-apical return time is clearly prolonged compared to the values in constrictive pericarditis [38].

In different studies in pediatric patients, it has been shown that the diastolic function described in cardiomyopathies in adults, including RCM, is not useful in children. Gewilling et al. state that in their series of six pediatric patients, the diastolic pattern behavior was different from the classical pattern in adults. The echocardiographic patterns were pseudonormal and not restrictive, showing an L wave [27].

Newer echocardiographic techniques such as speckle-track imaging, velocity vector imaging, can help differentiate constriction from restriction with high sensitivity and specificity. [39] The results shown by Dragulescu et al. suggest that among the variousdiastolic function (DF) echo parameters, mitral E wave deceleration time (DT), and left atrial volume indexed to body surface area (LAVi) are likely to be the most useful in the evaluation of DF in children with CM. They conclude that isolated delayed relaxation is seen in only a minority of HCM patients and not in DCM or RCM. And these results suggest that pediatric diastolic dysfunction (DD) does not follow the progression seen in adult patients and that new diagnostic criteria are needed in children [40].

In our series of 36 patients a greatly enlarged left atrial (LA) (X= 35 mm; range, 31 mm-40 mm) was observed, with a significantly elevated aorta/left atrium (AO/LA) ratio (2.4 ± 0.4) in all studies (Figure 4).

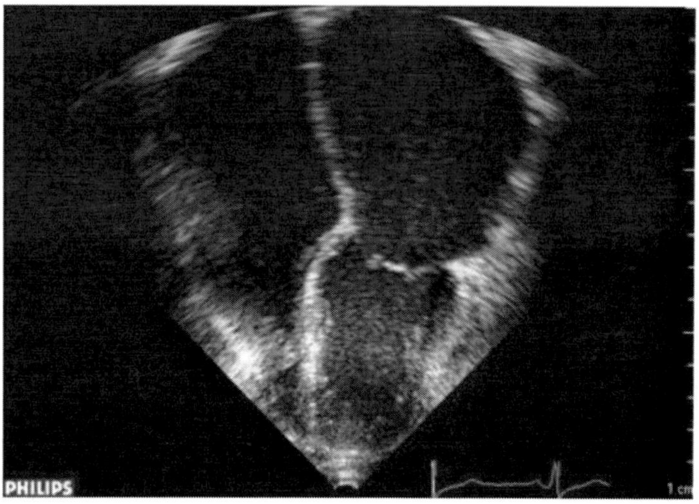

Figure 4. Apical four- chamber echocardiographic view. The right atrium and the left atrium are both seen to be markedly enlarged. The right and left ventricle are normal in size.

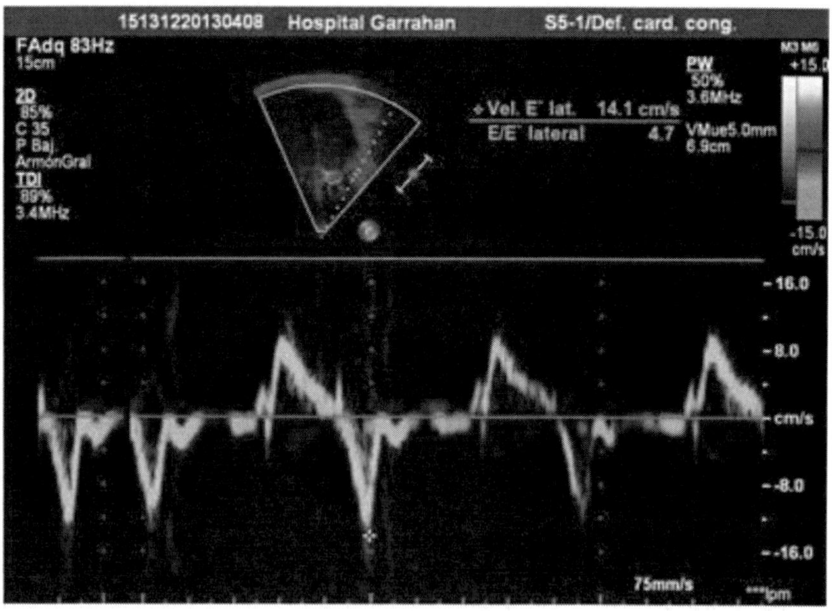

Figure 5. Pulsed tissue Doppler of the mitral ring.Mitral annular demonstrating velocities curves. Low late diastolic filling (A-wave) of the transmitral velocity suggesting of markedly impaired left ventricular diastolic function with elevated filling pressures.

The LV diastolic end diameter and posterior wall thickness were normal (Z score < 2) in 27/36 patients. Patients in the group with a mixed phenotype presented with bi-ventricular hypertrophy in seven patients and LV hypertrophy in two patients.

The evaluation of the systolic function of the LV showed a shortening fraction (SF) of 34% (range, 28-40%). Thirty patients presented with no or very mild valve insufficiency.

In the evaluation of ventricular filling three patterns of relaxation were identified: (Figure 5)

1. Restrictive pattern: seen in 19 patients, with an E/A relaxation ratio greater than 2.
2. Pseudonormalized pattern: seen in 12 patients, with an E/A relaxation ratio less than or equal to 2.
3. In five patients a pattern with three diastolic waves (E, L and A)was observed.

Cardiac Magnetic Resonance

CMR is helpful because it can detect the anatomy of any pericardial thickening, the haemodynamics of constriction and any abnormality of the underlying myocardium. The pericardium can be delineated on black-blood imaging and inflammation can be imaged using late gadolinium enhancement (LEG) (owing to the increased extracellular space associated with oedema and breakdown of cell walls). Tethering to underlying myocardium and lack of slippage can be seen using tagging, and real-time cine-CMR [19] may show ventricular–ventricular interaction (compression of the left ventricle by the right ventricle during deep inspiration), which is a hallmark of constriction.

Therapeutic Options

Preventing arrhythmias, sudden death and selecting the right candidates for cardiac transplantation instead of only offering to treat heart failure symptoms have become the present day therapeutic challenges for the cardiologist. Even though the diastolic alterations that these patients present generate pulmonary venous or systemic congestion and can be treated with diuretics, the use of these medications must be controlled, since they produce low cardiac output and require an adequate preload in order to preserve it. Spironolactone is the drug of choice and can be used as single medication or together with furosemide at low doses.

When the disease progresses, systolic dysfunction appears, but unlike the case of other pathologies, the use of vasodilators in RCM should be controlled, since these patients are unable to increase the ejection volume and this can lead to hypotension without increase in cardiac output. [41]

Concerning the patients that present with signs of ischemia as evidenced in the ECG or Holter monitor, beta blockers have been used, however controversial, provided they do not show sinus node disease or AV block.

In the case of patients with sudden cardiac events, such as sudden death episode, syncope or arrhythmias, the implantation of implantable cardioverter-defibrillators (ICDs) should be considered. In addition, different authors have described the development of AV block. Walsh et al. [41] showed a series of 17 patients that presented sudden events with the resulting death in 4 of them, 2 due to acute AV block. They observed that the patients who showed these events had a prolonged PR and a QRS of longer duration [42].

In our series of 36 patients with RCM, during the follow-up 2 patients presented AV block and they received a pacemaker. Two patients showed ventricular tachycardia (VT) and they died. One patient developed auricular flutter and was put under amiodarone therapy. Two patients that presented with signs of ischemia and frequent ventricular extrasystoles as evidenced in Holter monitoring received antiarrhythmic medication.

Children with RCM have a higher risk of developing thromboembolic events; the series published in the literature show between 12% and 32% of occurrence. According to the review by Chen et al., the risk factors for such events are: LA with Z score >3 and reduced systolic function. This group of patients should receive warfarin, and those with preserved systolic function should receive aspirin. Patients with arrhythmias should also be anticoagulated [43].

Heart transplant is the definitive treatment of choice for RCM, since survival rates and quality of life post transplant far exceed the natural history of the pathology. But when should transplant be the option? Consensus as to when it should be indicated has only been reached when considering patients that show severe signs of cardiac failure or a high pulmonary pressure and pulmonary vascular resistance, although some physicians enroll their patients on an early list for transplant [44].

But the greatest dilemma around this pathology arises when patients show mild symptoms or they are asymptomatic. What should be done in those cases? Webber et al. showed in their review that survival rates since diagnosis were almost the same in the case of patients that presented with symptoms or syncope as with those who were asymptomatic at diagnosis. They did not find any statistical correlation between pulmonary vascular resistance index (PVRI) and survival in their cohort. The authors suggest that the presence of cardiac symptoms should not be the key factor to determine when to enroll patients for transplantation, as is usually the case in other types of pediatric cardiomyopathies [45].

Furthermore, there is another controversy around transplantation: what levels of pulmonary vascular resistance (PVR) should a patient have to be listed for heart or cardiopulmonary transplant? A pulmonary vascular resistance index greater than 6 Wood units (WU) × m2 is often considered as a contraindication for heart transplant because there is a marked increase in PVR that can lead to right ventricular dysfunction during the postoperative time [46, 47].

However, Bograd et al. reported data on the evaluation of a group of patients with RCM and PVR> 6 UW, with a mortality rate of 86% per year and normalization of PVR in approximately 3 months. Nevertheless, these patients required extracorporeal membrane oxygenation (ECMO) after heart transplant [47, 48].

In our experience, 6 out of 45 patients with RCM were transplanted and 3 remain on a waiting list. Three of the 6 transplanted patients presented PVR> = 6 UW/m, with severe global heart failure; they received ventricular assistance (Berlin Heart) prior to being transplanted. Survival after one year of diagnosis was 83.3% for the 6 patients. We believe these patients must be closely controlled in order to follow the progression of PVR. Our patients are enrolled for transplantation when they present heart failure of elevated pulmonary pressure, since the lack of donors in our country is an important problem [49].

Discussion

RCM in children is an infrequent disease accounting for 2.5-5% of all pediatric cardiomyopathies. The clinical prognosis of RCM in children is very different from the adult phenotype. Survival rate two years after diagnosis is 50%.

In a study published by our team in 2002, we observed that the survival rate of our population was 42.8% during a mean follow-up of 4 years, and 13.8% of the cohort had a family history of cardiomyopathies [50].

The Pediatric Cardiomyopathy Registry (PCMR) analysis showed 152 cases of RCM, which accounts for 4.5% of all cardiomyopathies identified under PCMR. A fourth of them had a family history of cardiomyopathy. This highlights the need to perform genetic studies to further understand this rare form of cardiomyopathy. [45] In addition, it has been observed that patients with restrictive physiology have phenotypes for HCM and RCM overlapped in pediatric populations [45].

At present it is known that some patients with sarcomeric genetic mutations develop RCM [10-16] and that those mutations can produce different phenotypes even within one single family. Up to date, RCM has been associated with mutations in genes that codify for troponin I, troponin T β myosin heavy chain and αactin. [17-19] Several mutations within the desmin gene have also been associated with RCM. [20-22] However, the phenotype generally implies skeletal myopathy and conduction abnormalities. The new technologies have led to a better understanding of the genome and the identification of novel mutations that can cause RCM in childhood. The technological advances, such as the ICDs [42], ventricular assistance [49]and transplant have improved the therapeutic options and survival [44-46].

In our sample population, 3 patients received the Berlin Heart and were transplanted successfully. Nevertheless, there is not enough information to define when is timely to enroll patients for transplantation. Furthermore, the outcome of transplant has improved gradually, with a mean graft survival of 12 years or even greater (17 years) for children, exceeding the survival rate of the natural history of the disease [45].

Some asymptomatic patients pose especial challenges to the physician as to which therapy mode to use, since the risk of sudden death is real. Walsh et al. described anomalies of the conduction system that are produced in this patient population. Bradyarrhythmia and the development of sudden heart block may be the trigger for events of sudden death. The sudden death rate reported due to these events is 25% [8] in RCM in children [42].

Histopathological evidence for ischemia was found in most patients that died and Holter monitoring showed that ischemia predicted death. [5] Rivenes et al. [32] described that sudden death was due to lethal ventricular arrhythmia and showed examples of ventricular tachycardia/fibrillation associated to ischemia. Walsh et al. [41] also described that ischemia was associated to the appearance of AV block. It is worth noting that those patients with a long PR interval are bound to develop AV block, while those with a short PR interval tend to remain unchanged. Another potential disease mechanism of the conduction system could be related to the atrial and ventricular dilatation as a consequence of the progression of the disease. Moreover, many of these patients have structurally abnormal myocytes with abnormal gap unions that are believed to lead to the development of abnormalities [29].

Patients with long PR interval, wide QRS and left bundle branch block (LBBB) must be monitored and taken into account to receive ICD/pacemaker [42].

Other studies have analyzed the risk to stratify survival up to 8-12 years. [8-10] Other risk factors have been identified, such as cardiomegaly, young age, thromboembolic events, pulmonary vascular resistance, pulmonary venous congestion, syncope, chest pain. [26-28] Webber et al. found that the right and left ventricle, the diastolic pressure and the relationship LA/AO root during presentation of the disease have a negative correlation with the time of survival after diagnosis [51].

Up to date, no risk factors that can help detect risk populations in asymptomatic patients have been identified.

Conclusion

Restrictive cardiomyopathy in childhood is a rare entity with a poor prognosis and a high mortality rate. Of all the cardiomyopathies, RCM has been the most difficult to define, in part due to poorly defined criteria to categorize this entity.

Prospective large pediatric studies are needed to better understand the outcome of these patients and risk stratification for sudden death, congestive heart failure, pulmonary thromboembolism and increased pulmonary vascular resistance.

Identification of specific genetic mutations will help to better understand the molecular pathology of restrictive cardiomyopathy and create new therapies to delay or reduce the number of cardiac transplants.

References

[1] Elliott P, Andersson B, Arbustini E et al. Classification of the cardiomyopathies: a position statement from the european society of cardiology working group on myocardial and pericardial diseases. *Eur. Heart J.* 2008; 29: 270–76.

[2] Kushwaha S, Fallon JT, Fuster V. Restrictive Cardiomyopathy. *N. Engl. J. Med.* 1997; 336: 267–76.

[3] Nugent AW, Daubeney PE, Chondros P et al. The epidemiology of childhood cardiomyopathy in Australia. *N. Engl. J. Med.* 2003; 348: 1639–46.

[4] Angelini A, Calzolari V, Thiene G et al. Morphologic spectrum of primary restrictive cardiomyopathy. *Am. J. Cardiol.* 1997; 80:1046-50.

[5] Jacoby D, McKenna WJ. Genetics of inherited cardiomyopathy. *Eur. Heart J.* 2012; 33: 296–04.

[6] Gomes AV, Liang J, Potter JD. Mutations in human cardiac troponin I that are associated with restrictive cardiomyopathy affect basal ATPase activity and the calcium sensitivity of force development. *J. Biol. Chem.* 2005; 280: 30909-30915.

[7] Maron BJ, Towbin JA, Thiene G et al. Contemporary Definitions and Classification of the Cardiomyopathies. An American Heart Association Scientific Statement from the Council on Clinical Cardiology, Heart Failure and Transplantation Committee; Quality of Care and Outcomes Research and Functional Genomics and Translational Biology Interdisciplinary Working Groups; and Council on Epidemiology and Prevention. *Circulation* 2006; 113:1807-16).

[8] Mogensen J, Kubo T, Duque M et al. Idiopathic restrictive cardiomyopathy is part of the clinical expression of cardiac troponin I mutations. *J. Clin. Invest.* 2003; 111: 209–16.

[9] Peddy SB, Vricella LA, Crosson JE et al. Infantile restrictive cardiomyopathy resulting from a mutation in the cardiac troponin T gene. *Pediatrics* 2006; 117: 1830–33.

[10] Ware SM, Quinn ME, Ballard ET et al. Pediatric restrictive cardiomyopathy associated with a mutation in beta-myosin heavy chain. *Clin. Genet.* 2008; 73: 165–70.

[11] Kaski JP, Syrris P, Burch M et al. Idiopathic restrictive cardiomyopathy in children is caused by mutations in cardiac sarcomere protein genes. *Heart* 2008; 94: 1478–84.

[12] Pinto JR, Yang SH, Hitz MP et al. Fetal cardiac troponin isoforms rescue the increased Ca2_sensitivity produced by a novel double deletion in cardiactroponin T linked to restrictive cardiomyopathy. A clinical, genetic, and functional approach. *J. Biol. Chem.* 2011, 286: 20901-912.
[13] Ahmad F, Banerjee SK, Lage ML et al. The role of cardiac troponin T quantity and function in cardiac development and dilated cardiomyopathy. *PLoS One* 2008; 3(7): e2642. doi: 10.1371/journal.pone.0002642.
[14] Kubo T, Gimeno JR, Bahl A et al. Prevalence, clinical significance, and genetic basis of hypertrophic cardiomyopathy with restrictive phenotype. *J. Am. Coll. Cardiol.* 2007; 49: 2419–26.
[15] Richard P, Charron P, Carrier L et al. Hypertrophic cardiomyopathy: distribution of disease genes, spectrum of mutations, and implications for a molecular diagnosis strategy. *Circulation* 2003; 107: 2227–32.
[16] Olson TM, Karst ML, Whitby FG et al. Myosin light chain mutation causes autosomal recessive cardiomyopathy with mid-cavitary hypertrophy and restrictive physiology. *Circulation* 2002; 105: 2337–40.
[17] Hook S, Ratliff NB, Rosenkranz E et al. Isolated noncompaction of the ventricular myocardium. *Pediatr. Cardiol.* 1996; 17: 43–5.
[18] Ozkutlu S, Hascelik S, Yalnizoglu D et al. Familial isolated non-compaction of myocardium presenting as restrictive cardiomyopathy. *Pediatr. Int.* 2007; 49: 536–9.
[19] Biagini E, Ragni L, Ferlito M et al. Different types of cardiomyopathy associated with isolated ventricular noncompaction. *Am. J. Cardiol.* 2006; 98: 821–24.
[20] Peled Y, Gramlich M, Yoskovitz G et al. Titinmutación in familial restrictive cardiomyophaty. *Int. J. Cardiol.* 2014; 171: 24-30.
[21] Arbustini E, Pasotti M, Pilotto A et al. Desmin accumulation restrictive cardiomyopathy and atrioventricular block associated with desmin gene defects. *Eur. J. Heart Fail.* 2006; 8: 477–83.
[22] Dalakas MC, Park KY, Semino-Mora C et al. Desmin myopathy, a skeletal myopathy with cardiomyopathy caused by mutations in the desmin gene. *N. Engl. J. Med.* 2000; 342: 770–80.
[23] Zhang J, Kumar A, Stalker HJ et al. Clinical and molecular studies of a large family with desmin-associated restrictive cardiomyopathy. *Clin. Genet.* 2001; 59: 248–56.
[24] Goldfarb LG, Park KY, Cervenakova L et al. Missense mutations in desmin associated with familial cardiac and skeletal myopathy. *Nat. Genet.* 1998; 19: 402–03.
[25] Schwartz ML, Colan SD. Familial restrictive cardiomyopathy with skeletal abnormalities. *Am. J. Cardiol.* 2003; 92: 636–39.
[26] Denfield SW, Webber SA. Restrictive cardiomyopathy in childhood. *Heart Fail. Clin.* 2010; 6: 445–52.
[27] Gewillig M, Mertens L, Moerman P et al. Idiopathic restrictive cardiomyopathy in childhood. A diastolic disorder characterized by delayed relaxation. *Eur. Heart J.* 1996; 17: 1413-20.
[28] Denfield SW, Bricker JT, Gajarski Ret al. Restrictive cardiomyopathies in childhood: etiologies and natural history. *Tex. Heart Inst. J.* 1997; 24: 38–44.
[29] Cetta F, O'Leary PW, Seward JB et al. Idiopathic restrictive cardiomyopathy in childhood: diagnostic features and clinical course. *Mayo. Clin. Proc.* 1995; 70: 634–40.

[30] Hughes ML, Kleinert S, Keogh A et al. Pulmonary vascular resistance and reactivity in children with end-stage cardiomyopathy. *J. Heart Lung Transplant.* 2000; 19: 701-04.
[31] Denfield SW. Sudden death in children with restrictive cardiomyopathy. *Card. Electrophysiol. Rev.* 2002; 6: 163–67.
[32] Rivenes SM, Kearney DL, Smith EO et al. Sudden death and cardiovascular collapse in children with restrictive cardiomyopathy. *Circulation* 2000; 102: 876–82.
[33] Chen S, Balfour IC, Jureidini S. Clinical spectrum of restrictive cardiomyopathy in children. *J. Heart Lung Transplant.* 2001; 20: 90–2.
[34] Goldstein JA. Differentiation of constrictive pericarditis and restrictive cardiomyopathy. J Am Coll Cardiol, ACC Educ Highlights (Fall) 1998; 14 -22.
[35] Garcia MJ, Rodriguez L, Ares M. Differentiation of constrictive pericarditis from restrictive cardiomyopathy: assessment of left ventricular diastolic velocities in longitudinal axis by Doppler tissue imaging. *J. Am. Coll. Cardiol.* 1996; 27: 108-14.
[36] Garcia MJ, Thomas JD, Klein AL. New Doppler echocardiographic applications for the study of diastolic function. *J. Am. Coll. Cardiol.* 1998; 32: 865-75.
[37] Butz T, Piper C, Langer C. Diagnostic superiority of a combined assessment of the systolic and early diastolic mitral annular velocities by tissue Doppler imaging for the differentiation of restrictive cardiomyopathy from constrictive pericarditis. *Clin. Res. Cardiol.* 2010; 99:207-15.
[38] Rodriguez L, Ares M, Vandervoort P et al. Does color M- Mode flow propagation differentiate between patients with restrictive vs constrictive physiology?. *J. Am. Coll. Cardiol.* 1996; 27 (2s1): 268-268. doi:10.1016/S0735-1097(96)81961-9.
[39] Mookadam F, Jiamsripong P, Raslan SF et al. Constrictive pericarditis and restrictive cardiomyopathy in the modern era. *Future Cardiol.* 2011; 7: 471-83.
[40] Dragulescu A, Mertens L, Friedberg MK. Interpretation of left ventricular diastolic dysfunction in children with cardiomyopathy by echocardiography: problems and limitations. *Circ. Cardiovasc. Imaging* 2013; 6: 254-61.
[41] Bengur AR, Beekman RH, Rocchini AP, et al. Acute hemodynamic effects of captopril in children with a congestive or restrictive cardiomyopathy. *Circulation* 1991; 83: 523–27.
[42] Walsh MA, Grenier MA, Jefferies JL. Conduction abnormalities in pediatric patients with restrictive cardiomyopathy. *Circ. Heart Fail.* 2012; 5: 267-73.
[43] Chen K, Williams S, Chan AK et al. Thrombosis and embolism in pediatric cardiomyopathy. *Blood Coagul. Fibrinolysis.* 2013; 24: 221–30.
[44] Kimberling MT, Balzer DT, Hirsch R et al. Cardiac transplantation for pediatric restrictive cardiomyopathy: presentation, evaluation and short- term outcome. *J. Heart Lung Transplant.* 2002; 21: 455–59.
[45] Webber SA, Lipshultz SE, Sleeper LA et al. Outcomes of restrictive cardiomyopathy in childhood and the influence of phenotype: A report from the Pediatric Cardiomyopathy Registry. *Circulation* 2012; 126: 1237-44.
[46] Fenton MJ, Chubb H, McMahon AM et al. Heart and heart-lung transplantation for idiopathic restrictive cardiomyopathy in children. *Heart* 2006; 92: 85–9.
[47] Bograd AJ, Mital S, Schwarzenberger JC. Twenty-year experience with heart transplantation for infants and children with restrictive cardiomyopathy: 1986–2006. *Am. J. Transplant.* 2008; 8: 201–07.

[48] Murtuza B, Fenton M, Burch M et al. Pediatric heart transplantation for congenital and restrictive cardiomyopathy. *Ann. Thorac. Surg.* 2013; 95: 1675-84.
[49] Moreno G, Charroqui A, Pilan M et al. Clinical experience with Berlin Heart Excor in Pediatric Patients in Argentina: 1373 days of cardiac support. *Pediatr. Cardiol.* 2011; 32: 652-58.
[50] Villa A, Di Santo M, La Fuente V. Restrictive myocardiopathy in chilhood. Clinical and hemodynamic findings and outcome. *Arch. Argent. Pediatr.* 2003; 101: 245-49.
[51] Russo LM, Webber SA. Idiopathic restrictive cardiomyopathy in children. *Heart* 2005; 91: 1199–202.

In: Congenital Heart Diseases
Editor: Raúl Cayré and José Milei

ISBN: 978-1-61122-003-2

Chapter 10

Therapeutic Intervention in Congenital Heart Disease

Ana M. S. de Dios[1,*], Jesus Damsky Barbosa[2], Maria Fernanda Biancolini[3] and Julio Cesar Biancolini[4]

[1]Chief of Department,
[2]Chief Laboratory of Hemodynamics
[3]Staff Pediatric Cardiology
[4]Resident Pediatric Cardiology, Hospital Pedro de Elizalde

Abstract

TRANSCATHETER CLOSURE OF ASDs- PFOs: The type, size, and shape of atrial septal defects (ASDs) can vary greatly. Ostium secundum (OS) are the most common ASDs, are present in the region of the fossa ovalis, and account for 75% of all ASDs. The position and size of the ASDs, number of defects, distance between the defects, type of defects, and relationship with other structures must be determined to result in a successful procedure. ASDs that are not suitable for trans-catheter device closure are sinus venous defects (4-11%) and ostium primum ASDs (15-20%).

TRANSCATHETER CLOSURE OF VENTRICULAR SEPTAL DEFECTS (VSD): Common congenital heart disease (20%). Indications for VSD closure are: symptoms of heart failure; signs of volume overload in left heart chambers; history of endocarditis; and post-operatory residual VSD with volume overload. The procedure is not recommended in absence of the crista since this type of VSD has a deficient aortic and pulmonary margin. The risk factors for complications are age (<5 months) and weight (<5 kg), which are associated with a higher risk of early complications. The localization of the defect: pmVSD has an increased risk of complete cAVB after device implantation. The success rate was very high, as closure was successfully achieved in 95.3% of subjects in the follow-up.

AORTIC COARCTATION: Occurs in about 0.04% of live births and comprises about 7% of known congenital heart disease. Surgery is the best option in native coarctation in patients <25 kg and covered stent in patients >45 years old, to avoid

* E-mail: ana.dedios@gmail.com.

morbidity. In postsurgical residual gradient, the best option is angioplasty or stent, depending on age, type of defect, elasticity of the wall and other complications. If the aorta must be expanded to adult size, or when the initial measure requires a final diameter 3 times greater, covered stent is preferred.

Conclusion: Therapeutic intervention helps in congenital heart disease by solving an increasing number of pathologies and is complementary to other surgical lesions.

Transcatheter Closure of ASDs- PFOs

Atrial septal defects (ASD) are congenital cardiac defects that allow communication between the left and right atria and account for 10% of all congenital heart diseases (CHD). There are several different types of atrial septal defects. Ostium secundum (OS) are the most common ASDs [1], are present in the region of the fossa ovalis and account for 75% of all ASDs. They are due to deficiency in the septum primum or, rarely, to an "unguarded" foramen ovale from deficiency in the septum secundum. In the majority of the defects there is a complete absence, deficiency, or multiple fenestration of the septum primum. The type, size, and shape of the ASD can vary greatly. It is important to note that all these defects involve the fossa ovalis and do not include the vena cava, right pulmonary veins, or atrio-ventricular valves. The relationships to these structures should be recognized by echo when considering device closure. In the case of ASDs associated with an unroofed coronary sinus, there are publications where the authors describe closure with an Amplatzer device. However, there is no consensus on the best choice for closure of this defect. [2]

Echocardiography

Transthoracic echocardiography (TTE) is the primary diagnostic imaging modality for the diagnosis and description of ASD in children, but the most valuable information can be obtained from transesophageal echocardiography (TEE), especially in adult patients.

Rims required:

1. $\geq$ 7 mm around the defect for devices > 10 mm
2. $\geq$ 5 mm around the defect for devices < 10 mm
3. Aortic rim > 3 mm

Special considerations (Figure 1): The anatomic rims viewed from the right atria surface are:

1. The posterior-superior rim: the distance to the superior vena cava.
2. The anterior-superior rim: the distance to the aorta (Ao).
3. The posterior-inferior rim: the distance to the inferior vena cava (IVC).
4. The inferior rim: the distance to the tricuspid valve (TV) on the right and the mitral valve (MV) on the left atrium.
5. Other nearby structures important to avoid when closing with a device include: the coronary sinus (SC) and the right pulmonary veins (RPV), the left venous valve of

the inferior vena cava, and the Eustachian valve, since in some cases this can be mistaken for the inferior rim of an ASD.

The information required to close an ASD with a device are: Size of the ASD in mm in four chamber, short axis, and cava axis views using TTE. (Figure 1)

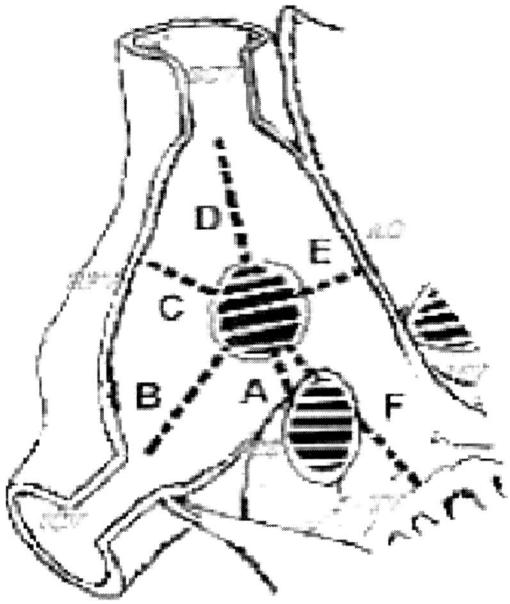

Figure 1. The anatomic rims viewed in a schematic drawing:

Reference:
A- The coronary sinus (SC).
B- The posterior and inferior rim: distance to the inferior vena cava (IVC).
C- The posterior rim: distance to the right pulmonary veins (RVP).
D- The posterior and superior rim: distance to the superior vena cava (SCV).
E- The anterior and superior rim: the distance to the aorta (Ao).
F- The tricuspid valves (TV) on the right and the mitral valve (MV) on the left.

The TEE angle to follow ASD closure is 40-60° in the medium esophagus. This offers the best view for balloon sizing and the position of the device during the procedure.

TEE allows the measurement of the distance to the atrioventricular valves in 0° and the distance between the defect and the top of the atrium; 35-40° is the best view to show the aortic rim; and 110-120° in the cava axis shows the distance between the defect and the superior and inferior vena cava. (Figure 2)

The following parameters should be assessed (2):

- Presence, type and number of defect/s by TTE and TEE.
- Exact defect size determined in at least two planes; the largest measure should be taken into account.
- Distance from the defect rims to other structures by TEE (atrioventricular valves, coronary sinus, superior and inferior vena cava, aorta, and pulmonary veins).

- Quality of the margin defects (rims) by TEE [3].
- Entry of the pulmonary veins into the left atria, to rule out anomalous venous return.
- Right ventricular size, its function, and signs of volume overload (paradoxical movement of the ventricular septum).
- Magnitude of the left to right shunts using non-invasive calculation of the pulmonary to systemic blood flow ratio (Qp/Qs).
- Pulmonary artery pressure derived from non-invasive calculation of the right ventricular systolic pressure in the presence of tricuspid regurgitation with no pulmonary stenosis.
- -Any other associated congenital anomalies, including another ASD, pulmonary stenosis, VSD, etc.
- Size and systolic and diastolic function of the left ventricle.
- Mitral valve prolapse and magnitude of mitral regurgitation.

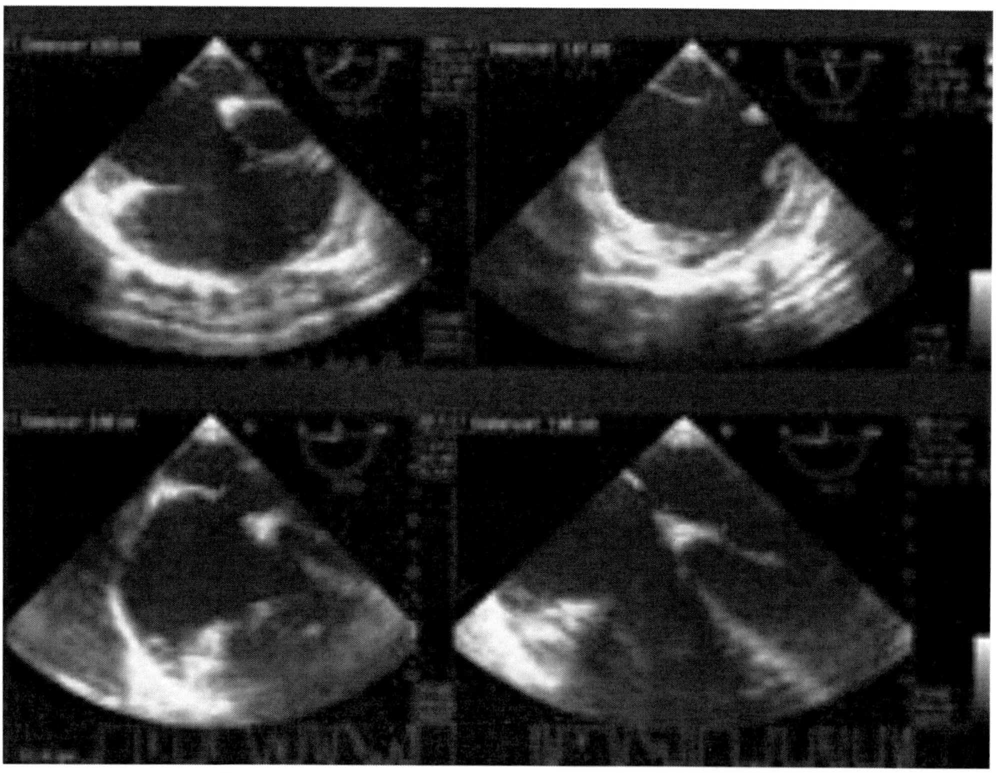

Figure 2. TEE showing the defect in 30-45º (minor axis view), in 90-120º (cava axis view), and in 0º (four-chamber view).

TEE helps to carry out the procedure in 4 basic times: (Figure 3)

1. First: to recognize localization and extension of the defect.
2. Second: to measure the ASD by balloon sizing.
3. Third: to recognize residual shunts and to stabilize the device.
4. Fourth: to decide when to release the device.

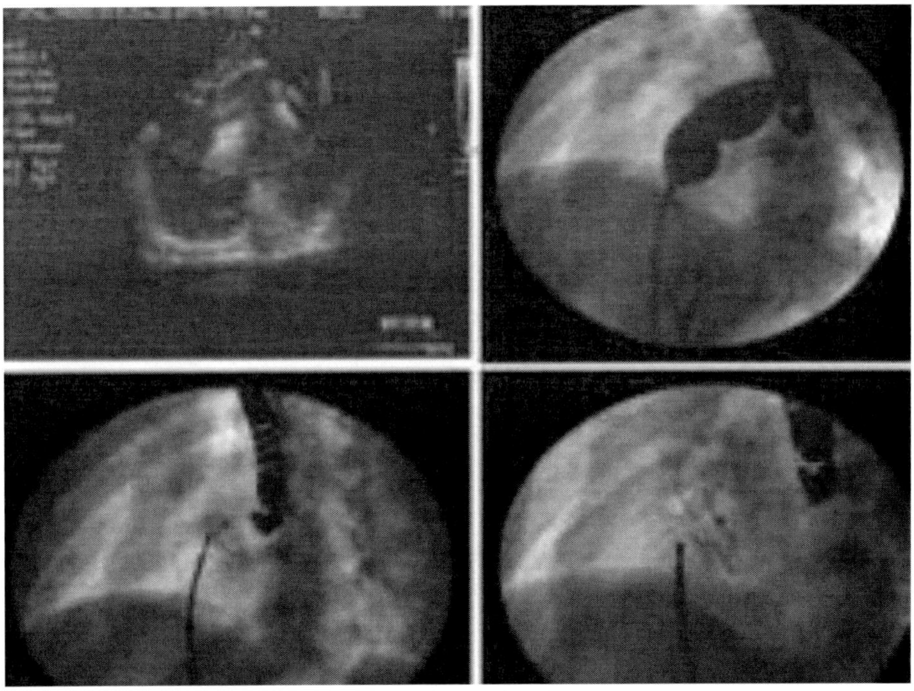

Figure 3. The four steps during the hemodynamic procedure. A: First: to recognize localization and extension of the defect. B: Second: to measure the ASD by balloon sizing. C: Third: to stabilize the device. D: Fourth: release of the device.

The most important points that should be considered during echo evaluation of ASD are:

- The location and size of the ASD, number of defects, distance between the defects, type of defect, and relationship with other structures. (Figure 4)
- It is necessary to evaluate how to close the defects: with one or two devices. Generally, if the defects are in close proximity, it is possible to close both of them with only one device. (Figure 5)

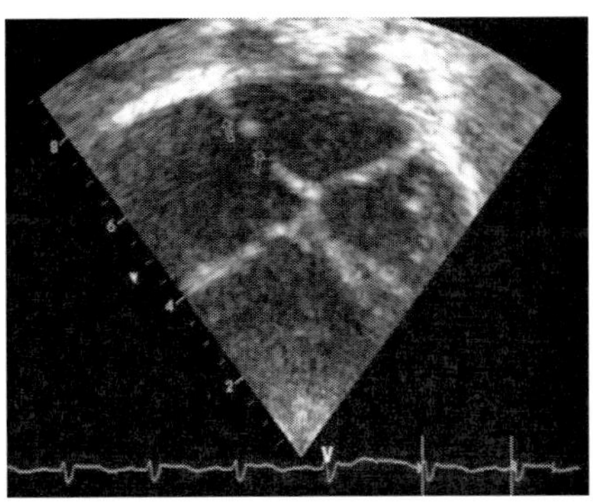

Figure 4. Two ASDs near each other (arrows).

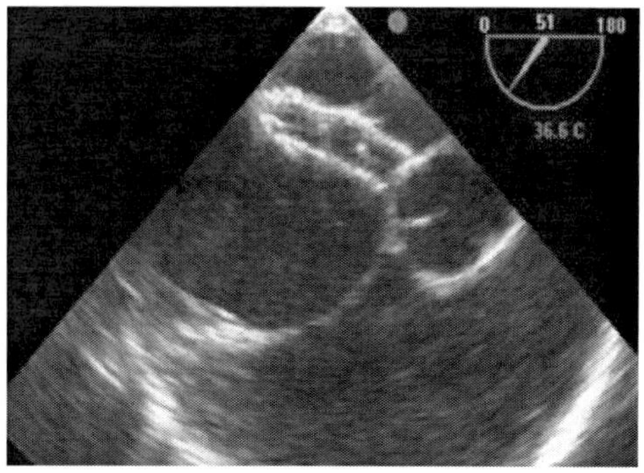

Figure 5. Both ASDs closed with only one device.

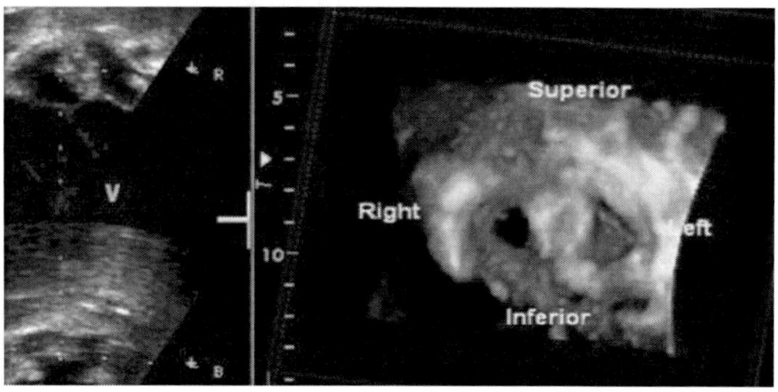

Figure 6. 3D echo: ASD closed with a Cardias device.

Post-procedure control should be done within 24 hours, after the 1st month, and then 6 months later (Figure 6). Antiplatelet therapy is required for six months following the procedure.

Complications: Device migration; device malposition; cardiac erosion/perforation leading to cardiac tamponade and death; atrioventricular heart block; and the usual complications encountered in a cardiac catheterization, including air embolism, thrombus formation, infection and hematomas. Thrombus formation is a rare complication, as the procedure is done under Heparin therapy (100UI/kg). However, as the devices are positioned into the heart through a delivery sheath (Cook® or AGA®), this can sometimes produce thrombus, generally near the valve, which can be delivered into circulation. (Figure7)

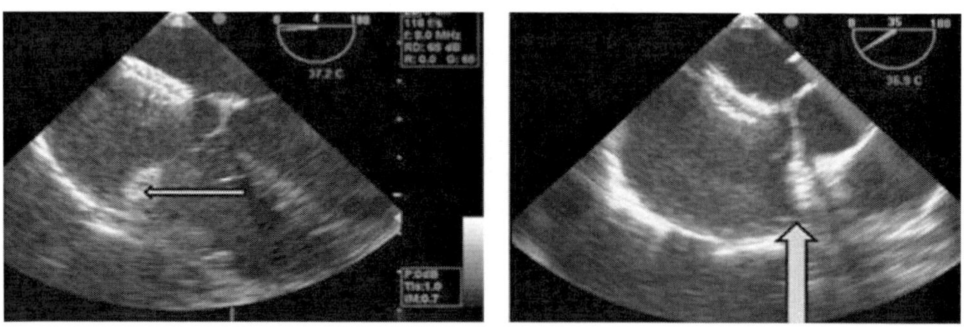

Figure 7. Complication during the procedure: thrombus (green arrow) inside the right atrium.

When embolization of the device occurs (0.8%), it may be retrieved and used to continue closing the ASD in the same procedure. (Figure 8)

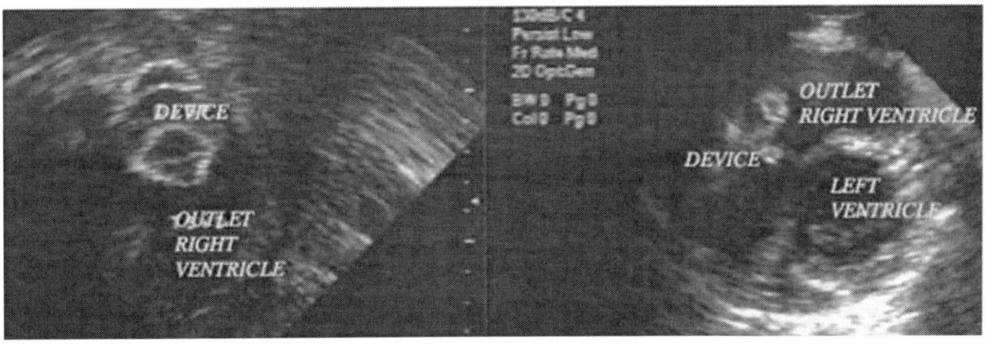

Figure 8. Device embolization and migration of the device into the pulmonary artery (on the left). The device was recovered and taken inside the right ventricle (on the right).

ASDs Not Suitable for Device Closure

Sinus venous defects (4-11%) and ostium primum (15-20%) are ASDs that are not suitable for trans-catheter device closure. For coronary sinus defects (<1%), we continue to recommend surgical treatment. Atrioventricular septal defects are contraindicated for trans-catheter device closure.

Partial or total anomalous venous return, insufficient rims, weight <10 kg, and deviation of septum primum are also situations where it is not possible to close the ASD with a device. Another problem might be not continent or weak ASD walls.

The size limit for device closure in ASDs is > 38mm, and in the aortic rim < 3 mm.

Patent Foramen Ovale (PFO)

PFO is a gap between the septum secundum, which forms the limbos of the fossa ovalis, and the septum primum, which forms the flap valve that covers the fossa ovalis. [4, 5, 6, 7] The PFO is circular to elliptical in shape and is located in the anterior-superior portion of the atrial septum. The size ranges from 1 to 19 mm, with a mean of 4.9 mm. [8] PFO length also referred to as tunnel length, ranges from 3 to 18 mm, with a mean of 8 mm. [9] Both the diameter and length increase with age. The effective size of the foramen ovale depends on the size of the space between the two septal components and the degree of valve competency. [10]. This valve competency can have 3 different situations: stretching of the superior limbos of the fossa ovalis (seen in atrial dilatation) with lack of apposition with the valve of fossa ovalis; aneurysm formation of the septum primum that prevents complete closure of atrial communication; or real deficiencies of septum primum resulting in a true ostium secundum ASD. PFO has become a subject of increasing interest in modern cardiovascular disease. This has been the result of several factors including, among others, description of paradoxical embolism, documentation of PFO with right to left shunt, the rather ubiquitous use of echocardiography, the issue of stroke prevention [11] and more recently, the relationship between patent foramen ovale and migraine. This last point is controversial.

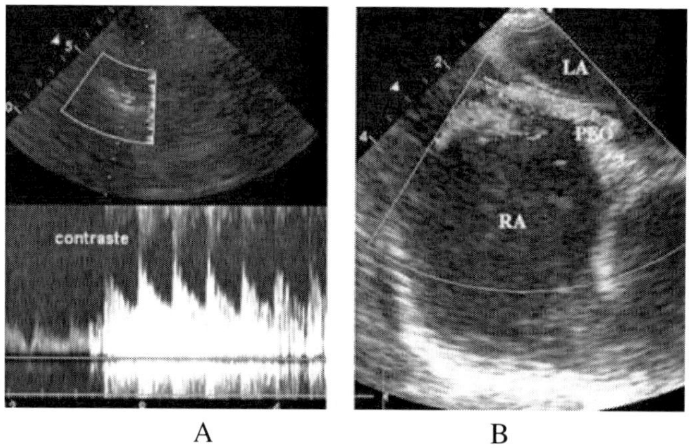

Figure 9. Intravenous shacked saline solution technique: A: Bubbles showing reversal shunt. B: Echo showing PFO tunnel length.

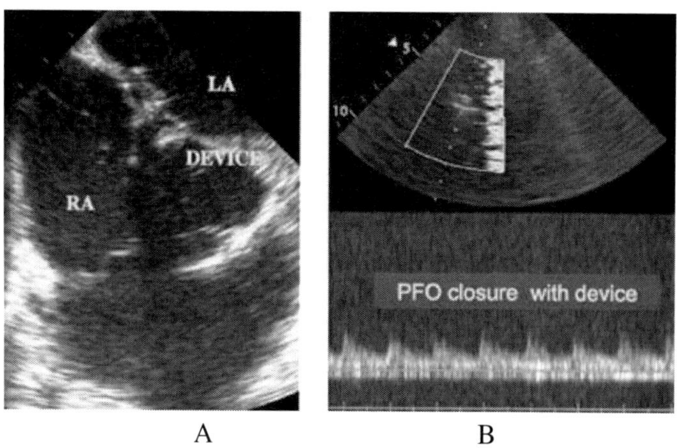

Figure 10. Intravenous shacked saline solution technique to prove no residual shunt: A: PFO closed with Helex device. B: Bubbles showing no reversal shunt.

Trans-cranial Doppler of the vertebro-basilar artery or the right middle cerebral artery with Valsalva maneuver aids in the clinical diagnosis of paradox reversal shunts [12]. The presence of 1 to 10 micro bubbles (MB) in the left atrium means minimal shunt, 11 to 25 MB means moderate shunt, and more than 25 MB means massive shunt.

Another procedure that proves the presence of reversal shunt is using intravenous shacked saline solution. (Figure 9-10)

Aneurysm of the atria septum (AAS): in this defect the valve of the fossa ovalis flaps more than 10 mm around the virtual line of the septum. (Figure11) It is associated with multi-fenestration of this lamina (2.5%), with no restrictive left to right shunt.

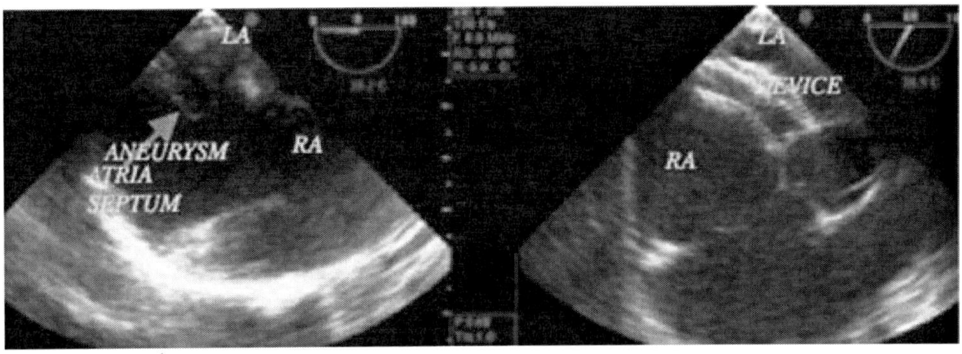

A B

Figure 11. A: AAS. B: Device closure.

PFO is present in 14.9% to 30% of the population. [13] The combination of PFO and aneurysm of the atria septum is associated with recurrent stroke in 15.2%. However, the recurrence of the stroke without AAS is only 4%. [14]

Indications for PFO closure are:

- -Recurrent stroke associated with the presence of a PFO and reversal shunt in patients under correct antiplatelet therapy.
- -Patients that had a stroke and have an AAS.
- -Patients with atrial fibrillation.
- -Patients with multi-fenestrated PFO and signs of volume overload.

Trans-Catheter Closure of Congenital Ventricular Septal Defects (VSD)

Ventricular septal defects (VSDs) are a common congenital heart disease (approximately 20%). [15]. According to their location within the septum, the defects can be classified as: muscular, perimembranous, and supracrystal. [16]

1. The most common are the perimembranous (Pm) VSD (around 70%), while completely muscular VSD may occur in approximately 15% of the cases.
2. Supracrystal defects are quite rare, accounting for 5% of all VSDs.
3. Rarely, multiple VSDs may be present in a single patient (the so-called Swiss cheese VSDs).

Indications for VSD closure are: symptoms of heart failure, signs of volume overload of left heart chambers, history of endocarditis, and post-operatory residual ventricular septal defect [17] with volume overload. In patients with volume overload of left heart chambers, closure is necessary in order to prevent pulmonary arterial hypertension, ventricular dysfunction, arrhythmias, and aortic regurgitation.

Inclusion and Exclusion Criteria for VSD Closure

The following **inclusion criteria** were used:

1. Congenital VSD.
2. Residual VSD (post-surgical repair of a congenital VSD).
3. Muscular or perimembranous location within the septum.
4. Hemodynamically significant VSD demonstrated by clinical data and/or echocardiography and/or hemodynamic study and/or angiography methods. [18, 19]
5. History of infective endocarditis.

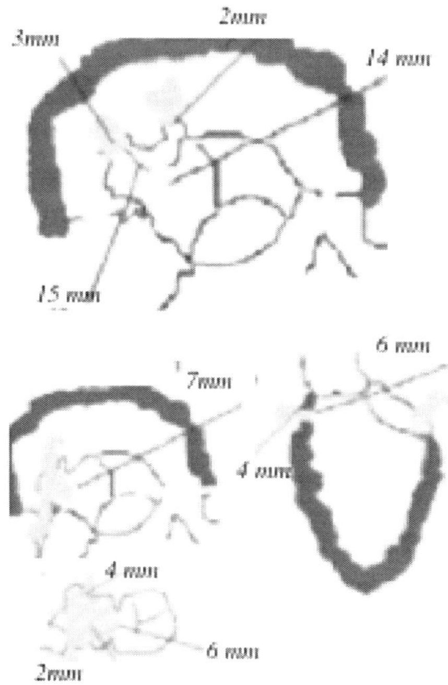

Figure 12. Short axis view and four-chamber view: Pm VSD with more than one orifice on the right side.

VSD Morphology: Percutaneous closure of perimembranous or muscular VSDs requires recognition of the type, size, shape and extension of the defect; the number of orifices on the right side (one, two or more orifices); the structures in proximity to the defect; other associated malformations; and tricuspid, mitral or aortic valve regurgitation. (Figure 12)

Exclusion criteria were [20, 21]:

1. presence of another cardiac lesion needing surgical approach; (2) irreversible pulmonary vascular disease (>7U/m2); (3) contraindication to antiplatelet therapy; (4) sepsis; (5) insufficient subaortic rim (less than 3 mm) in perimembranous VSD; (6) weight <5 kg.
2. Patient data considered:
3. Demographic details (date of procedure, age, gender, weight, height).
4. Echocardiographic data by TTE and TEE: location of VSD. (Figure 13)

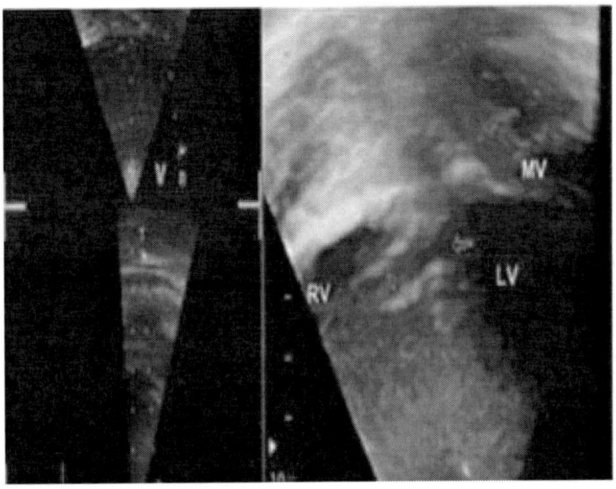

Figure 13. The image shows the closure mechanism in Pm VSD with 3D TT echo.

The anatomic types of VSD are muscular, perimembranous, multiple, or residual post-surgery. The defect must first be measured (Figure 13), and then the number of defects determined as well as their proximity to each other.

1. The sub-aortic rim (distance between the defect and the Ao valve) 3 mm or more are required in patients with perimembranous VSD (figure 14). Figure 14 B; type of closure mechanism (size and morphology). Other structures nearby to recognize are the mitral (MV) and tricuspid valve (TV) relationship with the defect.
2. Associated anomalies in: TV, MV, and Ao regurgitation.
3. Procedure details (vascular access, sheath size, pulmonary pressure, Qp/Qs, VSD size by angiography, type and size of device implanted, associated procedures, residual shunting, fluoroscopic and procedural times).
4. Trans-catheter closure of VSDs is achieved by implantation of the device into the defect, but in Pm VSDs the device is positioned inside of the closure mechanism when is necessary.

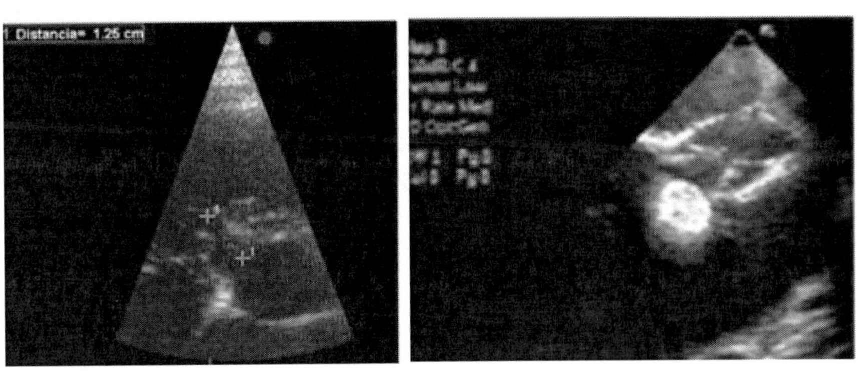

Figure14. Pm VSD sizing (A) and closure (B). A: Shows the closure mechanism of the Pm VSD by TTE, its size and morphology: orifice on the right and left ventricle and the total length. B: TEE: shows the distance between the device and the Aortic valve.

Additionally, when the closure fails, the reasons for failure must be recorded. Morphology of Perimembranous Ventricular Septal Defects (Pm VSD):

- By definition, a part of the margin of a PmVSD is the area of fibrous continuity abutting the central fibrous body that bears the atrioventricular conduction bundle. (Figure 15)

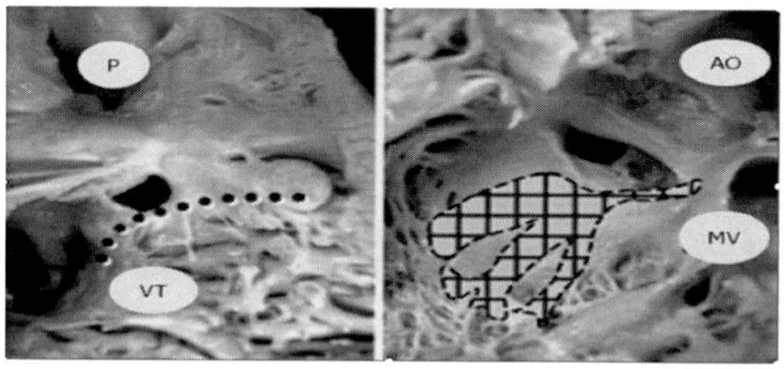

Figure 15. Pm VSD: shows the proximity with atrioventricular conduction bundle.

Pm VSD defect from the right ventricle (black points) and the left ventricle (cross lines).
P: pulmonary artery. AO: aortic artery. VT: Tricuspid valve. MV: Mitral valve.

- The remaining margins depend on the proximity of the extension of the defect [22] to the aortic, tricuspid or mitral valve. (Figure 16 A, B)

Device closure indications [23,24,25]:

- $Qp/Qs \geq 1.5$
- Restrictive VSD + hemodynamic repercussion
- Post-operatory residual VSD with hemodynamic repercussion
- Small VSD post-infectious endocarditis
- Pulmonary Hypertension (after therapy with sildenafil)

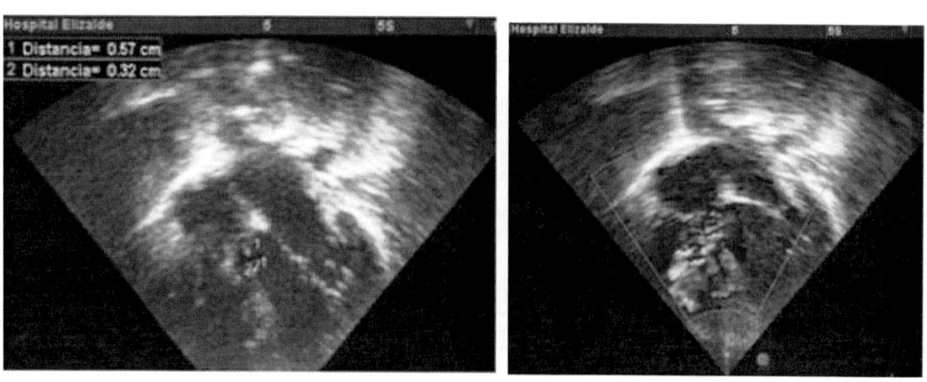

A B

Figure 16. 2D Echo measurement and morphology of Pm VSD: A: TTE Pm VSD sizing in black and white. B: VSD by color, relationship to TV and MV.

A better resolution is provided by 3D than with 2D echo, especially for analysis of the closure mechanisms or to differentiate types of defects. (Figure 17).

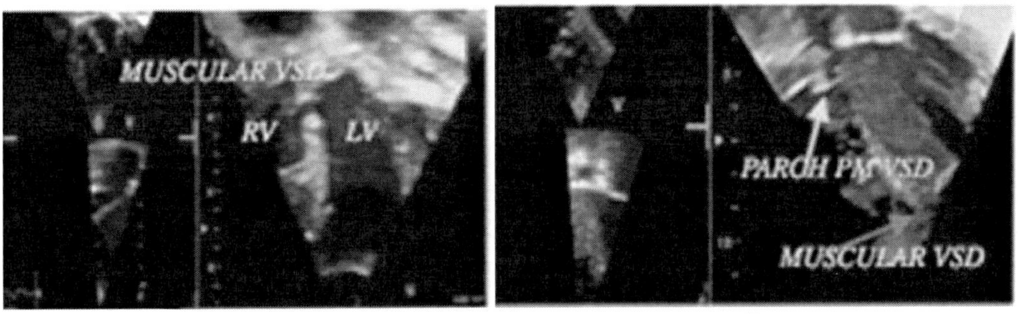

A B

Figure 17. 3D echo: muscular VSD. A: Muscular VSD (green arrow): 3D high muscular VSD, above and below muscular walls. B: Residual post surgery muscular apical VSD (red arrow), patch (yellow arrow).

Exclusion criteria:

- Weight <5 kg
- Non-reversible pulmonary hypertension (Pulmonary resistance >7 Woods)
- More than mild aortic regurgitation (aortic valve cusp prolapsed)
- Inlet extension
- Patients with anti-platelet therapy contraindications
- Not recommended in the absence of the crista, since this VSD has a deficient aortic and pulmonary margin, showing fibrous continuity of both arteries.

Complications

A major complication is defined as an event that results in death, long-term sequelae, requires immediate surgery, potentially life-threatening events, persistent arrhythmias needing long-term therapy (>6 months) or pacemaker placement, ongoing hemolysis requiring blood transfusion, thrombosis that requires thrombolytic therapy, or when increased valve regurgitation requires device removal or drug therapy. A minor complication is defined as an event that requires drug therapy but is not life- threatening and has no long-term sequelae (<6 months), or when it does not require long-term therapy. The following are also included in this group: device embolization with trans-catheter retrieval, hematomas of the groin, cardiac arrhythmias that require cardioversion with drug therapy during the procedure, minor degree atrio-ventricular blocks, and transient loss of peripheral pulse needing only Heparin therapy.

The *procedure* is *successful* when the device implantation is in the appropriate position and when there are no new reasons for surgery (for example, due to significant residual shunt or significant valve regurgitation).

Residual shunt is identified by color-Doppler flow mapping showing a left to right shunt across the ventricular septum. It is classified as: trivial (<1mm color jet width), small (1–2 mm color jet width), moderate (2–4 mm color jet width), or large (>4 mm color jet width).

Post-procedure *complete AV block (cAVB):* This can be transitory or definitive. When cAVB appears during the procedure, we prefer to remove the device to restore sinus rhythm. The procedure should be stopped and the closure programmed by surgery; the risk of cAVB after the device implantation in pmVSD is high. In our study cAVB was the most significant complication and required pacemaker implantation. [26] If this occurs after the procedure, we recommend corticoids to avoid definitive cAVB. In the literature, cAVBs needing pacemaker implantation are reported to occur in 0–8% of subjects. This complication is related to the proximity of the conduction system to the margins of the pm VSD. Therefore, both surgery and device implantation may interfere with atrio-ventricular conduction. Various mechanisms may be considered as causative. It is possible that the presence of the device may disturb atrio-ventricular conduction by direct traumatic compression. Furthermore, the device may raise an inflammatory reaction or scar formation in the conduction tissue. However, there is no specific data concerning the mechanisms involved in the occurrence of cAVB after percutaneous closure of a pm VSD. Larger studies are needed to clarify the real impact of arrhythmic problems in these patients and the mechanism of the events. Another dangerous complication is the rupture of the tricuspid valve chordae tendineae. [27]

Atrio-ventricular residual regurgitation with mild repercussion and non-significant residual shunt may be present after the procedure.

In our experience, total occlusion was obtained in 47% of patients at the end of the procedure, rising to 84% at discharge and 99% during the follow-up. The analysis of risk factors for complications showed that age and weight were associated with a higher risk of early complications. Residual shunt was trivial in 15% and mild in 2% of the subjects. Success rate was very high, as closure was successfully achieved in 95.3% of patients in the follow-up. This is in agreement with the data reported in the literature, where the success rate ranges between 87 and 100% of cases. Trans-catheter closure of congenital VSD offers encouraging results. More experience and long-term follow-up are mandatory to assess its safety and effectiveness.

Aortic Coarctation (Ao Co)

Coarctation of the aorta is typically a discrete stenosis of the proximal thoracic aorta. The apparent anatomic simplicity is misleading; however, coarctation varies considerably in its anatomy, physiology, clinical presentation, treatment options and outcomes. The pathophysiology of coarctation varies with the severity of the stenosis and is also affected by the presence of associated lesions, such as patent ductus arteriosus, ventricular septal defect and aortic or mitral stenosis. [28]. Coarctation of the aorta is a common form of congenital heart disease, accounting for 6 to 8% of all cardiac defects. The prevalence of coarctation is increased in certain disorders, such as Turner syndrome. [29] The most common associated cardiac anomaly is bicuspid aortic valve, which is present in 30 to 40% of all cases. The most important non-cardiac associated anomaly is intra-cerebral aneurysm (berry aneurysm), present in 10% of all cases.

Coarctation of the aorta (Ao Co) occurs in about 0.04% of live births and comprises about 7% of all known congenital heart disease (CHD). The reported natural history of untreated coarctation is poor. The mean age of death for patients with coarctation surviving the 1st year of life is 34 years (control: 72 years). [30]

The usual location of coarctation is juxtaductal, just distal to the left subclavian artery; less often, the coarctation is proximal to the origin of the left subclavian artery. The aortic coarctation may be a long-segment stenosis, and\or may be associated with hypoplasia of the transverse aortic arch. The abdominal presentation of the aortic coarctation is possible but fortunately is rare. When the location is abdominal, the coarctation can be associated with aortopathies with renal artery stenosis, such as Takayasu syndrome. [31]

In a collaborative work in 2007, Thomas J. Forbes et al. defined the coarctation of the aorta as "the presence of systemic hypertension with an upper to lower limb systolic blood pressure difference of 20 mmHg or an upper to lower extremity blood pressure differential of <20 mmHg in the presence of systemic hypertension or left ventricular hypertrophy, and confirmation of the coarctation should be done by computerized tomography (CT) scan, magnetic resonance imaging, or echocardiographic assessment." [32]

Discrete coarctation was defined as a coarctation segment measuring ≤5 mm. Extensive coarctation is present when it involves a long segment of coarctation measuring >5 mm. Forbes et al. add that when the obstruction occurred at the level of the transverse aortic arch, the ratio of the diameter of the narrowed segment to the diameter of the descending aorta at the level of the diaphragm of less than 0.6 was used to define coarctation in the presence of clinical evidence of coarctation.

Regarding the severity of the aortic coarctation, the Argentine Society of Cardiology (ASC) consensus of 2011 [33] based its definition on the systolic arm-to-leg blood pressure gradient:

- <20 mm Hg: mild Ao Co.
- 20-40 mm Hg: moderate Ao Co.
- 40 mm Hg: severe Ao Co.

Other signs and/or severity criteria were: hypertension during exercise, heart failure and/or severe left ventricular (LV) dysfunction.

Diagnosis

Transthoracic echocardiography confirms the diagnosis. Other imaging modalities (CT/MRI angiograms, cardiac catheterization) may not be obtained routinely unless the diagnosis is in doubt or additional information is needed to plan a surgical or catheter intervention; however, the information obtained by these studies will likely impact our long-term understanding of coarctation repair outcome. Noninvasive MRI/MRA and CT angiography provide a comprehensive view of the thoracic aorta, including the arch, coarctation site, and associated collateral vessels. MRI/MRA is particularly valuable in the follow-up of patients and permits monitoring of coarctation outcome.

Endovascular Treatment

Balloon Angioplasty

After experimental trials, percutaneous balloon angioplasty (BA) was established in 1982 as a treatment option both for native and recurrent postoperative aortic coarctation. [34-35]

The incidence of early and late aneurysms after balloon angioplasty has been reported to be between 5 and 11.5%. [36-37] Increasing age has been found to be a risk factor for a suboptimal outcome. [38] This has been attributed to the presence of fibrotic changes in the aorta secondary to long-standing obstruction [39] and to cystic medial necrosis observed after percutaneous balloon angioplasty of Ao Co, with both as potential factors contributing to adverse consequences, such as re-coarctation (RE-CO) of the aorta and aneurysms.

In 2003, the Task Force published [40] that BA of native aortic disease can often be achieved with excellent results, although failure to relieve stenosis (10–20%), aneurysm formation (5–10%) and restenosis (5–10%) have all been reported. BA of previous patch aortoplasty carries the highest risk of aortic rupture and should be performed with surgical standby.

In 2012, the American Heart Association published [41] that BA for native coarctation can also be performed safely and successfully beyond the neonatal period. Young patients (>1 month but <6 months of age) with discrete narrowing and no evidence of arch hypoplasia may benefit from BA.

This criterion applies to relatively few patients in this age group, because arch hypoplasia commonly accompanies coarctation of the aorta. However, the recurrence rate is higher for younger patients (<6 months of age), and there is a small but important incidence of aneurysm formation after balloon dilation of native coarctation at any age.

Our experience covered the years from 1984 to 2005, when we carried out 47 BA in patients (p) with Ao Co. The mean age was 8 years old ± 8 months (20 days-19 years old). The procedure was effective in 81% of the cases, reducing the gradient from X: 50±17 mmHg to 14±10mmHg; 19% had no reduction in gradient.

Postsurgical: 17p (13.3%) (Figure: 1-4). 1p died due to a dissection of the aorta (patch aortoplasty with PTFE).

Native: 30p (86.7%): 21p with heart failure (HF), 3p with cardiomyopathy and 6p without collateral circulation. 1p died during the procedure: a newborn with heart failure (HF).

Follow up: re-coartation (67%) and sacular aneurysms (4.2%) (Figure 19). Due to these complications, since 2005 we have indicated BA only in:

1. Patients over 18 kg with a localized coarctation of the aorta.
2. Patients under 18 kg without collateral circulation.
3. Postsurgical re-coarctation. (Figure 18)

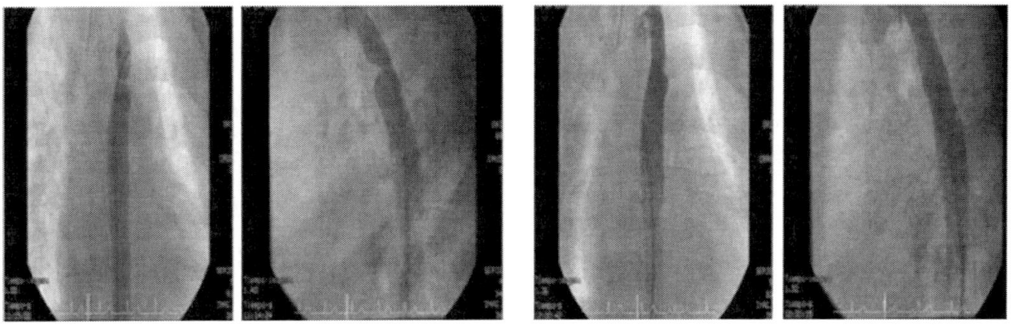

Figure 18. A-B-C-D. Postsurgical re-coarctation. A: Co Ao Antero posterior view. B: Co Ao lateral view. C Post BA: Antero posterior view. D: lateral view.

Newborn with Ao Co and heart failure or cardiomyopathy with contraindications for surgery (palliative).

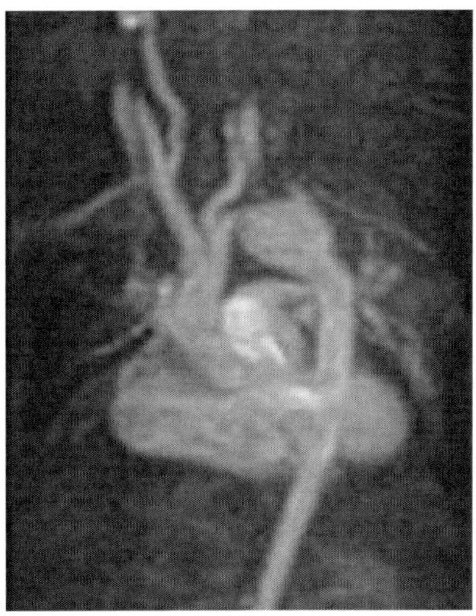

Figure19. Sacular aneurysm after BA.

Angioplasty with Stent

Since 1980, stent implantation has evolved as an important therapeutic strategy for coarctation of the aorta. It provides the potential for long-term repair with less chance of coarctation recurrence or aneurysm formation. Of course, long-term benefit has yet to be proven. Stents provide a homogenous framework for smooth endothelial growth along the aortic wall that reduces the risk of thrombosis, neo-intimal hyperplasia and subsequent restenosis. [42]. However, at an early age, restenosis by intimal growth may develop. In addition, while the incidence of aneurysm formation is low (7%), it is not eliminated by the use of stents compared to balloon angioplasty alone. [43] Stent implantation for native coarctation or re-coarctation of the aorta has also emerged as a beneficial therapeutic option for patients who can receive a stent that can be expanded to an adult size. The morbidity associated with stent implantation for coarctation of the aorta is lower than with surgery or balloon dilation alone. [44] Our experience began with the Palmaz stent in 1993. Before 2000 we were using the Cheatam-Platinum (CP) stent (NuMED, Hopkinton, NY) and, after 2002, the CP covered stent (PTFE). The measurements obtained from the angiography were: (1) diameter and length of the stenotic area; (2) diameter of the descending aorta at the level of the diaphragm; (3) diameter of the aorta at the level of the subclavian artery; and (4) diameter of the transverse arch.

Experience with Palmaz Stent

In our experience with 35 cases, aged between 6 to 38 years old, the results were acceptable. The complications that we experienced were:

- 4 balloon punctures.
- 2 balloon migrations during inflation.
- 1 peri-stent hematoma.
- 1 small saccular aneurysm.

Experience with CP stent

Bare stent

1. Native coarctation of aorta, weight permitted: > 25 kg
2. Mild native aortic coarctation with exaggerated hypertensive response to stress
3. Postsurgical re-coarctation with recoil

Covered Stent

1. If the relationship between the initial diameter and the required final diameter is greater than 3, the best option is to employ the covered stent due to the risk of damaging the aortic artery. (Figures 20, 21 and 22)

Picture 20- 21-22: Severe aortic coarctation.

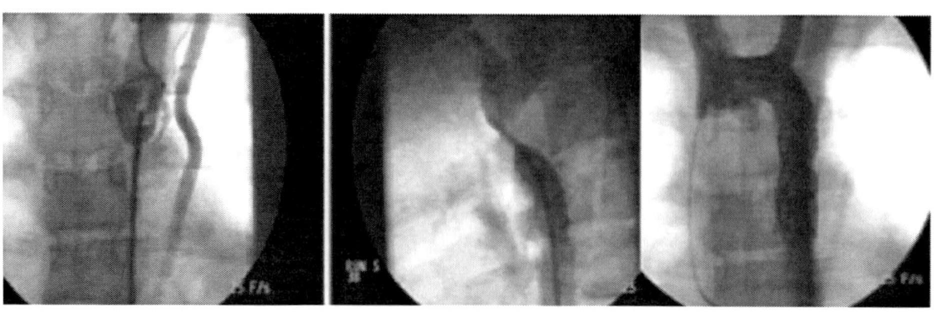

Picture 20. Antero-posterior view. Picture 21. Lateral view .Picture 22. Stent anterior-posterior view.

2. Association with native (Figures: 23, 24, 25, 26, 27, 28) or postsurgical (Figures: 29, 30) aneurysm. Covered stents are preferred because the sick aortic wall has not been previously removed by surgery and, therefore, the covered stent will prevent wall rupture, dissection or similar complications.

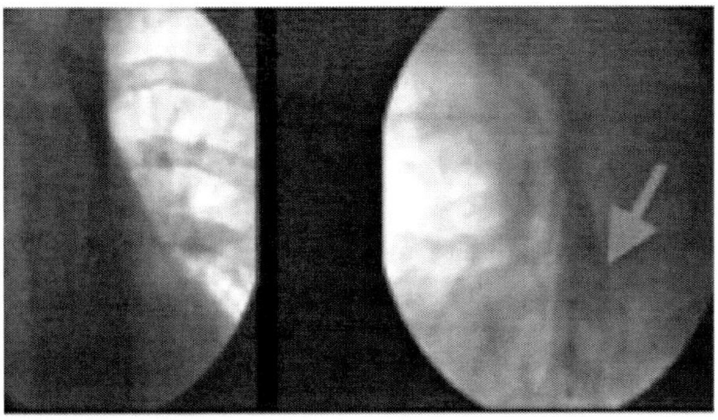

Antero-posterior view.

Figure 23. Severe aortic coarctation.

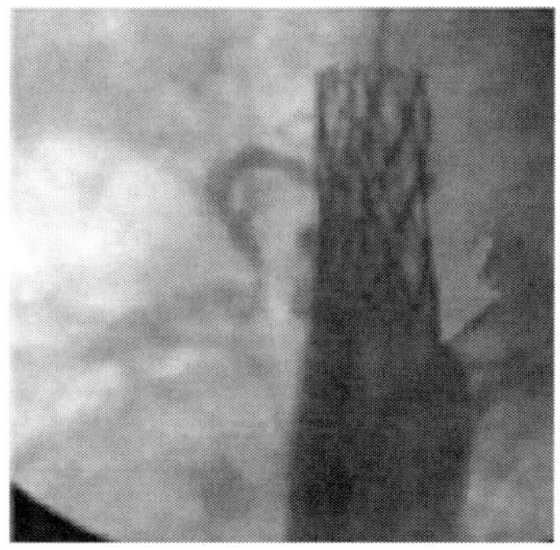

Lateral view 1st covered stent. Red arrow: native sacular aneurism.

Figure 24. Severe aortic coarctation.

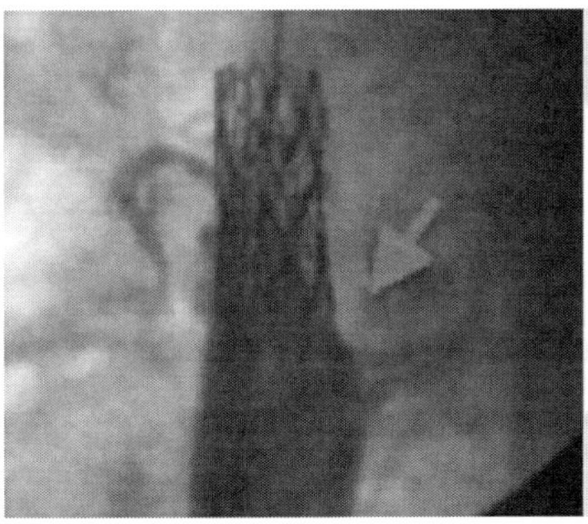

Lateral view 1st covered stent.

Figure 25. Severe aortic coarctation.

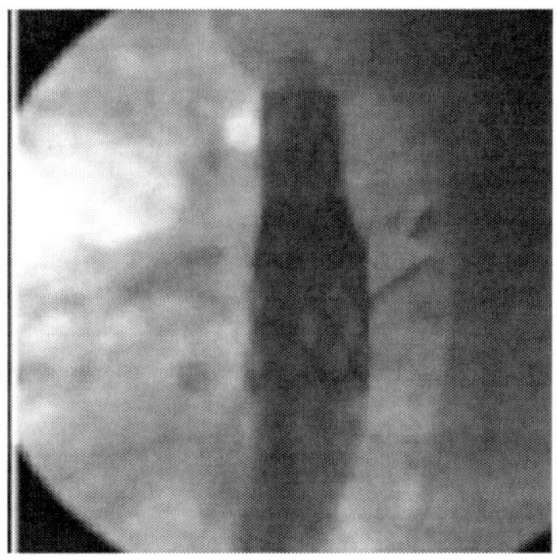

Lateral view 2nd covered stent.

Figure 26. Severe aortic coarctation.

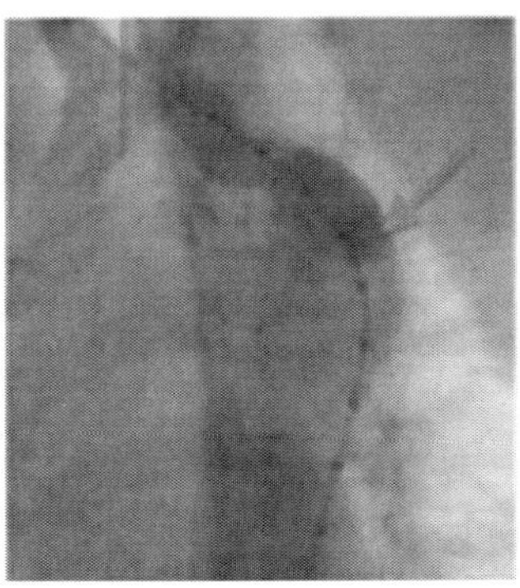

Figure 27. Coarctation of the aorta with isthmus hypoplasia and post- Operatory. aneurysm.

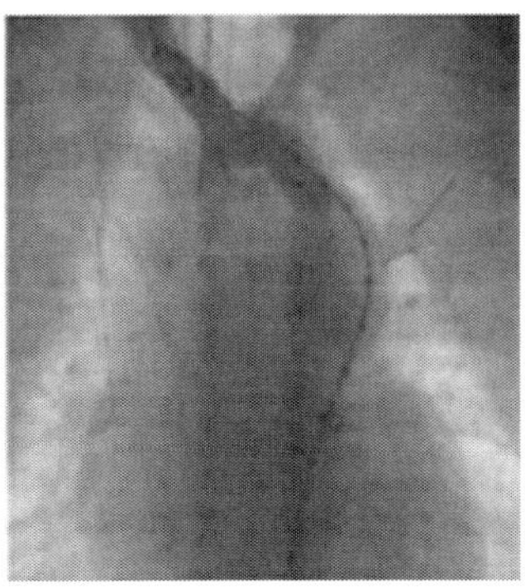

Figure 28. Coarctation of the aorta intra procedure showing aneurysm

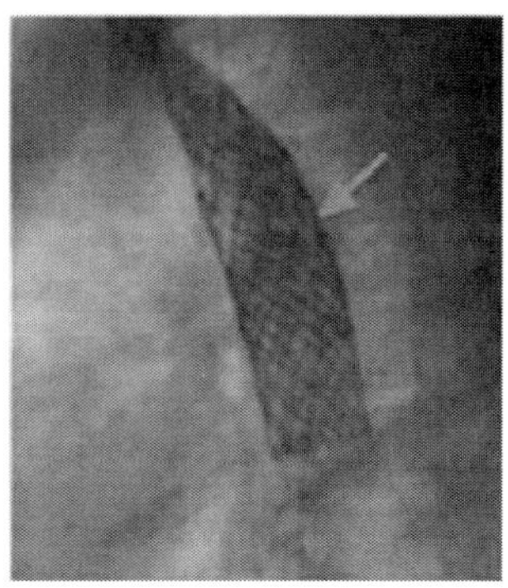

Figure 29. Coarctation of the aorta treated with 3 covered stents.

3. In patients > 45 years old, to avoid bleeding and other major complications.
4. What should we consider in a patient with coarctation of the aorta?
    1. Age and weight: surgery is the best option in patients <25 Kg, and covered stent in patients >45 years old, to avoid morbidity.
    2. Native or postsurgical: in postsurgical patients the best solution is catheter angioplasty with or without stent, depending on the age, type of defect, elasticity of the wall and other complications.
    3. Severity: When it is necessary to expand the aorta to adult size, or when the initial diameter is less than 3 times the required final diameter, the covered stent is preferred.
    4. Localized or extensive membranous type, or tubular type even with hypoplasia of the isthmus.
    5. Re-coarctation after balloon angioplasty or stent.
    6. Compromise of any of the neck vessels.
    7. Acquired interruption.
    8. Presence of native or postsurgical aneurysm.
    9. Indemnity of femoral arteries (history of other procedures).

References

[1] Anderson RH, Brown NA, Webb S. Development and structure of the atrial septum. *Heart*. 2002:88(1): 104-110.

[2] Santoro G, Gaio G and Russo MG. *Transcatheter Treatment of Unroofed Coronary Sinus on and Cardiovascular Interventions* 2013; 81:849–852

[3] Feltes TF, Bacha E, Beekman III RH, et al; On behalf of the American Heart Association Congenital Cardiac Defects Committee of the Council on Cardiovascular Disease in the Young, Council on Clinical Cardiology, and Council on Cardiovascular Radiology and Intervention. Indications for Cardiac Catheterization and Intervention in Pediatric Cardiac Disease. A Scientific Statement From the American Heart Association. *Circulation*. 2011;123: 2607-2652.

[4] Ziyad M Hijazi, Feldman Ted, Mustafa H, et al. Transcatheter closure of ASD san PFOs. *Cardiotext Book* 2011. Part II and III. Page. 97-229.

[5] Hijazi ZM, Cao Q-L, Patel HT, Rhodes J, et al. Transesophageal echocardiographic results of catheter closure of atrial septal defect in children and adults using the Amplatzer device. *Am J Cardiol*. 2000; 85(11): 1387-1390.

[6] Mc Kenzie JA, Edwards WD, Hagler DJ. Anatomy of the patent foramen ovale for the interventional list. *Cathet Cardiovasc Intervent*. 2009; 73(6):821-826.

[7] Hagen P, Scholz D, Edwards W. Incidence and size of patent foramen ovale during the first 10 decades of life: an autopsy study of 965 normal hearts. *Mayo Clin Proc*. 1984;59:17-20.

[8] Ho SY, Mc Carthy KP, Rigky ML. Morphological features pertinent to interventional closure of patent foramen ovale in patents oval foramen. *J Interv Cardiol*. 2003:16:303-307.

[9] Marshall AC, Lock JE. Structural and complicant anatomy of the patent foramen ovale in patients undergoing transcatheter closure. *Am Heart J.* 2000: 140:303-307.
[10] Holmes Jr, Cohen HA. and Ruiz C. Patent foramen ovale, systemic embolization, and closure. *Curr. Probl. Cardiol.* 2009;34:483-530.
[11] Spencer MP, Moehring MA, Jesurum J. et al. Power m-mode transcranial Doppler for diagnosis of patent foramen ovale and assessing transcathter closure. *J. Neuroimaging* 2004;14:342-9.
[12] Del Sette M, Dinia L, Rizzi D, et al. Diagnosis of right to left shunt with trans cranial Doppler and vertebro basilar recording. *Stroke* 2007; 38:2254-6.
[13] Ditullio MR, Sacco RL, Sciacca RR, et al. Patent foramen ovale and the risk of ischemic stroke in a multiethnic population. *J Am Coll Cardiol* 2007: 49:797-802.
[14] Mas JL, Arquizan C, Lamy C, et al. Recurrent cerebrovascular events associated with patent foramen ovale, atrial septal aneurysm or both. *N Engl J Med* 2001; 345:1740-6.
[15] Carminati M. et al. Transcatheter closure of congenital ventricular septal defects: results of the European Registry. *European Heart Journal* (2007) 28, 2361–2368.
[16] Pedra AC, Pedra SRF, Esteves CA, Pontes SC, Braga SL, Arrieta SR, Santana MV, Fontes VF, Masura J. Percutaneous closure of perimembranous ventricular septal defects with the Amplatzer device: technical and morphological considerations. *Catheter Cardiovasc Interv* 2004;61: 403– 410.
[17] Knauth AL, Lock JE, Perry SB, McElhinney DB, Gauvreau K, Landzberg MJ, Rome JJ, Hellenbrand WE, Ruiz CE, Jenkins KJ. Transcatheter device closure of congenital and post-operative residual ventricular septal defect. *Circulation* 2004;110:501–507.
[18] Thanopoulos BD, Rigby ML. Outcome of transcatheter closure of muscular ventricular septal defects with the Amplatzer ventricular septal defect occluder. *Heart* 2005; 91:513–516.
[19] Ralf Holzer, Jo de Giovanni, Kevin P. Walsh, Andrew Tometzki, TH Goh, Fakhri Hakim, Carlos Zabal, Jose Suarez de Lezo, Qi-Ling Cao, Ziyad M. Hijazi. Transcatheter closure of perimembranous ventricular septal defects using the Amplatzer membranous VSD occluder. *Catheter and Cardiov. Interv* 2006. 68:620-628.
[20] Hijazi ZM, Hakim F, Al Fadley F, Abdelhamid J, Cao QL. Transcatheter closure of single muscular ventricular septal defects using the Amplatzer muscular VSD occluder: initial results and technical considerations. *Catheter Cardiovasc Interv* 2000;49:167–172.
[21] Chessa M, Carminati M, Cao QL, Butera G, Giusti S, Bini RM, Hijazi Z. Transcatheter closure of congenital and acquired muscular ventricular septal defects using the Amplatzer device. *J Invasive Cardiol* 2002;14:322–327.
[22] Siew Yen Ho, Path Karen, Mc Carthy B, Rigby Michael. Morphology and perimembranous ventricular septal defects: Implications for transcatheter device closure. *J. Interv Cardiol* 2004; 17: 99-108.
[23] Bass JL, Kalra GS, Arora R, Masura J, Gavora P, Thanoupoulos B, Torres W, Sievert H, Carminati M, Fisher G, Ewert P. Initial human experience with the Amplatzer perimembranous ventricular septal occluder device. *Catheter Cardiovasc Interv* 2003;58:238–245.
[24] Masura J, Gao W, Gavora P, Sun K, Zhan AO, Jiang S, Tiang-Liang C, Wang Y. Percutaneous closure of perimembranous ventricular septal defects with the eccentric Amplatzer device: multicenter follow-up study. *Pediatr Cardiol* 2005;26:216–219.

[25] Fu YC, Bass J, Amin Z, Radtke W, Cheatham JP, Hellenbrand WE, Balzer D, Cao QL, Hijazi ZM. Transcatheter closure of perimembranous ventricular septal defects using the new Amplatzer membranous VSD occluder. Results of the U.S. phase I trial. *J Am Coll Cardiol* 2006;47: 319–325.

[26] Gianfranco Butera, Mario Carminati, Massimo Chessa, Luciane Piazza, Angelo Micheletti, Diana Gabriella Negura, Raul Abella, Alessandro Giamberti, Alessandro Frigiola. Transcatheter Closure of Perimembranous Ventricular Septal Defects. *J Am Coll Cardiol.* 2007;50(12):1189-1195.

[27] Yun-Ching Fu, MD, PhD; John Bass, MD; Zahid Amin, MD; Wolfgang Radtke, MD; John P. Cheatham, MD; William E. Hellenbrand, MD; David Balzer, MD; Qi-Ling Cao, MD; Ziyad M. Hijazi. *J Am Coll Cardiol.* 2006;47(2):319-325.

[28] Robert H. Beekman III. Coarctation of the Aorta. Allen, Hugh D.; Driscoll, David J.; Shaddy, Robert E.; Feltes, Timothy F. Title: Moss and Adams' Heart Disease in Infants, Children, and Adolescents: Including the Fetus and Young Adults, 7th Edition. 2008 Lippincott Williams & Wilkins. Page. 988-1004.

[29] Gotzsche CO, Krag-Olsen B, Nielsen J, Sørensen KE, Kristensen BO. Prevalence of cardiovascular malformations and association with karyotypes in Turner's syndrome. *Arch Dis Child.* 1994;71:433– 436.

[30] Campbell M. Natural history of coarctation of the aorta. Br Heart J 1970;32:633–640.

[31] Jesús María Damsky Barbosa, Victorio Lucini, Adelia Marques Vitorino, Carola Canteros, Ana De Dios. Covered stent in the treatment of aortic coarctation in a Takayasu arteritis. *Revista Argentina de Cardio-angiología* 2012, Vol 3 (4), 220-222.

[32] Thomas J. Forbes, Swati Garekar, Zahid Amin, Evan M. Zahn, David Nykanen, Phillip Moore, Shakeel A. Qureshi, John P. Cheatham, Makram R. Ebeid, Ziyad M. Hijazi, Satinder Sandhu, Donald J. Hagler, Horst Sievert, Thomas E. Fagan, Jeremy Ringewald, Wei Du, Liwen Tang, David F. Wax, John Rhodes, Troy A. Johnston, Thomas K. Jones, Daniel R. Turner, Carlos A.C. Pedra, and William E. Hellenbrand, Congenital Cardiovascular Interventional Study Consortium (CCISC). Procedural Results and Acute Complications in Stenting Native and Recurrent Coarctation of the Aorta in Patients Over 4 Years of Age: A Multi-Institutional Study. *Catheterization and Cardiovascular Interventions.* 2007; 70:276–285.

[33] de Dios A, Sardella A, Peirone A et al. *Rev Argent Cardiol* 2011; 79:62-78.

[34] Singer MI, Rowen M, Dorsey TJ. Transluminal aortic balloon angioplasty for coarctation of the aorta in the newborn. *Am Heart J.* 1982; 103:131–132.

[35] Hijazi ZM, Fahey JT, Kleinman CS, Hellenbrand WE. Balloon angioplasty for recurrent coarctation of aorta. Immediate and long-term results. *Circulation.* 1991; 84:1150–6.

[36] Hellenbrand WE, Allen HD, Golinko RJ, Hagler DJ, Lutin W, Kan J. Balloon angioplasty for aortic recoarctation: Results of Valvuloplasty and Angioplasty of Congenital Anomalies Registry. *Am J Cardiol.* 1990; 65:793–7.

[37] Ovaert C, Benson LN, Nykanen D, Freedom RM. Transcatheter treatment of coarctation of the aorta: A review. *Pediatr Cardiol.* 1998; 19:27–44. Discussion 45-7.

[38] Forbes TJ, Garekar S, Amin Z, Zahn EM, Nykanen D, Moore P, et al. Procedural results and acute complications in stenting native and recurrent coarctation of the aorta in patients over 4 years of age: A multi-institutional study. *Catheter Cardiovasc Interv.* 2007; 70:276–85.

[39] McCrindle BW, Jones TK, Morrow WR, Hagler DJ, Lloyd TR, Nouri S, et al. Acute results of balloon angioplasty of native coarctation versus recurrent aortic obstruction are equivalent. Valvuloplasty and Angioplasty of Congenital Anomalies (VACA) Registry Investigators. *J Am Coll Cardiol.* 1996; 28:18.

[40] Task Force members, Chairperson, John Deanfield*, Erik Thaulow, Carol Warnes, Gary Webb, Frantizek Kolbel, Andreas Hoffman, Keld Sorenson, Harald Kaemmerer, Ulf Thilen, Margreet Bink-Boelkens, Laurence Iserin, Luciano Daliento, Eric Silove†, Andrew Redington, Pascal Vouhe. Management of Grown Up Congenital Heart Disease The Task Force on the Management of Grown Up Congenital Heart Disease of the European Society of Cardiology *European Heart Journal* (2003) 24, 1035–1084.

[41] Timothy F. Feltes, MD, FAHA, Chair; Emile Bacha, MD; Robert H. Beekman III, MD, FAHA; John P. Cheatham, MD; Jeffrey A. Feinstein, MD, MPH; Antoinette S. Gomes, MD, FAHA; Ziyad M. Hijazi, MD, MPH, FAHA; Frank F. Ing, MD; Michael de Moor, MBBCh; W. Robert Morrow, MD; Charles E. Mullins, MD, FAHA; Kathryn A. Taubert, PhD, FAHA; Evan M. Zahn, MD; on behalf of the American Heart Association Congenital Cardiac Defects Committee of the Council on Cardiovascular Disease in the Young, Council on Clinical Cardiology, and Council on Cardiovascular Radiology and Intervention. Indications for Cardiac Catheterization and Intervention in Pediatric Cardiac Disease. A Scientific Statement From the American Heart Association. *Circulation*. 2011; 123:2607-2652.

[42] De Lezo JS, Pan M, Romero M, et al. Balloon-expandable stent repair of severe coarctation of the aorta. *Am Heart J* 1995; 129:1002–8.

[43] Magee AG, Brzezinska-Rajszys G, Qureshi SA, et al. Stent implantation for aortic coarctation and re-coarctation. *Heart* 1999; 82:600–6.

[44] Carr JA. The results of catheter-based therapy compared with surgical repair of adult aortic coarctation. *J Am Coll Cardiol* 2006; 47:1101–1107.

In: Congenital Heart Diseases
Editor: Raúl Cayré and José Milei
ISBN: 978-1-61122-003-2

Chapter 11

Hybrid Procedures for Congenital Heart Disease: Palliation of Hypoplastic Left Heart Syndrome, Closure of Muscular Ventricular Septal Defect and Stenting of Branch Pulmonary Arteries

Alejandro R. Peirone[*1] *and Carlos A. C. Pedra*[†2]
[1]Catheterization Laboratory Children Hospital of Córdoba,
Division of Pediatric Cardiology, Private Hospital of Córdoba,
Córdoba, Argentina
[2]Catheterization Laboratory for Congenital Heart Disease,
Instituto Dante Pazzanese de Cardiología,
Hospital do Coração da Associação Sanatório Sírio,
Sao Paulo, Brazil

Abstract

Evolving surgical and catheter-based techniques and a collaboration environment between surgeons and interventionalists resulted in the advent of the so-called hybrid procedures in congenital heart disease. Although the hybrid approach starts with a collaborative effort between surgeons and interventionalists, it continues with careful planning among different subspecialties such as imaging, intensive care and anesthesia. The goals of hybrid therapies include reduction of morbidity and mortality in patients with more complex diseases, mitigation of the negative cumulative effects of multiple procedures, improvement in quality of life and delivery of a more cost-efficient care. Also the hybrid environment encourages the sharing of expertise, ideas, equipment and techniques, which is crucial to introduce novel therapies for challenging patients. These procedures have significantly expanded the therapeutic options for several patients with

[*] E-mail: alepeirone@yahoo.com.
[†] E-mail: cacpedra@uol.com.br, carlosacpedra@hotmail.com.

complex congenital heart disease in the last 10 years. In this chapter we will discuss the application of the hybrid approach in the management of hypoplastic left heart syndrome, muscular ventricular septal defects and pulmonary artery stenosis.

Introduction

Surgical and catheter-based interventions for congenital heart disease (CHD) have evolved remarkably over the past 50 years. Corrective surgery for intracardiac defects was introduced in the 1950s with the advent of cardiopulmonary bypass (CPB). Since then, surgical techniques have been refined progressively resulting in complete repair of more complex defects in infants, neonates and even in low-birth-weight premies. Transcathteter procedures have also evolved, mainly in the 1980s and 1990s, allowing the treatment of a variety of lesions without the use of CPB. In the 2000s, an increasingly collaborative environment between interventional cardiologists and cardiothoracic surgeons led to the development of the so-called "hybrid procedures" [1], in which the combined expertise of both professionals specialists is used to deliver optimal quality of care and achieve better outcomes. The goals of hybrid therapies include reduction of morbidity and mortality in patients with more complex diseases such as Hypoplastic Left Heart Syndrome (HLHS) and Muscular Ventricular Septal Defects (MVSD), mitigation of the negative cumulative effects of multiple procedures, improvement in quality of life and delivery of a more cost-efficient care. Also the hybrid environment encourages the sharing of ideas, equipment and techniques, which is crucial to introduce novel therapies for challenging patients. Although the hybrid approach starts with a collaborative effort between surgeons and interventionalists, it continues with careful planning among other subspecialties such as imaging, intensive care, anesthesia and others. These procedures have undoubtedly expanded the therapeutic options for many patients with more complex CHD. This new therapeutic modality has been rapidly growing as recently reported by the C3PO registry [2].

In this chapter we will review the indications, techniques and outcomes of some common forms of hybrid therapies such as palliation of HLHS [3], perventricular closure of MVSD [4] and intraoperative stent placement for pulmonary artery stenosis [5].

Hypoplastic Left Heart Syndrome (HLHS)

HLHS is a relatively common cardiac malformation, accounting for 4-9% of all children born with CHD. Since 1981, the Norwood operation and its variants have been considered the gold-standard approach for the treatment of this disease. Despite remarkable improvements in surgical techniques and post-operative care, the overall short and long-term outcomes have remained disappointing in the majority of centers. Cumulative attrition is the rule with an estimated 5-year survival of only 54% [6]. The classic Norwood procedure with placement of a modified Blalock-Taussig (MBT) shunt results in a delicate circulation in which balancing the systemic and pulmonary blood flow may be challenging. Diastolic runoff associated with increased flow through the shunt and resultant "coronary steal" may increase the risks of this operation [7]. To overcome these limitations, a modification of the classic operation was proposed by Dr Sano and co-workers in Japan [8]. In the Norwood-Sano operation a right ventricle–pulmonary artery (RV-PA) shunt in lieu of the MBT shunt to provide sufficient pulmonary flow. This technical modification has minimal effects in systemic blood pressure and coronary perfusion, which may potentially lead to a lower perioperative and interstage mortality [8]. In this regard, a recent randomized multicenter study comparing both types of surgical approaches showed that the classic Norwood procedure with a MBT shunt had overall higher short and long-term morbidity and mortality rates [9]. The transplantation-free survival at 12 months of follow up was 64% and 74% for the classic Norwood and the Sano variation, respectively [9]. Also, a significant incidence of neurodevelopmental disabilities and low motor scores has been commonly reported during follow up [10]. All the above limitations led to the exploration of other alternatives for the palliation of this challenging disease.

Although ductal stenting and banding the pulmonary arteries (PAs) was first reported in the UK for initial palliation of HLHS [11], the Giessen group in Germany perfected the procedure with excellent short and long-term outcomes, comparing favorably with those observed after the Norwood operation [12]. This strategy was popularized by the group from Columbus, Ohio, USA under the leadership of Drs. Cheatham and Galantowicz [13].This strategy is reproducible and was subsequently employed at other centers [14, 15].

In institutions with extensive experience with the Norwood operation, the application of the hybrid approach to HLHS is still limited to high-risk neonates for a standard Norwood operation and prolonged CPB (i.e.: prematures and/or with other associated conditions). More often, the hybrid approach has been applied for most patients with HLHS irrespective of the presence of additional risk factors. It shifts the risks of a major operation with the need of CPB from the neonatal to a later period when the infant is more mature [13]. Despite the increasing use of this approach, data on long-term outcomes is still limited.

The stage I hybrid palliation for HLHS is usually performed in the first days of life and includes three steps: bilateral PA banding, stent placement in the ductus and balloon atrial septostomy. In most centers, the initial procedure is performed in a hybrid room via a limited median sternotomy and combines bilateral PA banding and ductal stenting. Prostaglandins are usually discontinued when the neonate is anesthetized. The bands are configured using a 1-mm-wide ends cut from a 3.5 mm Gore-Tex tube graft and adjusted in such a way to result in a postductal systemic saturation of 75-80% and a mild increase in the systemic blood pressure of about 10 mmHg [13]. Other techniques such as an adjustable banding system have also been described [16]. After bilateral PA banding, a short 6-7 F sheath is positioned in the main pulmonary artery (MPA) immediately above the level of the pulmonary valve and secured by a purse string suture. An angiogram is obtained in the lateral view with a hand injection through the side arm of the sheath (Figure 1A). Proper measurements are made with regards to minimal and maximal ductal diameter and length. The selected stent is advanced over a wire through the sheath and should cover the full length of the ductus, between the proximal MPA at the point of the take-off of the right and left PAs and the distal ductal-aortic arch junction (Figure 1B). Incomplete coverage of ductal tissue may result in repeated procedures [17]. Usually stents of 8-10 mm in diameter and 20 mm in length are used in the full term neonate. Occasionally, longer stents or 2 stents in tandem are necessary in a longer duct. Self-expandable stents are preferred over balloon-expandable stents because they do not interfere with ductal flow and hemodynamics during deployment.

This approach is applicable for the initial palliation of most patients with HLHS and also for patients with multiple left sided obstructions.

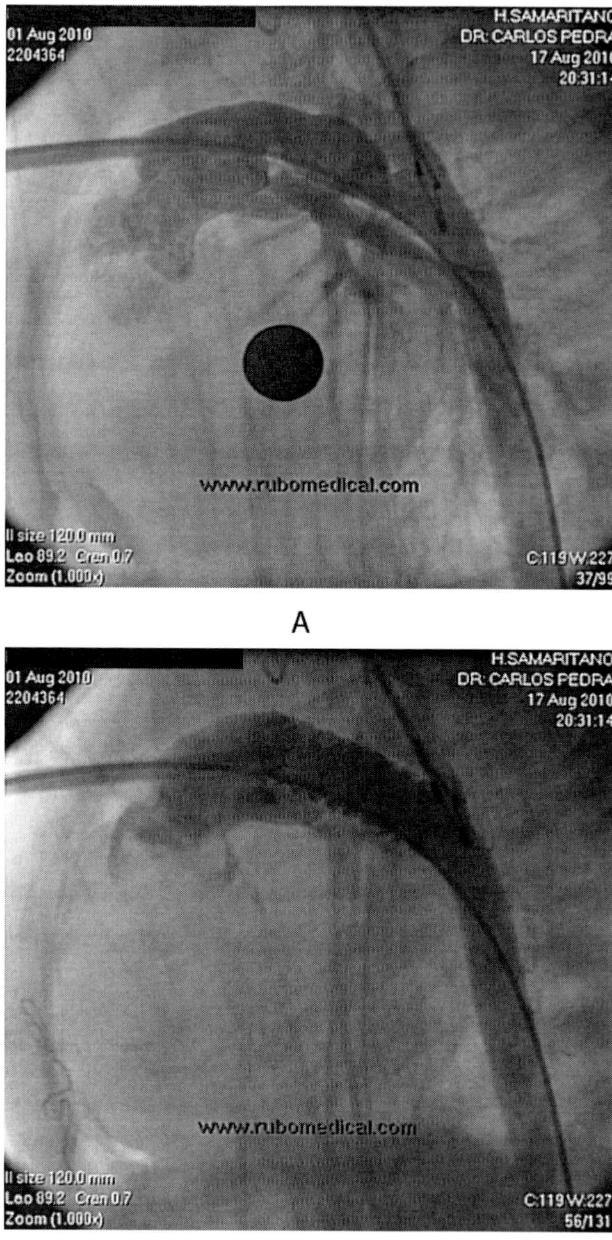

Figure 1. Ductal stenting in a patient with a Hypoplastic Left Heart Syndrome variant. **A**: Angiogram taken in lateral view after bilateral pulmonary artery banding with the sheath secured in the main pulmonary artery showing a tortuous patent ductus arteriosus with unobstructed right-left shunt. The banded left pulmonary artery can also be appreciated in this picture. **B**: Same view as before after balloon expandable stent implantation. The length of the stent covered the whole extension of the ductus without significant protrusion towards the descending aorta. The stent is well apposed on the ductal wall. There is no retrograde aortic arch obstruction.

A relative contraindication of the hybrid procedure in HLHS, especially in those patients with aortic atresia, is the presence of a severely restricted retroaortic blood flow at the level of the distal aortic arch in baseline conditions [13]. Placement of a stent in this setting could further impair the retrograde flow to the aortic arch, neck vessels, ascending aorta and coronary arteries resulting in acute ischemia and right ventricular dysfuntion. To overcome this problem and secure adequate coronary flow, an alternative technique was proposed by the group in Toronto [18, 19] and consists of placement of a 3-4 mm Goretex shunt between the MPA and the innominate artery at the same time of PA banding and stent insertion.

Also, an unrestrictive atrial septal defect (ASD) is required for ideal hemodynamics and prevention of pulmonary hypertension. Typically, a balloon atrial septostomy is performed in the catheterization laboratory just before hospital discharge. This is performed irrespective of the gradient across the ASD and should be considered as an integral part of the hybrid approach for HLHS. The use of new, non-compliant balloons such as the Z 5 (Numed, Canada) has greatly increased procedural success and reduced the need for repeated interventions in the interatrial septum. However, in an occasional patient, gradients across the interatrial septum may increase overtime, requiring additional interventions with alternative technique such as static balloon atrial septoplasty (using cutting and standard balloons), radio-frequency perforation and/or stent insertion in the atrial septum [20, 21].

The interstage period requires close periodic surveillance. The infant is generally evaluated every other week with emphasis on weight gain and saturation levels. Arm-leg blood pressure and an EKG are also part of the clinical evaluation. Failure to thrive is common in infants with HLHS and those with poor growth may be at risk for worse surgical and neurodevelopmental outcomes. The Feeding Work Group of the National Pediatric Cardiology Quality Improvement Collaborative has recently published nutrition algorithms for infants suffering from this heart lesion [22] and the Columbus group [23] highlighted that interstage home monitoring significantly improved weight gain and outcomes in patients undergoing the hybrid procedure. Potential complications in the interstage period may include retrograde aortic arch obstruction (RAAO), ASD restriction and ductal stent stenosis and are best diagnosed using transthoracic echocardiography.

RAAO after PDA stenting can be life-threatening especially in patients presenting with the aortic atresia variant [24]. Careful echocardiographic evaluation should be performed looking for increasing retrograde gradients across the arch, progressive deterioration in right ventricular function and appearance or worsening of tricuspid regurgitation, which are all associated with myocardial ischemia and possible new EKG changes. Patients with smaller aortic roots, higher retrograde aortic flow velocities on initial echocardiogram and a more acute angle between the arch and the ductus on the initial angiogram are at highest risk for developing RAAO [24]. The treatment for this complication is either an earlier comprehensive stage II procedure (when the patient is 3-5 months of age) or retrograde stent placement through the cells of the previously implanted ductal stent. Recurrent or residual ductal stent stenosis is another potential problem that might occur during the interstage period. If this complication is observed during the echocardiographic Doppler assessment, it is best managed implanting a second ductal stent [17]. The balloon expandable stent is usually preferred in this setting because the higher radial forces necessary to expand a residual obstruction. Recurrent ASD obstruction may occur but it has been unusual using the current techniques and materials. Alternative techniques such as those outlined above are used to manage this intersatge complication.

The comprehensive stage II palliation is usually performed at 6 months of life when the patient weighs $\geq$ 5-6 kg [13]. This big operation includes debanding and reconstruction of the branch PAs, atrial septectomy, bidirectional Glenn anastomosis, aortic arch reconstruction and incorporation of the small native ascending aorta into the newly created neo-aorta using a variety of techniques. Although most centers advocate complete removal of the ductal stent, the Toronto group suggested a modified arch reconstruction leaving part of the stent as a retained stented ductus patch [25]. Typically these patients behave as post-operative Glenn patients with more stable hemodynamics. Possible complications of this operation include pulmonary artery stenosis and distortions, which may be associated with local thrombus formation. Early diagnosis using exit angiography [26] and aggressive treatment with intra operative stenting (see below) or in the first days after the operation may be required.

Although some have raised some concerns with regards adequate pulmonary artery growth after the hybrid strategy for HLHS palliation, Honjo et al [27] from the Hospital of Sick Children in Toronto showed that the hybrid palliation does not have a significant adverse impact on pulmonary artery development, with similar pulmonary artery growth, hemodynamics, survival and diminished hospital utilization when compared with Norwood strategies. Finally, the same group has recently reported their experience comparing hybrid versus Norwood strategies for single-ventricle palliation [28]. A longitudinal evaluation was undertaken since the two strategies differ substantially in terms of the stage II palliative procedures. Freedom from death / transplant after stage II palliation was equivalent between groups although hybrid patients had a higher pulmonary artery reintervention rate and lower Nakata index at pre-Fontan evaluation. Aortic arch and atrioventricular valve reinterventions were not different between the groups and the ventricular end-diastolic pressure, mean pulmonary artery pressure, and ventricular function were equivalent. Survival after stage II palliation and subsequent Fontan completion was equivalent between both groups.

It seems that more and more centers are embracing the hybrid approach for the initial palliation of neonates born with HLHS. With increasing number of patients and longer follow-up, a prospective multicenter trial comparing both strategies would be ideally required for proper assessment of outcomes. However, this is unlikely to occur in the real world since there is a wide variation of institutional policies and preferences. Also, it should be acknowledged that there are institutions that perform better doing Norwoods and others doing Hybrids. Customization and offering the patient what you do best are crucial to achieve optimal outcomes.

Perventricular Closure of Muscular Ventricular Septal Defects

Muscular ventricular septal defects (MVSDs) accounts for about 20% of all congenital ventricular septal defects [29]. They can be located in the trabecular, apical or anterior region of the interventricular septum and are usually distant from the atrioventricular node. When the defect is restrictive, the natural history usually shows spontaneous closure in most patients within the first 4-5 years of life. Treatment is indicated when the defect results in heart failure in infancy or when there is volume overload of the left ventricle on echocardiography [29]. Percutaneous closure of such defects was introduced in the late 80s [30] but was fraught with technical limitations inherent to the available devices at that time. With evolving device technology and the advent of nitinol devices to close intracardiac defects the results of percutaneous closure of the MVSD improved significantly. A multicenter experience showed that closure of such defects with a nitinol self-expandable double-disc device was feasible resulting in excellent outcomes in patients from infancy to adulthood [31]. However, its application to the small infant < 5-6 kgs was associated with a higher risk for complications including hemodynamic compromise, arrhythmias, cardiac perforation, tamponade and death [31]. The concept of intraoperative closure of VSDs via a perventricular approach was introduced by Amin and co-workers in the late 90s [32]. In this procedure, after a standard median sternotomy is performed by the surgical team, a delivery sheath is advanced through the anterior wall of the right ventricle (RV) (Figure 2) across the defect into the left ventricle (LV). Under transesophageal echocardiographic (TEE) guidance, an intracardiac device is implanted through the delivery sheath by the interventionalist. Initial and subsequent experiences documented its feasibility, reproducibility, safety and efficacy in this high risk age group [4, 29, 33].

Perventricular closure of MVSDs is mainly indicated for the small infant (<6 kgs) with large and unrestrictive MVSDs, suffering from intractable heart failure, pulmonary hypertension and failure to thrive [29]. These patients are too fragile to undergo a long cardiac catheterization procedure in which the need to establish an arterio-venous wire loop results in hemodynamic compromise. Also vascular issues may be an additional limiting factor. Small infants with associated lesions that require surgical repair, such as coarctation of the aorta, double outlet right ventricle, transposition of great arteries and status-post pulmonary artery banding, may also benefit from the perventricular approach. After device closure of the MVSD, the associated lesion can be surgically repaired at the same session in the operating room (OR). Avoidance of CPB or limiting its time is a major advantage of the perventricular approach resulting in less morbidity, both in the short and long term, and faster recovery.

Technically, the procedure is performed under general endotraqueal anesthesia. A median sternotomy or a limited subxiphoid incision is performed and under continuous TEE guidance, the RV free wall is punctured through a purse string using an 18-gauge needle in a location that is perpendicular to the plane of the MVSD. Sometimes, a gentle manual or instrumental RV compression is helpful to determine the ideal location of the puncture. A variety of wires can be used to cross the VSD but the "J"-tipped short wire that comes with the short sheath is the most frequently employed. It is important to measure the distance between the RV free wall and the LV posterior wall to avoid injury of the LV posterior wall caused by sheath and dilator progression (Figure 3). Once the short sheath is properly visualized by echocardiography in the LV cavity, the selected self-expandable double-disc device (with a waist 1-3 mm larger than the largest diameter of the defect measured in diastole by TEE) is advanced. The distal disc is carefully deployed in the free LV cavity (away from the mitral valve apparatus). After minimal deployment of the central waist the whole system is pulled back as a unit against the interventricular septum until some resistance is felt. Further retraction of the sheath and advancement of the delivery cable using a two-hand technique is required to fully deploy the waist within the defect and the RV disc in the RV (Figure 4). After ruling out any significant AV valve regurgitation or residual shunt, the device is released, the short sheath is removed and the purse string is closed. Finally, surgical closure of the sternotomy is performed.

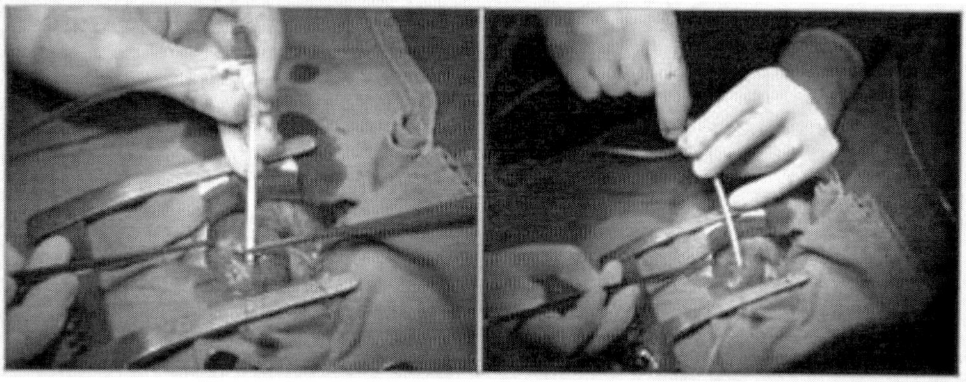

Figure 2. Perventricular device closure of a large muscular ventricular septal defect in a small infant. Sheath positioning across the right ventricular free wall. Left panel: An 8 F Standard short sheath is positioned through the right ventricular free wall. Note the suture on the sheath abutting the right ventricular wall. Right panel: After the device is transferred from the loader to the short sheath, implantation is performed with gentle movements, pulling on the sheath and pushing on the delivery cable.

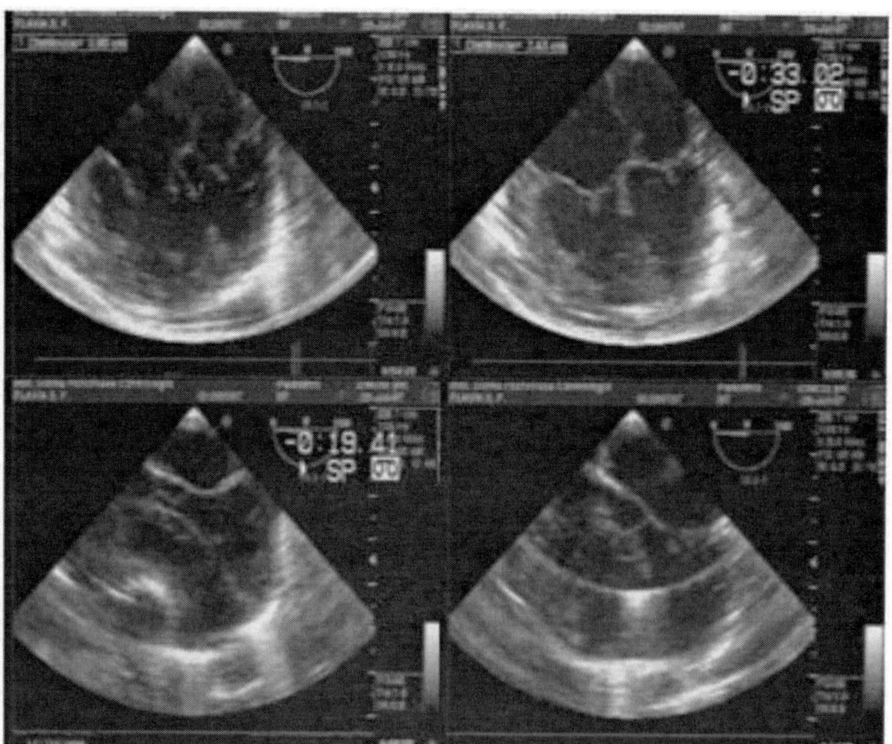

Figure 3. Transeophageal echocardiographic monitoring during perventricular closure of a muscular ventricular septal defect. Four-chamber view. Left upper panel: Single muscular ventricular septal defect located in the mid-trabecular area of the sepum measuring 9-10 mm. Right upper panel: The distance between the anterior right ventricular free wall and the posterior left ventricular wall is measured (35 mm). Left lower panel: Internal bulging of the anterior right ventricular free wall after it is gently pushed using the index finger. Right lower panel: A J-tip 0.038” echogenic guide wire is seen across the defect into the left ventricle.

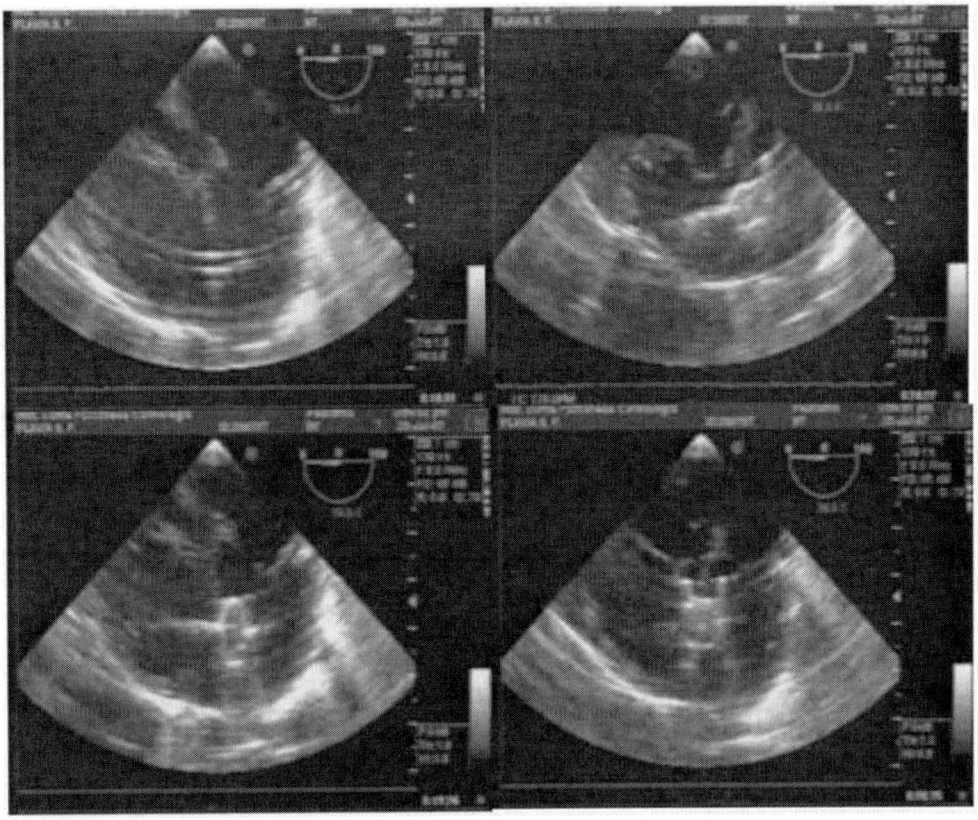

Figure 4. Transeophageal echocardiographic monitoring during implantation. Four-chamber view. **Left upper panel**: The short 8 F sheath is seen across the defect. The tip is located in the mid left ventricular cavity, away from the posterior wall. Right upper panel: The left disc and the waist of a 12 mm device are deployed in the mid left ventricular cavity. Left lower panel: The left disc is approaching the interventricular septum. Right lower panel: Adequate device positioning within the septum.

In an occasional patient, the defect cannot be crossed from the RV free wall, especially when it is located below the moderator band in the heavily trabeculated area of the interventricular septum. In this setting, the creation of an arterio-venous loop followed by wire snaring through the perventricular sheath may facilitate sheath progression through the defect [34]. In more apical defects, there may not be enough room for complete RV disc reconfiguration. In such cases a patent ductus arteriosus device can be used instead and/or the pin of the RV disc sutured in the RV wall to provide optimal stability [29].

Hybrid Approach to Branch Pulmonary Artery Stenosis

Treatment of PA stenoses continues to be challenging for patients with a variety of lesions, particularly those with conotruncal anomalies such as tetralogy of Fallot, truncus arteriosus, as well as pulmonary atresia and ventricular septal defects. Surgical patch angioplasty and transcatheter stent therapy are the current treatment options for PA stenoses.

Generally, surgical patch angioplasty is fraught with vessel distortions and tissue scarring resulting in suboptimal outcomes. The use of endovascular stents for the treatment of such stenoses, pioneered by Dr. Charles E. Mullins, improved the immediate results and the rates of restenosis [35]. However, percutaneous delivery of large stents that can be redilated to adult size requires high profile delivery systems, is technically demanding and not without complications. Due to these drawbacks, the idea of intraoperative delivery of endovascular stents in the operating room emerged as an alternative treatment option to increase the safety, ease and effectiveness of these procedures. The experience with the hybrid intraoperative PA stenting has increased significantly in the recent era, accounting for about 11% of all hybrid interventions [2]. Not every patient and not every lesion are suitable for intraoperative stent placement, and the choice of the appropriate treatment strategy should be tailored to the individual patient.

The first description of this technique was reported by Mendelsohn et al in 1993 [5] and since then, many centers have adopted this strategy with reproducible outcomes in terms of safety and the efficacy [36, 37]. Hybrid stent delivery is commonly performed in the operating room under direct or cardioscopic vision with an opened PA under CPB or through a sheath inserted in the PAs or in the right ventricular outflow tract before or after the initiation of CPB under angiographic guidance (Figure 5). Although this procedure can be done using a portable fluoroscopic C-arm, a well-equipped hybrid suite should be considered the ideal environment to perform such complex interventions (Figure 5).

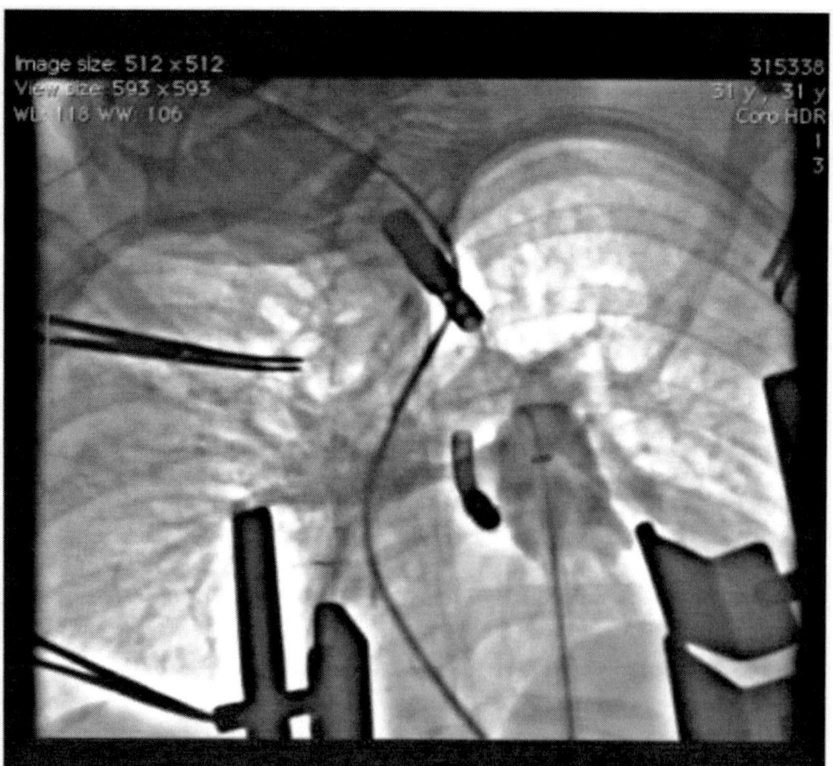

A

Figure 5. (Continued)

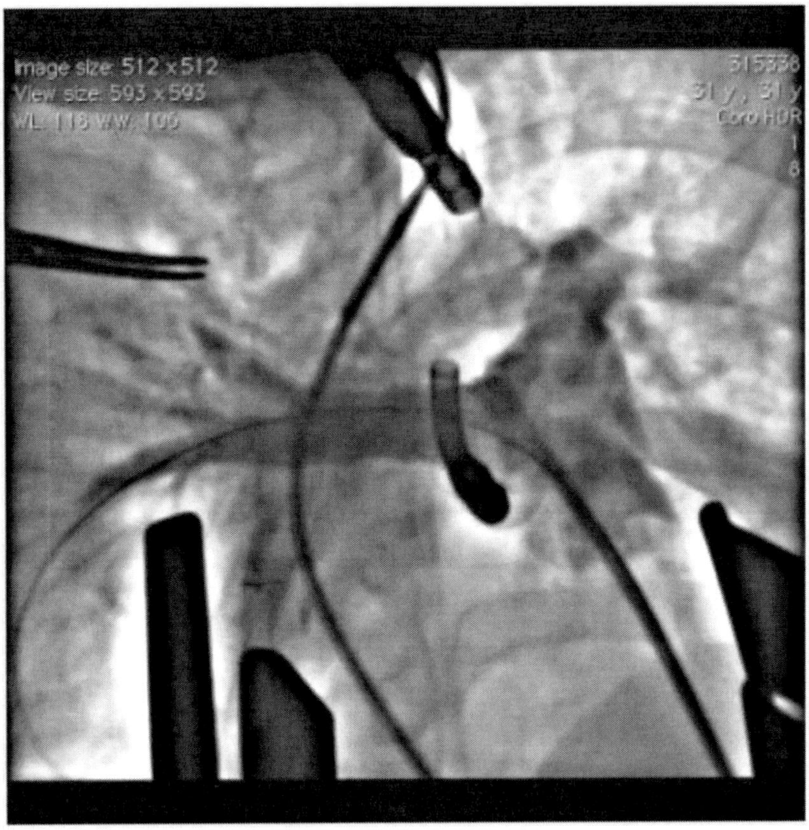

B

Figure 5. Intraoperative pulmonary artery stenting in a patient status post Tetralogy of Fallot repair with free pulmonary insufficiency and bilateral pulmonary artery stenosis. A: After a bioprosthetic valve was placed in the pulmonary valve position and the proximal left pulmonary artery was patch repaired, an angiogram performed in the main pulmonary artery after discontinuation of cardiopulmonary bypass showed significant proximal right pulmonary artery stenosis. The stenosis is related to the position of the vessel behind the dilated ascending aorta. Surgical instruments are evident in the picture. B: Stent implantation through a sheath positioned in the main pulmonary artery resulted in optimal stenosis relief in an angiogram obtained immediately after implantation. This strategy was planned before the patient was brought to the operating room and resulted in speedy recovery with hospital discharge in 5 days.

The target lesions should be initially assessed using integrated imaging modalities [26] with the use of angiograms of previous caths, magnetic resonance imaging and computed tomography. The optimal delineation of the underlying anatomy beforehand allows to select a proper size stent expediting the procedure, saving time and contrast injections. Also, new software protocols allow beautiful digital imaging fusion in modern hybrid suites.

The advantages of hybrid stent delivery include no size restrictions for sheaths, catheters and stents, avoidance of tortuous courses and better catheter and stent navigation, no need for stiff wires and long sheaths, no interference with tricuspid and pulmonary valve function that might cause hemodynamic compromise, possibility of manually cutting the stent to adjust for individual requirements, shorter procedural time, fluoroscopy time and radiation exposure, and better control of complications such as stent migration, or mal position, balloon rupture and vascular injuries.

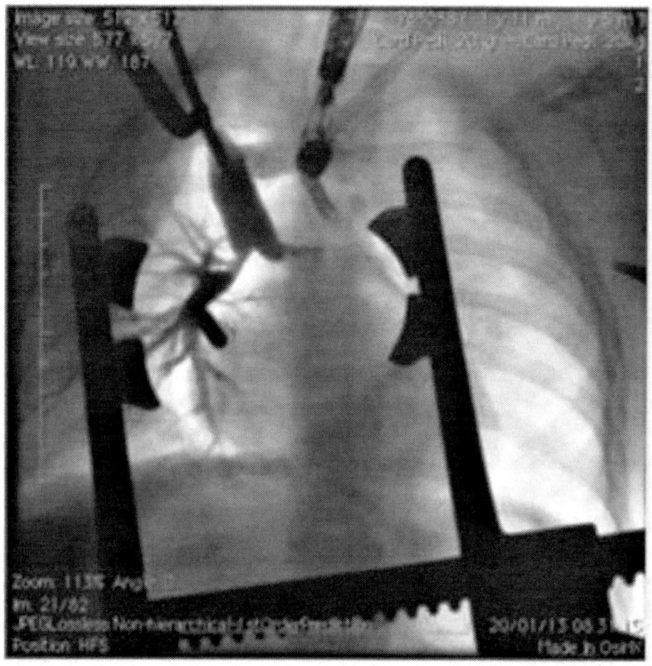

A

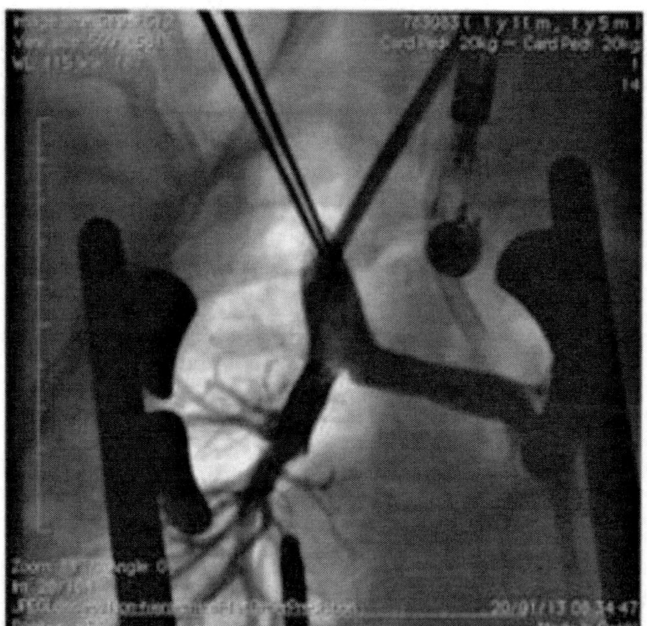

B

Figure 6. Exit angiography and intraoperative stent implantation in a patient with univentricular heart and multiple stenosis in the pulmonary arteries. A: Exit angiogram after a Glenn operation and patch enlargement of both pulmonary arteries was performed. Significant stenosis at the origin of both pulmonary arteries is appreciated in this angiogram performed in right anterior oblique with caudal angulation view. B: Bilateral stent implantation was undertaken through a sheath positioned in the superior vena cava. Optimal relief of stenosis was achieved, which resulted in speedy recovery and early extubation. Because of the presence of surgical instruments, the lesion should be profiled using variations of usual projections in the hybrid room.

The need for sternotomy and/or CPB should not be considered a disadvantage because these patients are usually brought to the OR for concomitant intra cardiac surgical repairs.

The decision as to whether implant the stents under direct or cardioscopic vision or angiographic guidance on the beating heart depends on the type of surgical procedure performed, the need for CPB, the availability of a cardioscope, the presence of comorbidities that may increase the risks of contrast induced renal injury and institutional policies. Pre-existing landmarks and measurements should be assessed and taken in previous angiographic and imaging studies (if available) no matter what the employed technique is. Fluoroscopic guided stenting is usually applied for patients that require an exit angio to assess immediate surgical results for whatever reason. Patients with pre-operative abnormal PAs, regardless of the underlying disease, who also require repair of associated intra cardiac lesions are common candidates for hybrid stent implantation. When there is bilateral central PA stenosis requiring kissing stents, the surgeon can bend the proximal stents struts towards the carina under direct vision in order to secure free access in future catheter procedures. Also, dilatation of a stent cell may be performed under direct or cardioscopic vision to secure access to a branch vessel in future cath procedures. Finally, transapical access for hybrid stent delivery is an additional technique that can be used for patients who do not need a median sternotomy for surgical repair of associated lesions. A limited subxiphoid incision is performed and a purse string suture placed at the right ventricular apex in order to facilitate a more straight progression of sheaths, catheters and stent. This has been employed in very small patients with vascular size restrictions and in those with very tortuous venous course that could preclude percutaneous catheter progression. Immediate results of intraoperative stent implantation are assessed by serial angios or direct cardioscopic vision. The ability to treat any residual PA lesion before transferring the patient to the intensive care unit is crucial for a speedy recovery and better in-hospital outcomes (Figure 6).

In conclusion, exit angios and hybrid stent delivery to the PAs has changed the landscape of the treatment options for PA stenosis. The collaboration between surgical and interventional teams resulted in better outcomes for these challenging patients.

References

[1] Hjortdal V. E., Redington A. N., de Leval M. R., Tsang V. T. Hybrid approaches to complex congenital cardiac surgery. *Eur. J. Cardiothorac. Surg.*, 2002; 22: 885-890.

[2] Holzer R., Marshall A., Kreutzer J., Hirsch R., Chisolm J., Hill S., Galantowicz M., Phillips A., Cheatham J., Bergerson L. Hybrid procedures: adverse events and procedural characteristics--results of a multi-institutional registry. *Congenit. Heart Dis.*, 2010; 5: 233-242.

[3] Michel-Behnke I., Akintuerk H., Marquardt I., Mueller M., Thul J., Bauer J., Hagel K. J., Kreuder J., Vogt P., Schranz D. Stenting of the ductus arteriosus and banding of the pulmonary arteries: basis for various surgical strategies in newborns with multiple left heart obstructive lesions. *Heart,* 2003; 89: 645-650.

[4] Bacha E. A., Cao Q. L., Starr J. P., Waight D., Ebeid M. R., Hijazi Z. M. Perventricular device closure of muscular ventricular septal defects on the beating heart: technique and results. *J. Thorac. Cardiovasc. Surg.*, 2003; 126: 1718-1723.

[5] Mendelsohn A. M., Bove E. L., Lupinetti F. M., Crowley D. C., Lloyd T. R., Fedderly R. T., Beekman R. H. 3rd. Intraoperative and percutaneous stenting of congenital pulmonary artery and vein stenosis. *Circulation*, 1993; 88 (5 Pt 2): II210-217.

[6] Ashburn D. A., McCrindle B. W., Tchervenkov C. I., Jacobs M. L., Lofland G. K., Bove E. L., Spray T. L., Williams W. G., Blackstone E. H. Outcomes after the Norwood operation in neonates with critical aortic stenosis or aortic valve atresia. *J. Thorac. Cardiovasc. Surg.*, 2003; 125: 1070-1082.

[7] Norwood W. I., Lang P., Casteneda A. R., Campbell D. N. Experience with operations for hypoplastic left heart syndrome. *J. Thorac. Cardiovasc. Surg.,* 1981; 82: 511-519.

[8] Sano S., Ishino K., Kado H., Shiokawa Y., Sakamoto K., Yokota M., Kawada M. Outcome of right ventricle-to-pulmonary artery shunt in first-stage palliation of hypoplastic left heart syndrome: a multi-institutional study. *Ann. Thorac. Surg.*, 2004; 78: 1951-1957.

[9] Ohye R. G., Devaney E. J., Hirsch J. C., Bove E. L. The modified Blalock-Taussig shunt versus the right ventricle-to-pulmonary artery conduit for the Norwood procedure. *Pediatr. Cardiol.*, 2007; 28: 122-125.

[10] Tabbutt S., Nord A. S., Jarvik G. P., Bernbaum J., Wernovsky G., Gerdes M., Zackai E., Clancy R. R., Nicolson S. C., Spray T. L., Gaynor J. W. Neurodevelopmental outcomes after staged palliation for hypoplastic left heart syndrome. *Pediatrics*, 2008; 121: 476-483.

[11] Gibbs J. L., Wren C., Watterson K. G., Hunter S., Hamilton J. R. Stenting of the arterial duct combined with banding of the pulmonary arteries *Br. Heart J.*, 1993 Jun.;69(6):551-5.

[12] Akintuerk H., Michel-Behnke I., Valeske K., Mueller M., Thul J., Bauer J., Hagel K. J., Kreuder J., Vogt P., Schranz D. Stenting of the arterial duct and banding of the pulmonary arteries: basis for combined Norwood stage I and II repair in hypoplastic left heart. *Circulation,* 2002; 105: 1099-1103.

[13] Galantowicz M., Cheatham J. P. Lessons learned from the development of a new hybrid strategy for the management of hypoplastic left heart syndrome. *Pediatr. Cardiol.,* 2005; 26: 190-199.

[14] Pilla C. B., Pedra C. A., Nogueira A. J., Jatene M., Souza L. C., Pedra S. R., Ferreiro C., Ricachinevsky C. P., Lucchese F. A. Hybrid management for hypoplastic left heart syndrome: an experience from Brazil. *Pediatr. Cardiol.*, 2008; 29: 498-506.

[15] Caldarone C. A., Benson L., Holtby H., Li J., Redington A. N., Van Arsdell G. S. Initial experience with hybrid palliation for neonates with single-ventricle physiology. *Ann. Thorac. Surg.,* 2007; 84: 1294-1300.

[16] Assad R. S., Zamith M. M., Silva M. F., Thomaz P. G., Miana L. A., Guerra V. C., Pedra C. A., Marcial M. B. A novel adjustable pulmonary artery *Ann. Thorac. Surg.*, 2007 Dec;84(6):2081-4.

[17] Baba K., Chaturvedi R., Lee K. J., Caldarone C. A., Benson L. N. Fate of the ductal stent after hybrid palliation for hypoplastic left heart syndrome. *Ann. Thorac. Surg.*, 2013; 95: 1660-1664.

[18] Caldarone C. A., Benson L. N., Holtby H., Van Arsdell G. S. Main pulmonary artery to innominate artery shunt during hybrid palliation of hypoplastic left heart syndrome. *J. Thorac. Cardiovasc. Surg.*, 2005; 130: e1-2.

[19] Baba K., Honjo O., Chaturvedi R., Lee K. J., Van Arsdell G., Caldarone C. A., Benson L. N. "Reverse Blalock-Taussig shunt": application in single ventricle hybrid palliation. *J. Thorac. Cardiovasc. Surg.,* 2013; 146: 352-357.

[20] Holzer R. J., Wood A., Chisolm J. L., Hill S. L., Phillips A., Galantowicz M., Cheatham J. P. Atrial septal interventions in patients with hypoplastic left heart syndrome. *Catheter Cardiovasc. Interv.,* 2008; 72: 696-704.

[21] Pedra C. A., Neves J. R., Pedra S. R., Ferreiro C. R., Jatene I., Cortez T. M., Jatene M., Souza L. C., Assad R., Fontes V. F. New transcatheter techniques for creation or enlargement of atrial septal defects in infants with complex congenital heart disease. *Catheter Cardiovasc. Interv.*, 2007; 70: 731-739.

[22] Slicker J., Hehir D. A., Horsley M., Monczka J., Stern K. W., Roman B., Ocampo E. C., Flanagan L., Keenan E., Lambert L. M., Davis D., Lamonica M., Rollison N., Heydarian H., Anderson J. B.; Feeding Work Group of the National Pediatric Cardiology Quality Improvement Collaborative. Nutrition algorithms for infants with hypoplastic left heart syndrome; birth through the first interstage period. *Congenit. Heart Dis.*, 2013; 8: 89-102.

[23] Miller-Tate H., Stewart J., Allen R., Husain N., Rosen K., Cheatham J. P., Galantowicz M., Cua C. L. Interstage weight gain for patients with hypoplastic left heart syndrome undergoing the hybrid procedure. *Congenit. Heart Dis.*, 2013; 8: 228-233.

[24] Egan M. J., Hill S. L., Boettner B. L., Holzer R. J., Phillips A. B., Galantowicz M., Cheatham J. P., Kovalchin J. P. Predictors of retrograde aortic arch obstruction after hybrid palliation of hypoplastic left heart syndrome. *Pediatr. Cardiol.*, 2011; 32: 67-75.

[25] Caldarone C. A., Honjo O., Benson L. N., Van Arsdell G. S. Modification of stage II procedure after hybrid palliation (bilateral pulmonary artery banding and ductal stenting) for hypoplastic left-sided heart syndrome: Modified arch reconstruction with retained stented ductus patch. *J. Thorac. Cardiovasc. Surg*., 2007; 134: 1588-1589.

[26] Pedra C. A., Fleishman C., Pedra S. F., Cheatham J. P. New imaging modalities *Curr. Opin. Cardiol.*, 2011 Mar;26(2):86-93.

[27] Honjo O., Benson L. N., Mewhort H. E., Predescu D., Holtby H., Van Arsdell G. S., Caldarone C. A. Clinical outcomes, program evolution, and pulmonary artery growth in single ventricle palliation using hybrid and Norwood palliative strategies. *Ann. Thorac. Surg.,* 2009; 87: 1885-1892.

[28] Baba K., Kotani Y., Chetan D., Chaturvedi R. R., Lee K. J., Benson L. N., Grosse-Wortmann L., Van Arsdell G. S., Caldarone C. A., Honjo O. Hybrid versus Norwood strategies for single-ventricle palliation. *Circulation,* 2012; 126 (11 Suppl 1): S123-131.

[29] Pedra C. A., Pedra S. R., Chaccur P., Jatene M., Costa R. N., Hijazi Z. M., Amin Z. Perventricular device closure *Expert Rev. Cardiovasc. Ther.*, 2010 May;8(5):663-74.

[30] Lock J. E., Block P. C., McKay R. G., Baim D. S., Keane J. F. Transcatheter closure of ventricular septal defects. *Circulation,* 1988; 78: 361-368.

[31] Holzer R., Balzer D., Cao Q. L., Lock K., Hijazi Z. M.; Amplatzer Muscular Ventricular Septal Defect Investigators. Device closure of muscular ventricular septal defects using the Amplatzer muscular ventricular septal defect occluder: immediate and mid-term results of a U.S. registry. *J. Am. Coll. Cardiol.,* 2004; 43: 1257-1263.

[32] Amin Z., Berry J. M., Foker J. E., Rocchini A. P., Bass J. L. Intraoperative closure of muscular ventricular septal defect in a canine model and application of the technique in a baby. *J. Thorac. Cardiovasc. Surg.,* 1998; 115: 1374-1376.

[33] Bacha E. A., Cao Q. L., Galantowicz M. E., Cheatham J. P., Fleishman C. E., Weinstein S. W., Becker P. A., Hill S. L., Koenig P., Alboliras E., Abdulla R., Starr J. P., Hijazi Z. M. Multicenter experience with perventricular device closure of muscular ventricular septal defects. *Pediatr. Cardiol.*, 2005; 26: 169-175.

[34] Diab K. A., Hijazi Z. M., Cao Q. L., Bacha E. A. A truly hybrid approach to perventricular closure of multiple muscular ventricular septal defects. *J. Thorac. Cardiovasc. Surg.*, 2005;130(3):892-3.

[35] O'Laughlin M. P., Perry S. B., Lock J. E., Mullins C. E. Use of endovascular stents in congenital heart disease. *Circulation*, 1991; 83: 1923-1939.

[36] Holzer R. J., Chisolm J. L., Hill S. L., Olshove V., Phillips A., Cheatham J. P., Galantowicz M. "Hybrid" stent delivery in the pulmonary circulation. *J. Invasive Cardiol.*, 2008; 20: 592-598.

[37] Menon S. C., Cetta F., Dearani J. A., Burkhart H. A., Cabalka A. K., Hagler D. J. Hybrid intraoperative pulmonary artery stent placement for congenital heart disease. *Am. J. Cardiol.*, 2008; 102: 1737-1741.

In: Congenital Heart Diseases
Editor: Raúl Cayré and José Milei
ISBN: 978-1-61122-003-2

Chapter 12

Strategy for Biventricular Outflow Tract Reconstruction for the Transposition of the Great Arteries with Ventricular Septal Defect and Left Ventricle Outflow Tract Obstruction: "Rastelli Procedure" and the "Newer Aortic Translocation Techniques"

Claudia Natalia Villalba, Mariela Mouratian *
and Horacio A. Capelli
Department of Cardiology, Hospital de Pediatría
"Prof. Dr. Juan P. Garrahan"-Buenos Aires, Argentina

Abstract

The surgical management of transposition of the great arteries with ventricular septal defect and left ventricle outflow tract obstruction is a true challenge in congenital heart surgery. Different surgical techniques such as the Rastelli procedure, "Reparation a` l'Etage ventriculaire", the Metras modification, Nikaidoh operation and its modifications were defined.

Although the Rastelli operation has been the most widely performed surgical procedure over the past decades, several studies have shown suboptimal long-term prognosis after its practice. A newer operation described by Bex and Nikaidoh has been performed with promising outcomes. The anatomical characteristics usually enable biventricular repair, though in some hearts univentricular palliation may be the only surgical option.

* E-mail: marumouratian@yahoo.com.ar.

Introduction

Transposition of the great arteries (TGA) with a ventricular septal defect (VSD) and left ventricular outflow tract obstruction (LVOTO) represents 0.67% of all congenital heart defects [1]. Although unusual, this lesion remains a surgical challenge.

The optimal treatment strategy for these patients is controversial due to high anatomical variability and unsatisfying long-term results. The anatomic correction of these lesions requires complete reconstruction of the biventricular outflow tract.

The arterial switch is contraindicated when pulmonary stenosis (PS) would be converted to significant aortic stenosis.

Three major surgical techniques have been developed during the past three decades: the Rastelli procedure, “Réparation a l'étage ventriculaire” (REV) and the aortic root translocation with biventricular outflow tract reconstruction (Nikaidoh procedure).

Surgical Procedures: A Journey towards the Corrective Surgery

Rastelli Procedure

In 1969 Giancarlo Rastelli of the Mayo Clinic proposed the surgical procedure that bears his name for the treatment of patients with transposition of the great arteries (TGA) with VSD and LVOTO. [2, 3, 4]

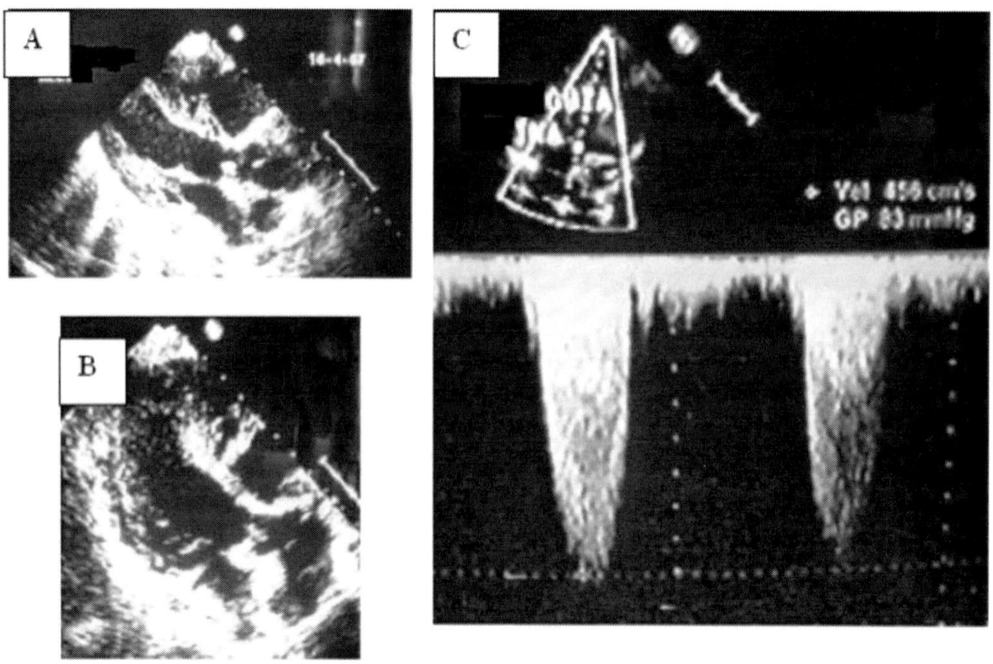

Figure 1. Echocardiographic image of a patient with DORV, subaortic VSD and PS undergoing the Rastelli procedure at the age of 3 years and 7 months, who developed severe subaortic stenosis 5 years after surgery. A and B: subaortic stenosis and the left ventricular baffle to the aorta with anterior and right orientation in the left parasternal long axis view. C: gradient of severe subaortic stenosis in a five-chamber apical view.

This procedure soon became the standard surgical treatment for this pathology and its practice extended to other congenital heart defects as double outlet right ventricle (DORV) with pulmonary stenosis as well.

Rastelli procedure includes an intraventricular rerouting to create a left ventricular outflow tract by the use of an intracardiac patch that directs the blood from the left ventricle (LV) to the aorta through the VSD. The right ventricular outflow tract is reconstructed and continuity between the right ventricle (RV) and the pulmonary artery (PA) is achieved by means of an extracardiac valved conduit.

This technique has the clear benefit of preserving the function of both ventricles (biventricular repair) with left ventricular baffling to the aorta. [5]

The Rastelli operation has been the method of choice over the past four decades. [6]. The procedure can be performed with low early mortality. However it is a complex procedure with marked morbidity and mortality in the medium and long-term follow-up. [7, 8, 9, 10, 11, 12]

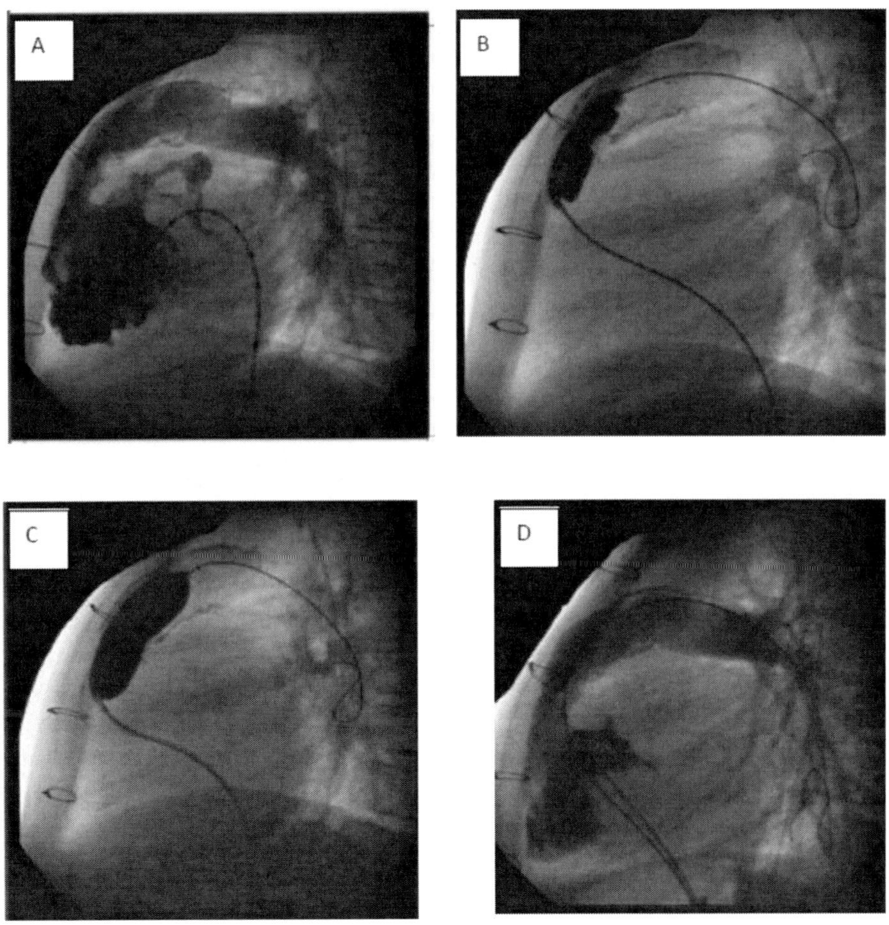

Figure 2. Interventional catheterization procedure of a patient with DORV, VSD and LVOTO who underwent Rastelli procedure at the age of 4 years and 8 months. Eight years after surgery he developed severe stenosis of the homograft. A: stenosis of the homograft in pulmonary artery position. B and C: balloon angioplasty dilatating the stenosis. D: angiography following the successful procedure.

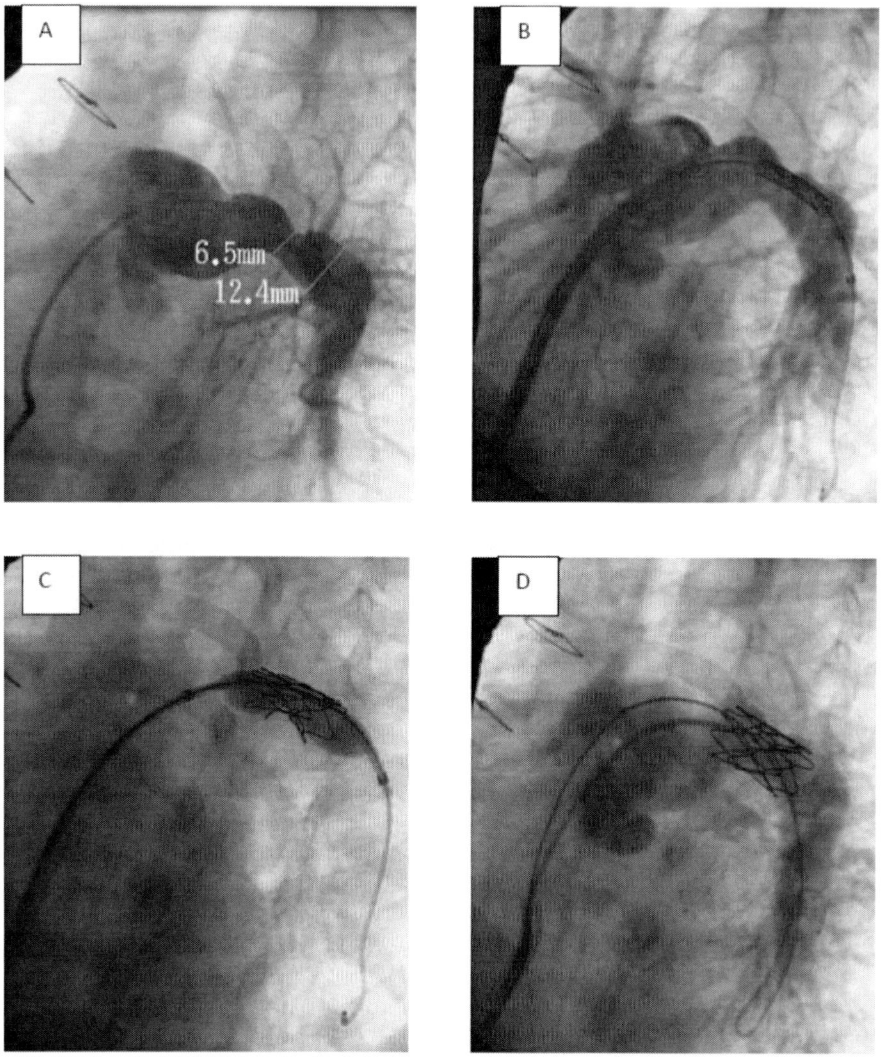

Figure 3. Angiography of a patient with DORV who underwent systemic-to-pulmonary artery shunt at the age of 7 months and Rastelli procedure at 3 years and 7 months old. Balloon angioplasty of the right pulmonary artery and stent implantation in the left pulmonary artery (images) were required 7 months after surgery.

The most frequent complications are residual VSD, development of left ventricular outflow tract obstruction, stenosis or insufficiency of the right ventricle-pulmonary artery conduit (RV-PA), ventricular arrhythmias and dysfunction. [13, 14]. Accordingly, reintervention and reoperation rates following the Rastelli procedure were frequently needed. [15]

Replacement of the extracardiac conduit is usually required. Extracardiac RV-PA homografts appear to be less durable than homografts in an orthotopic pulmonary position. [16, 17] Reoperation has been frequently informed for residual or recurrent LVOTO.

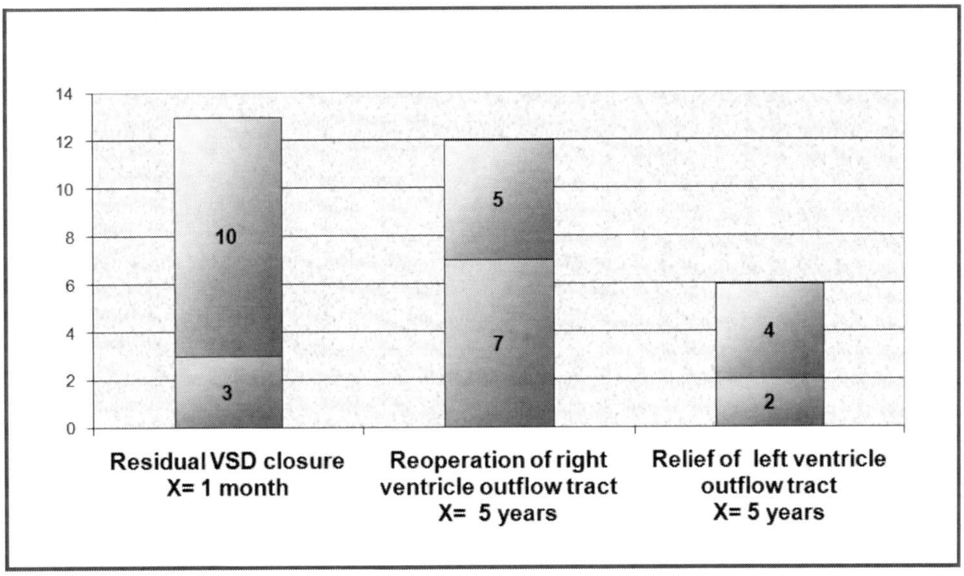

Figure 4. Surgical reinterventions in 47 patients operated with Rastelli surgery in the Hospital de Pediatría "J.P. Garrahan".

We reported our experience with Rastelli repair in 47 patients with a mean follow-up of 6 years post-op (15 months-14 years) [8]. Thirty nine reinterventions were performed (1 day - 13 years): 12 interventional catheterization procedures in 9 patients and 27 reoperations in 22.

The causes of reoperation are shown in Figure 4 and they were more frequent when the VSD was anatomically remote or non-committed to the aorta.

Several procedures have been reported as alternative to the Rastelli repair with varying results.

"Reparation a l'etage ventriculaire" (REV)

The "Reparation a l'etage ventriculaire" described by Lecompte in 1982 [18] entails resection of the infundibular septum along with reconstruction of the pulmonary outflow tract without using a prosthetic conduit by wide mobilization of the pulmonary arteries and reimplantation of the pulmonary trunk to the RV [19]

This surgical technique has the potential to decrease the incidence of LVOTO what preserves left ventricular function and improves long-term outcome [20]

However, the free pulmonary regurgitation following RV outflow reconstruction remains a concern in the early and the late postoperative period. [21]

Nikaidoh Procedure

The presence of a non-committed or restrictive VSD, a straddling mitral or tricuspid valve, cone-shaped implants of the tricuspid valve or the anterior implant of the mitral valve, a small right ventricular and/or an unusual coronary anatomy are anatomic variables that complicate the performance of a Rastelli/REV operation. [8, 9, 22, 23, 24, 25, 26, 27, 28, 29, 30, 31].

Aortic translocation becomes an attractive alternative when anatomy does not allow intraventricular rerouting (Rastelli/REV repair).

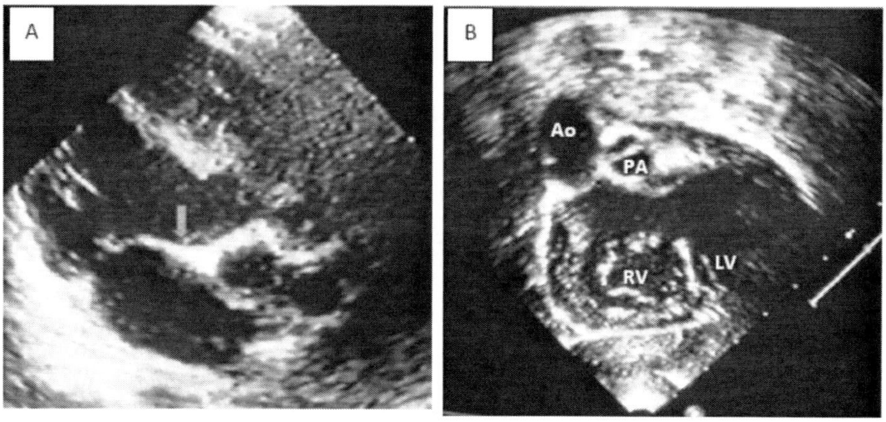

Figure 5. Patient with DORV, right anterior aorta and PS. A) Parasternal view showing mitral-semilunar valve discontinuity (arrow). B) Anatomic view (short axis of ventricles): VSD and both vessels emerging from the right ventricle (RV) with the aorta (Ao) in the right and anterior side. The pulmonary artery (PA) is of small size with a stenotic bicuspid valve. Both images show non-committed VSD.

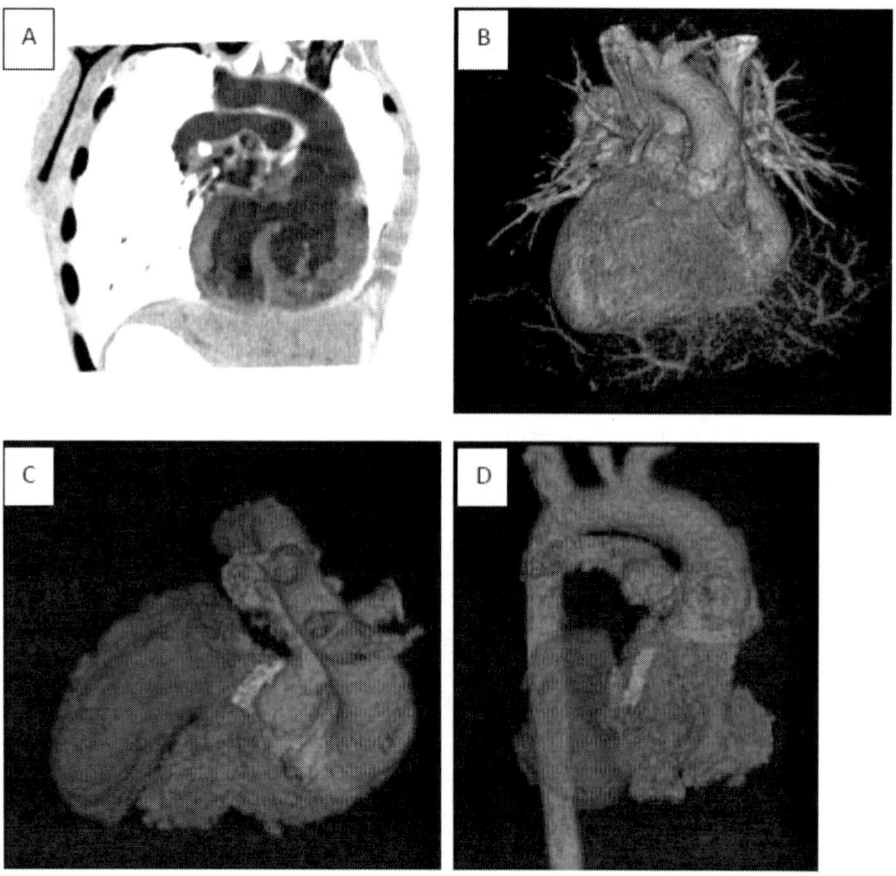

Figure 6. Multislice angiotomography of a patient with situs inversus, dextroposition and DORV type TGA with PS. C and D: tridimensional reconstruction. Both vessels (aorta in red, pulmonary artery in blue) arise from the right ventricle (in gray). Note the remote VSD (in yellow).

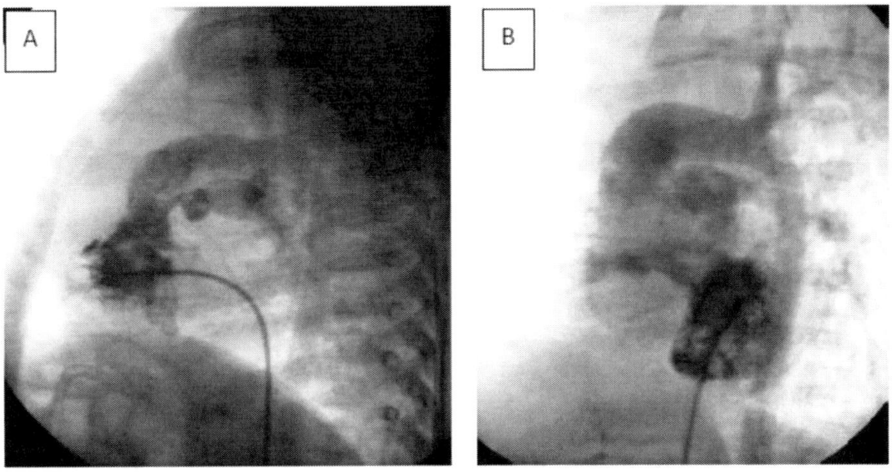

Figure 7. Angiography of a patient with DORV type TGV with PS. A) Right ventriculography. B) left ventriculography: both great arteries emerge from the right ventricle. Note the remote VSD.

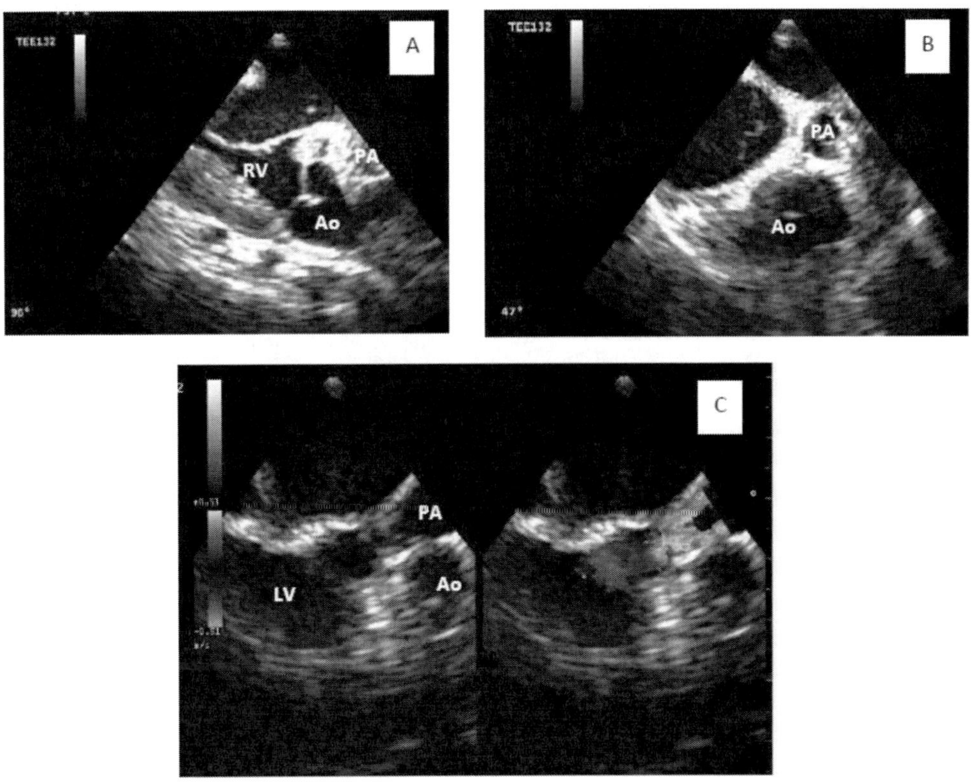

Figure 8. Patient with TGA, VSD and LVOTO. Transesophageal echocardiography in the operating room before surgery. A) Mid esophageal view at 85°: the aortic artery (Ao) emerges from the RV. B) Mid esophageal short axis view at 45°: relationship between the great arteries and the aorta in the right and anterior side. C) Mid esophageal long axis view at 120°: a stenotic pulmonary artery (PA) emerges from the left ventricle (LV).

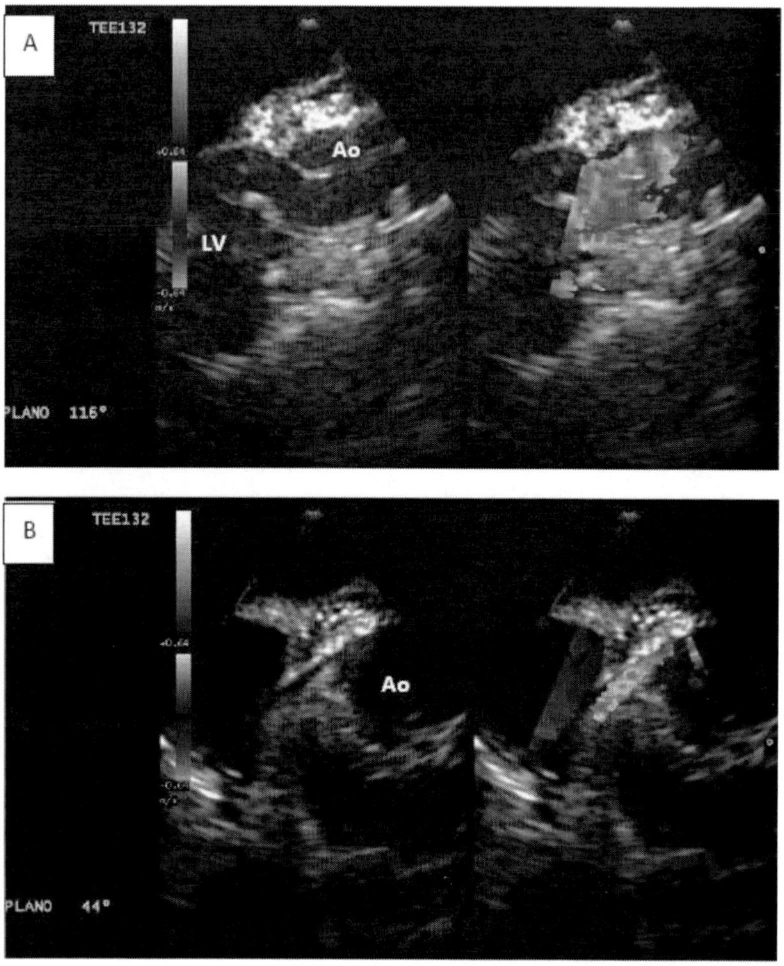

Figure 9. Transesophageal echocardiography of the same patient in the operating room after Nikaidoh surgery. A) Mid esophageal long axis view at 120° shows the translocated aortic artery to the expanded LVOTO. Notice a laminar flow without any obstruction and competent aortic valve. B) Mid esophageal short axis view at 45° shows normal flow in the reimplanted coronary arteries. (Ao= aortic artery; LV= left ventricle).

This new surgical approach for the TGA, VSD and SP denominated "aortic translocation and biventricular outflow tract reconstruction" was proposed by Hisahi Nikaidoh of the Children's Medical Center of Dallas in 1984. [32]

This repair consists of harvesting the aortic root and attached coronary arteries from the right ventricle and relieving the LVOTO (the outlet septum is divided and the pulmonary valve is excised). The left ventricular outflow tract (with the posteriorly translocated aortic root and the VSD patch) and the right ventricular outflow tract (with a pericardial patch) are both reconstructed.

Nikaidoh´s original technique described a direct mobilization of the aortic root without detaching the coronary arteries. Several modifications were introduced later: coronary transfers preventing coronary insufficiency, Lecompte maneuver and homograft interposition connecting the RV infundibulum to the pulmonary trunk to improve reconstruction of the right ventricular outflow tract. [21, 23, 30, 33, 34, 35, 36, 37]

Though technically demanding, the Nikaidoh procedure theoretically has several advantages: it can be performed early in life avoiding multiple palliations, cavity and volume of the RV are not reduced, a straight alignment of both outflows is created likely improving LV and RV function, LV is 'anatomically' connected to the aorta and the RV- PA conduit is orthotopical and the right ventricle is preserved [20, 31]

Despite the small number of patients and follow-up data, the Nikaidoh procedure and its various modifications have been performed with promising outcomes.

The midterm follow-up for LVOTO has not been reported. Frequent complications are: stenosis or insufficiency of the pulmonary artery or the RV- PA conduit, aortic regurgitation, ventricular arrhythmias and dysfunction. [20, 21, 23, 30, 33, 34, 35, 36, 38, 39, 40]

Aortic valve regurgitation which is not progressive and usually appears in the immediate postoperative period is a matter of concern [30, 40]. An adequate surgical technique of aortic root transfer avoids this complication.

Since 2005 we have been using the Nikaidoh procedure in our hospital with encouraging preliminary results so far.

Nine patients with TGA + VSD + LVOTO and two patients with DORV + SP have already been operated. The surgery consisted on aortic translocation, reimplantation of coronary arteries and right ventricle-to-pulmonary artery connection using homografts. The 11 patients had a non-committed VSD and one of them had a mildly hypoplastic RV.

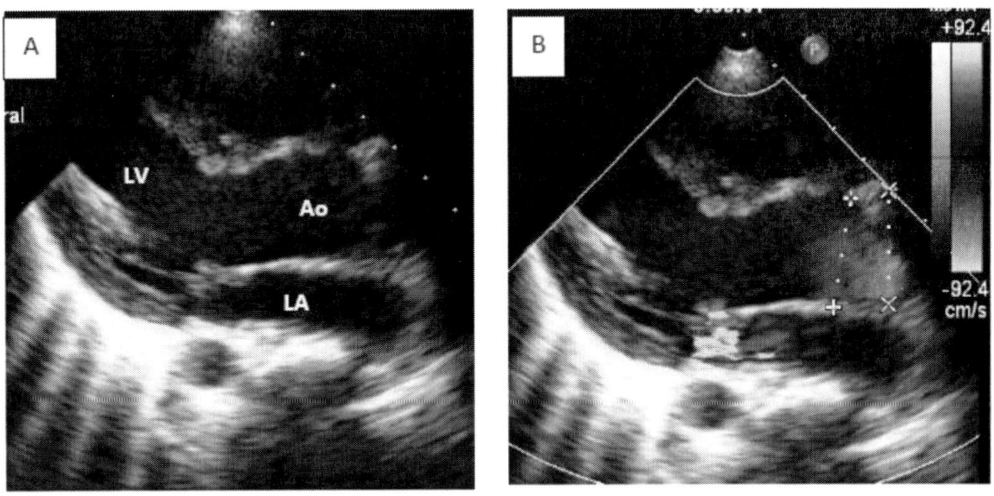

Figure 10. Color Doppler echocardiography 4 years after the Nikaidoh surgery of a DORV type TGV with PS. Notice the normal LV outflow, properly aligned and without obstruction in the long axis parasternal view (LV=left ventricle; Ao=aortic artery; LA=left atrium).

No deaths have occurred after this procedure. After 4.3 years on average (2–5.6 years) from surgery, all patients are in NYHA functional class I with neither arrhythmias nor LVOTO and have normal biventricular function. Only mild aortic insufficiency has been observed. There was one reoperation in a patient who developed post-surgery infective endocarditis and needed a mitral valve and RV-PA homograft replacement. Another patient underwent balloon angioplasty of the stenotic homograft RV-PA. Figures 11 and 12 respectively show immediate and mid-term surgical results.

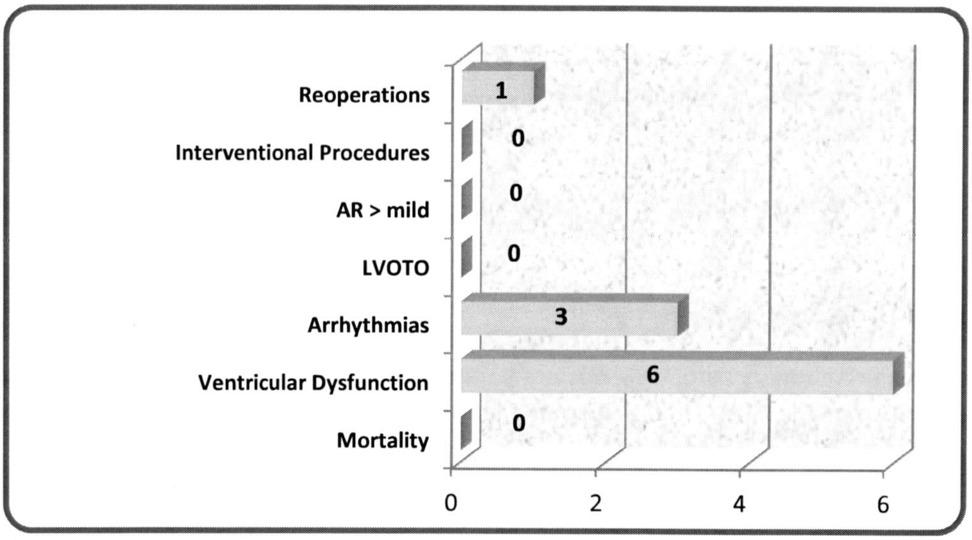

Figure 11. Immediate postoperative outcome of 11 patients operated with Nikaidoh procedure at the Hospital de Pediatría "J P Garrahan".

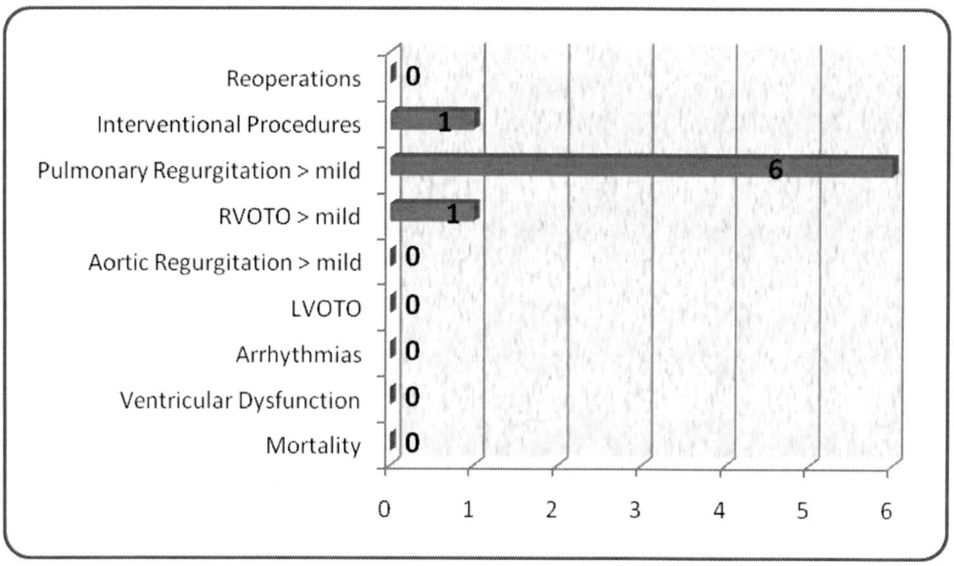

Figure 12. Mid-term outcome of 11 patients operated with Nikaidoh procedure at the Hospital de Pediatría "J P Garrahan" 3 years follow-up on average (2 - 5.6 years).

Aortic translocation and biventricular outflow tract reconstruction result in a more normal anatomic repair, which could result in improved cardiac performance and long-term survival.

The risk of subaortic obstruction is reduced because left ventricular outflow tracts are properly aligned.

The RV-PA conduit originates normally from the right ventricle and is therefore less susceptible to sternal compression. It may last for a long time with a decreased incidence of reoperation. [30, 36].

In patients with TGA + VSD + LVOTO who are inadequate for an intraventricular rerouting (Rastelli/REV operation) the Nikaidoh procedure arises as the best surgery option due to its mid-term results. [23, 31, 34, 40].

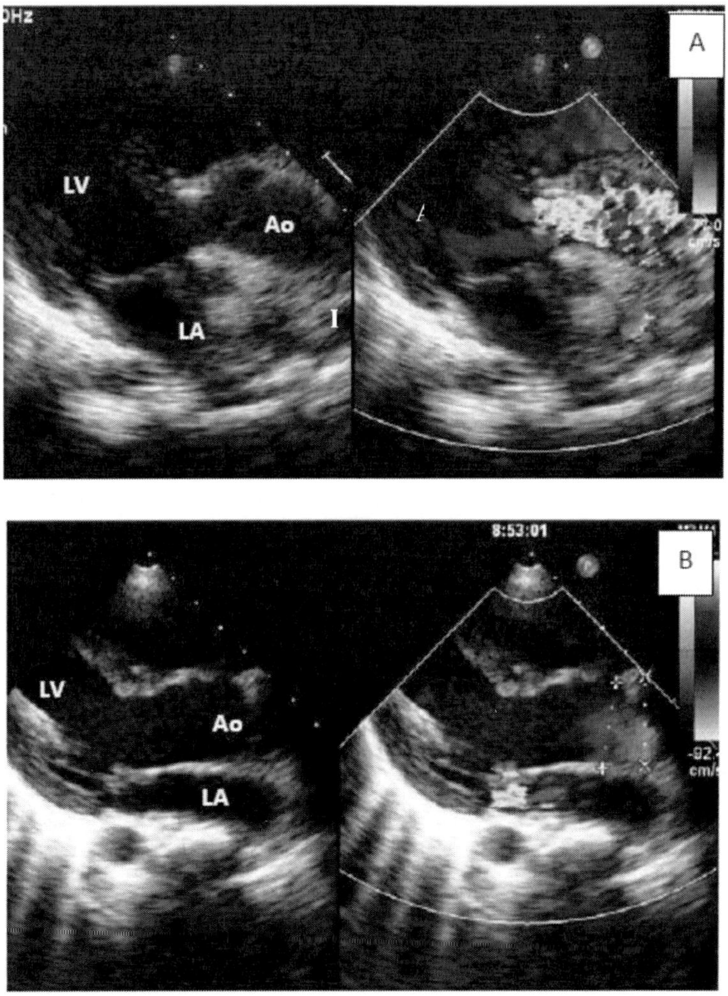

Figure 13. Echocardiographic image ofa patient with DORV with VSD and PS undergoing the Rastelli procedure (A) and the Nikaidoh procedure (B). A: notice the wrong alignment between the left ventricular (LV) and the aortic artery (Ao) with an elongated and stenotic baffle. B: notice the properly aligned LVOTO without obstruction.

Univentricular correction should be considered when surgical repair is not possible. The Fontan-Kreutzer procedure might be superior to the high-risk biventricular repair despite the well-known long-term problems associated with single ventricle circulation. [31]

Conclusion

The transposition of the great arteries with ventricular septal defect and left ventricular outflow tract obstruction, regardless of its low prevalence among congenital heart diseases, represents a serious challenge for pediatric cardiac surgeons.

The optimal surgical treatment of these patients is controversial.

Up to now the Rastelli procedure has been the most frequent surgical treatment even though its long-term results are not optimal.

In the subgroup of patients with TGA + VSD + LVOTO who are inadequate for an intraventricular rerouting (Rastelli/REV operation), the Nikaidoh procedure emerges as the best surgery option in terms of the immediate hemodynamic results and the comparatively fewer complications in the medium and long-term.

Although the Nikaidoh operation and its modifications have been performed with promising outcomes, a larger number of patients and longer follow-ups are required to evaluate the long-term benefits.

Finally, univentricular palliation can be the only surgical option in some hearts.

References

[1] Keith J, Rowe R, Vlad P. *Heart disease in infancy and childhood.* New York: MacMillan, 1978.

[2] Rastelli G. A new approach to anatomic repair of transposition of the great arteries. *Mayo Clin Proc* 1969; 44: 1-12.

[3] Rastelli G, McGoon D, Wallace R. Anatomic correction of transposition of the great arteries with ventricular septal defect and subpulmonary stenosis. *J Thorac Cardiovasc* Surg 1969; 58: 545-52.

[4] Lewis Backer C: Mauvroudis C: The Rastelli operation. *Operative Techniques in Thoracic and Cardiovascular Surgery*, 2003; 8: 121-130.

[5] Sato Y, Ayusawa, Komatsu S et al. MCDT evaluation of a double oulet right ventricle after the Rastelli procedure. *Int J Cardiol* 2007; 117: 430-2.

[6] Rastelli G, Wallace R, Ongley P. Complete repair of transposition of the great arteries with pulmonary stenosis: a review and report of a case corrected by using a new surgical technique.*Circulation.* 1969; 39: 83-95.

[7] Kreutzer C, De Vive J, Oppido G, et al. Twenty-five year experience with Rastelli repair for transposition of the great arteries. *J Thorac Cardiovasc Surg* 2000; 120: 211—23.

[8] Villalba C, Woloszyn M, Mouratian M, et al. Cirugía de Rastelli: impacto adverso de la comunicación interventricular no relacionada con los grandes vasos en los resultados quirúrgicos. *Revista Argentina de Cardiología* 2010; 78: 315-322.

[9] Dearani J, Danielson G, Puga F, et al. Late results of the Rastelli operation for transposition of the great arteries. *Semin Thorac Cardiovasc Surg Pediatr Card Surg Annu* 2001; 4: 3—15.

[10] Vouhé P, Tamisier D, Leca F, et al. Transposition of the great arteries, ventricular septal defect, and pulmonary outflow tract. *J Thorac Cardiovasc Surg* 1992; 103: 428-36.

[11] Brown J, Ruzmetov M, Okada Y, et al. Surgical results in patients with double oulet right ventricle: a 20-year experience. *Ann Thorac Surg* 2001; 72: 1630-5.

[12] Hörer J, Schreiber C, Dworak E, et al. Long-term results after the Rastelli repar for transposition of the great arteries. *Ann Thorac Surg* 2007; 83: 2169-75.

[13] Capelli H, Faella H. Cardiopatías congénitas. En: Bertolasi CA, Barrero C, Gimeno G, Liniado G, Mauro V, editores. *Transposición completa de los grandes vasos*. Buenos Aires: Editorial Médica Panamericana; 2000. p 2507.

[14] Moss and Adams' Heart Disease in Infants, Children, and Adolescents: Including the Fetus and Young Adults, 7th Edition. Copyright ©2008 Lippincott Williams & Wilkins.

[15] Giardini A, Donti A, Gargiulo G, et al. Trascatheter residual ventricular septal defect closure after Rastelli operation. *Cathet Cardiovasc Interv* 2005; 64: 209-12.

[16] Selamet Tierney E, Gersony W, Altmann K, et al. Pulmonary position cryopreserved homografts: durability in pediatric Ross and non-Ross patients. *J Thorac Cardiovasc Surg* 2005; 130: 282.

[17] Takeuchi K, Murakami A, Sekiguchi A, et al. Fate of equine pericardial roll conduit for Rastelli operation during long-term follow-up. *Congenit Heart Dis* 2007; 2: 121-4.

[18] Lecompte Y, Neveux JY, Leca F, et al. Reconstruction of thepulmonary outflow tract without a prosthetic conduit. *J Thorac Cardiovasc Surg* 1982; 84: 727–33.

[19] Borromee L, Lecompte Y, Batisse A, et al. Anatomic repair of anomalies of ventriculoarterial connection associated with ventricular septal defect. II. Clinical results in 50 patients with pulmonary outflow tract obstruction. *J Thorac Cardiovasc Surg* 1988; 95: 96 –102.

[20] Weyand K, Haun C, Blaschczok H, et al. Surgical Treatment of Transposition of Great Arteries With Ventricular Septal Defect and Left Ventricular Outflow Tract Obstruction: Midterm Results. *World Journal for Pediatric and Congenital Heart Surgery* 2010; 1: 163.

[21] Hernandez V, Marx G, Bacha E, et al. Aortic Root Translocation Plus Arterial Switch for Transposition of the Great ArteriesWith Left Ventricular Outflow Tract Obstruction Intermediate-Term Results. *JACC* 2007; 49: 485–90.

[22] Lee J, Lim H, Kim Y, et al. Repair of transposition of the great arteries, ventricular septal defect and left ventricular outflow tract obstruction. *Eur J Cardiothorac Surg* 2004; 25: 735-741.

[23] Hu SS, Liu ZG, Li SJ, et al. Strategy for biventricular outflow tract reconstruction: Rastelli, REV, or Nikaidoh procedure?. *J Thorac Cardiovasc Surg*. 2008; 135: 331-338.

[24] Fujii Y, Kotani Y, Takagaki M, et al. The impact of the length beteen the top of the interventricular septum and the aortic valve on the indications for a biventricular repair in patients with a transposition of the great arteries or a double oulet rigth ventricle. *Interactive Cardiovascular and thoracic surgery* 2010: 900-905.

[25] Navabi M., Shabanian R, Kiani A, et al. The effect of ventricular septal defect enlargement on the outcome of Rastelli or Rastelli-type repair. *J Thorac Cardiovasc Surg* 2009; 138: 390-396.

[26] Imamura ES, Morikawa T, Tatsuno K, et al. Surgical consideration of ventricular septal defect associated with complete transposition of the great arteries and pulmonary stenosis: with special reference to the Rastelli operation. *Circulation* 1971; 44: 914-23.
[27] Niinami H, Imai Y, Swatari K, et al. Surgical management of tricuspid malinsertion in the Rastelli operation: Conal Flap Method. *Ann Thorac Surg* 1995; 59: 1476-80.
[28] Huhta JC, Edwards WD, Danielson GK, et al. Abnormalities of the tricuspid valve in complete transposition of the great arteries with ventricular septal defect. *J Thorac Cardiovasc Surg* 1982; 83: 569-76.
[29] Villagra F, Quero-Jimenez M, Maitre-Azcarate MJ, et al. Transposition of the great arteries with ventricular septal defect: Surgical considerations concerning the Rastelli operation. *J Thorac Cardiovasc Surg* 1984; 88:1004-11.
[30] Morell V, Jacobs J, and Quintessenza J. Aortic Translocation in the Management of Transposition of the Great Arteries with Ventricular Septal Defect and Pulmonary Stenosis: Results and Follow-Up. *Ann Thorac Surg* 2005; 79: 2089 –93.
[31] Hazekamp M, Portela F, Bartelings M. The optimal procedure for the great arteries and left ventricular outflow tract obstruction. An anatomical study. *Eur J Cardiothorac Surg* 2007; 31: 879—87.
[32] Nikaidoh H. Aortic translocation and biventricular outflow tract reconstruction: a new surgical repair for transposition of the great arteries associated with a ventricular septal defect and pulmonary stenosis. *J Thorac Cardiovasc Surg* 1984; 88: 365–72.
[33] Morell V, Jacobs P, Quintessenza J. The Rol of Aortic translocation in the Management of Complex Transposition of the Great Arteries. *Pediatric Cardiac Surgery anual of the Seminars in thoracic and Cardiovascular Surgery* 2004; 7: 80-84.
[34] Emani S, Beroukhim R, Zurakowski D, et al. Outcomes after Repair for D-Transposition of the Great Arteries with Left Ventricular Outflow Tract Obstruction. *Circulation* 2009; 120 (suppl1): S53-S58.
[35] Sayin OA, Ugurlucan M, Saltik L, et al. Modified Nikaidoh procedure for transposition of great arteries, ventricular septal defect and left ventricular outflow tract obstruction. *Thorac Cardiovasc Surg* 2006; 54: 558–560.
[36] Ugurlucan M, Sayin O, Tireli E. Modified Nikaidoh procedure in a patient with transposition of the great arteries, ventricular septal defect, and left ventricular outflow tract obstruction with unusual coronary anatomy. *Cardiology in the Young* 2011; 21: 703–706.
[37] Nikaidoh Procedure for the Correction of Transposition of the Great Arteries, Ventricular Septal Defect, and Pulmonary Stenosis To the Editor. *Rev Esp Cardiol.* 2008; 61:1100-10.
[38] Shengshou H, Yongquan X, Shoujun L, et al. Double-Root translocation for Double-Oulet Right Ventricle with Noncommitted Ventricular Septal Defect or Double-Oulet Right Ventricle With Subpulmonary Ventricular Defect Associated With Pulmonary Stenosis: An Optimized Solution. *Ann Thorac Surg* 2010; 89: 1360-5.
[39] Sheng-Shou H, Zhi-Gang L, Shou-Jun L et al. Strategy for biventricular outflow tract reconstruction: Rastelli, REV, or Nikaidoh procedure? *The Journal of Thoracic and Cardiovascular Surgery* 2008; 135: 331-338.
[40] Yeh TJ, Ramaciotti C, Leonard S et al. The aortic translocation (Nikaidoh) procedure: Midterm results superior to the Rastelli procedure. *J Thorac Cardiovasc Surg* 2007; 133: 461-9.

[41] Delius RE, Rademecker MA, de Leval MR et al. Is a high risk biventricular repair always preferable to conversion to a single ventricle repair? *J Thorac Cardiovasc Surg* 1996; 112: 1561-1568.

In: Congenital Heart Diseases
Editor: Raúl Cayré and José Milei
ISBN: 978-1-61122-003-2

Chapter 13

Adult Congenital Heart Disease: Problems and Perspectives

Horacio Capelli and Mariela Mouratian *
Department of Cardiology, Hospital de Pediatría
Buenos Aires, Argentina

Abstract

Major advances and refinement in the diagnosis and surgical treatment of congenital heart defect in the last four decades has resulted in an increasing number of adult survivors [1, 2].

The incidence of congenital heart diseases is around 1%. Nearly 6000 children are born with one congenital heart defect in Argentina per year [3]. Two thirds of them require surgical treatment mostly within the first year of life. Fortunately, surgical mortality has been reduced to low single figures in the last 20 years and 90% of the operated patients are expected to reach adulthood. It is noteworthy that congenital heart surgery is "reparative" and not curative. Except for the ligated patent ductus arteriosus in the first months of life, all congenital heart lesions whether operated on or not will require lifelong control. Even the Atrial Septal Defect (ASD) operated upon in the first years of life may be exposed to the development of atrial fibrillation or sick sinus disease in the fourth decade.

Population Profile

We are facing two groups of adult patients with congenital heart disease: those operated on in infancy or childhood and patients who reached adulthood without diagnosis or surgical treatment.

* E-mail: marumouratian@yahoo.com.ar.

The operated group makes up a growing population not only in size but also concerning with the complexity of their heart defects. Most of them are diagnosed and treated in hospitals or pediatric institutions by the pediatric cardiac team.

The untreated patients are those who were not diagnosed in childhood due to the absence of symptoms or the presence of mild clinical signs that might have been overlooked. In this regard, the ASD typically accounts for about 30% of congenital heart defects diagnosed in adulthood.

There are also certain heart lesions within this group that may have a rather late clinical manifestation regardless of their complex morphology. Examples of these are the Ebstein´s disease or the congenitally corrected transposition of great vessels (atrioventricular and ventriculoarterial discordance).

The majority of the untreated patients usually attend the cardiology department at public hospitals. We have been collecting data of these adult patients in Garrahan and Argerich Hospitals for the last 25 years and keep a data base of 1520 patients coming from all over the country and neighboring countries as well (Figure1).

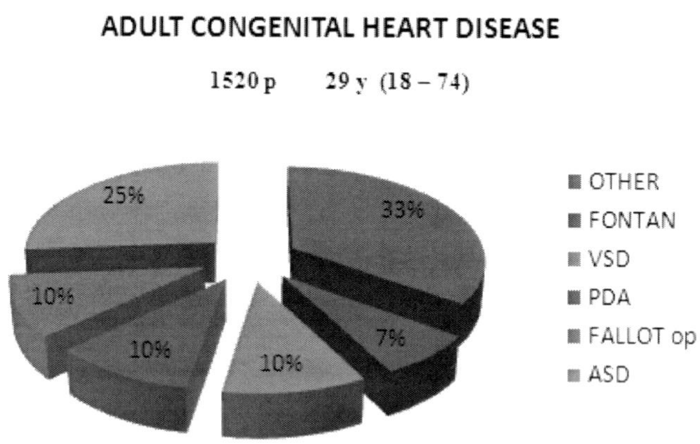

Figure 1. Database of Adult Congenital Heart Disease (ACDH).Outpatient´s long term follow-up at Garrahan and Argerich Hospitals (1987-2013).

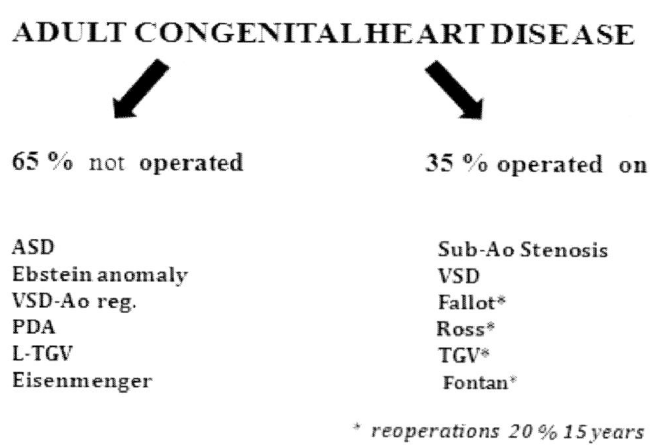

Figure 2. Population Profile, obtained from ACHD. Database Garrahan and Argerich Hospitals.

Unoperated patients make up 65% of the whole population and received medical care at the Argerich Hospital or other public hospital for adults (Figure 2). Most of the operated adults in our database come from the Garrahan Hospital where over 500 patients are operated yearly with an overall mortality of less than 5%.

Problems and Needs

The most frequent ensuing adverse events are the development of arrhythmias, right ventricular failure, pulmonary hypertension and infective endocarditis. Patients look for advice on additional special topics such as pregnancy, contraception, genetic transmission, physical exercise, work activity, health and life insurances. Hereafter we will briefly address some of the adverse events above mentioned [4].

Arrhythmias

Arrhythmias are a very common cause of symptoms and may trigger serious hemodynamic events. They may emerge as part of the natural history of the underlying disease or they may be related to the surgical procedure or acquired later during the long-term follow-up. Arrhythmias usually have an underlying anatomic or hemodynamic substrate which should be identified and treated [5].

Atrial arrhythmias like atrial fibrillation, flutter or re-entrant atrial tachycardia are usually associated with dilation of the right atrium due to chronic volume overload or fibrosis secondary to surgical scars. These may appear late in the follow-up in complex lesions such as the Fontan-Kreutzer surgery in patients with univentricular physiology, the Senning procedure in transposition of the great arteries or Ebstein´s disease. Nevertheless, they may occur also in simple defects like the ASD which is the most frequent congenital heart defect diagnosed in adulthood [6]. Eighteen percent of the unoperated patients and 2% of the operated patients had atrial fibrillation at age 55 on average in the follow-up of 350 adult cases with ASD from our database (Figure 3).

The most serious and life threatening ventricular arrhythmias are related to surgical ventriculotomies, fibromuscular resections, obstructive outlet tracts or pressure and/or volume overload of the right ventricle.

The typical case is that of patients with Tetralogy of Fallot after surgery. In our experience with 236 adult patients undergoing surgery, 29 years old on average (range 18 yrs-64 yrs) and followed over 25 years, ventricular arrhythmias were present in 25% of the population.

Most of them had extensive ventriculotomies and pressure and volume overload associated to distorted and stenotic pulmonary branch arteries following aortopulmonary shunts.

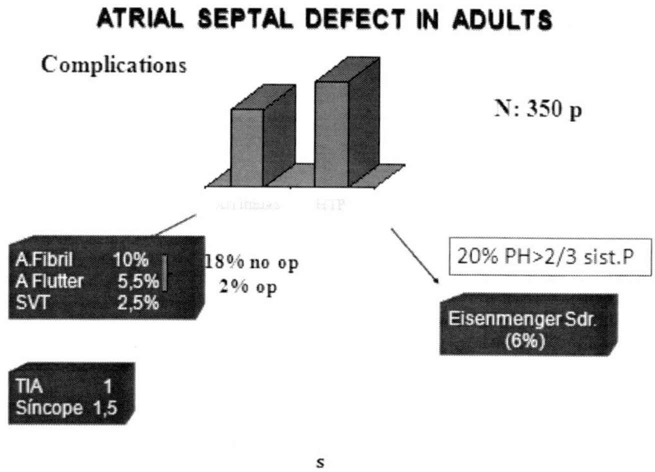

Figure 3. Eighteen percent of the unoperated patients and 2% of the operated patients had atrial fibrillation at age 55 on average in the follow-up of 350 adult cases with ASD from our database.

In surgical patients with Tetralogy of Fallot, the pressure and/or volume overload of the right ventricle associated to large ventriculotomies is the morphologic substrate for developing life threatening ventricular arrhythmias.

Likewise, there is an intimate relationship between the electrical disorders secondary to residual structural defects and the development of right ventricular dysfunction.

Dysfunction of the Right Ventricle

Right ventricular failure is a frequent cause of late morbidity and mortality in patients with congenital heart disease. This may happen in cases when the right ventricle is normally located in the subpulmonary position as it is in Fallot´s tetralogy. Chronic pulmonary regurgitation secondary to a transannular patch leads to right ventricular failure in the long run. Severe pulmonary insufficiency after the third or fourth decades of life is the most frequent cause of reoperation in adults with this condition [4, 7].

Currently, cardiac magnetic resonance is the gold standard diagnostic modality for the evaluation of volumes and function of the right ventricle. It allows referring confidently asymptomatic patients to surgically restore pulmonary competence before heart failure ensues.

On the other hand, dysfunction of the right ventricle may arise in those pathologies where the right ventricle sustains the systemic circulation. The best examples of this situation are the transposition of the great arteries with a previous physiologic surgical procedure which involves a rerouting of the systemic and pulmonary venous returns (Senning or Mustard procedures) and the congenitally corrected transposition. The capacity of the right ventricle to function as the systemic pump over time has gained growing concern since the beginnings of congenital cardiovascular surgery. There is evidence that, in the absence of tricuspid insufficiency, the right ventricle could function properly up to 20 or 25 years after surgery.

However, when it is associated to a progressive tricuspid regurgitation, as usually observed in patients with congenitally corrected transposition, the right ventricular failure appears earlier [8]. In this regard, the arterial switch operation for transposition of the great arteries that reconnects each large vessel to its corresponding ventricle has become by now the procedure of choice. Likewise, in order to avoid the dysfunction of a systemic right ventricle, there is currently a growing tendency to perform a double *switch procedure* (atrial and arterial) in children born with a congenitally corrected transposition [9].

Pulmonary Vascular Disease

It is a serious complication that may occur in either unoperated or operated patients with left-to-right shunts or late when the pulmonary artery resistances have already increased to systemic or supra systemic levels and thus, an Eisenmenger syndrome (ES) develops reversing the shunt and the patient turns cyanotic. We have seen 55 patients, aged 18 to 66 years (28 yrs on average) in our experience at the Argerich and Garrahan Hospitals. They present multiple and complex problems related to chronic cyanosis and represent a challenge to cardiologists at the time of relevant decisions, such as the indication of phlebotomy, contraception, or heart transplantation [10]. This topic will be covered in depth in the Eisenmenger Syndrome's chapter in this book.

Conclusion

Adult Congenital Heart Disease: An Unprotected Community

This special and increasing group of patients should be treated in specialized centers for adult congenital heart disease. These centers could be located in an adult general hospital or in a special center created in a pediatric hospital largely experienced in medical and surgical treatment of complex heart lesions and reoperations. Nowadays many pediatric hospitals in USA treat these adult patients routinely such as is the case of the children's hospitals in Houston, San Francisco, Boston, etc. In our experience, better surgical results were achieved when patients underwent surgery in pediatric hospitals with staff trained for congenital cardiology. On the other hand, this community is not a priority for adult cardiovascular surgeons who have been rarely exposed and much less trained in congenital heart defects and are highly demanded by coronary or valvular heart surgery. Additionally most of our adult population has no health or life insurance. These patients either find it hard to get a job due to their pre-existent illness history or they are systematically rejected when the scar of a previous sternotomy is detected in the physical exam.

The creation of a multidisciplinary team should include: 1) pediatric and adult cardiologists trained in adult congenital heart disease; 2) experts in the different imaging modalities to deal with the whole spectrum of congenital cardiac lesions and the surgical techniques as well, v.g.: transesophageal and three dimensional echocardiography, cardiac magnetic resonance and multislice computed tomography; 3) an interventional cardiologist trained in all the procedures inherent to this specialty; 4) a cardiovascular surgeon expert in complex congenital heart surgery and reoperations and an adult surgeon to attend to the potential associated coronary artery disease; 5) experts in cardiovascular postoperative care trained both to treat children and adults; 6) electrophysiologists familiarized with the anatomical and surgical variants of congenital defects; 7) gynecologists capable to cope with high risk pregnancy cases, etc. This specialized center would treat a considerable number of adults with congenital heart disease with good surgical results. The larger the amount of adult patients the shorter the learning curve. It also would be the ideal institution to train both pediatric and adult cardiologists in adult congenital heart medicine.

References

[1] Perloff JK, Warnes C. Congenital heart disease in adults: a new cardiovascular speciality.*Circulation* 2001; 84: 1881-90.

[2] Warnes CA, Liberthson R, Danielson GK, et al. Task force 1: the changing profile of congenital heart disease in adult life. *J Am Coll Cardiol* 2001; 37:1170-75.

[3] Magliola R, Laura JP, Capelli H. Current situation of children with congenital heart disease in Argentina. *Arch Argent Pediatr.* 2000; 98:130-33.

[4] Capelli H. Grown-up congenital heart disease: The problem of late arrhythmia and ventricular dysfunction. *Prog Pediatr Cardiol* 2006; 22: 165-73.

[5] Kanter R, Garson A. Atrial arrhythmias during chronic follow-up of surgery for complex congenital heart disease. *Pacing Clin Electrophysiol* 1997; 20: 502-11.

[6] Gatzoulis MA, Freeman MA, Siu SC, Webb GD, Harris L. Atrial arrhythmia after surgical closure of atrial septal defects in adults. *N Engl J Med* 1999; 340: 839-46.

[7] Bonhoeffer P, Boudjemline Y, Saliba Z, et al. Transcatheter implantation of a bovine valve in pulmonary position. A lamb study. *Circulation* 2000; 102: 813-16.

[8] Graham TP, Bernard YD, Mellen BG, et al. Long-term outcome in congenitally corrected transposition of great arteries: A multi-institutional study. *J Am Coll Cardiol* 2000; 36: 255-61.

[9] Yagihara T, Kishimoto H, Isobe F, et al. Double switch operation in cardiac anomalies with atrioventricular and ventriculoarterial discordance. *J Thorac Cardiovasc Surg* 1994; 107:351-58

[10] Somerville J. How to manage the Eisenmenger syndrome. *Int J Cardiol* 1998; 63:1-8.

In: Congenital Heart Diseases
Editor: Raúl Cayré and José Milei

ISBN: 978-1-61122-003-2

Chapter 14

Management of Cardiac Emergencies in Children with Congenital Heart Disease

Guillermo A. Kohn Loncarica*[1,*] *and Guillermo E. Moreno [2]
[1]Attending physician in the pediatric emergency department.
Hospital Nacional de Pediatría "Dr. Juan P. Garrahan". Buenos Aires, Argentina
[2]Attending physician in the pediatric cardiac intensive care unit.
Hospital Nacional de Pediatría "Dr. Juan P. Garrahan". Buenos Aires, Argentina

Abstract

Children with congenital heart disease require adequate clinical support. Intensive care units (neonatal and cardiovascular) and pediatric emergency departments have a vital role in the care of these patients. This chapter presents the key aspects for proper management of these children: early diagnosis, timely treatment, clinical support and prevention and treatment of complications.

1. Introduction

CHD are not preventable diseases at this time. The only way to currently improve the prognosis lies in early diagnosis and this is essential to the successful treatment of these patients. One third of all children with CHD will suffer a serious critical illness during the first year of life and will either die or receive surgical intervention [1, 2]. Surgical delay impairs the patient's clinical condition and is associated with a high morbidity and mortality. The more common scenarios include children with large ventricular septal defects, heart failure and respiratory infections while waiting for surgical repair.

* E-mail: guillecarekids@fibertel.com.ar.

The success of surgery in infants with CHD has led to an increasing number of patients who will require monitoring for the development of residual complications. In some cases, reoperation is required. If the CHD is not repaired, it may result in progressive and irreversible damage of the heart (e.g. myocardial hyperplasia, coronary angiogenesis), lungs with abnormal vascular bed/alveolar development and abnormal neurocognitive development.

2. The Emergency Physician and Congenital Heart Diseases. When Should CHD be Clinically Suspected?

The emergency department is a good setting to identify children with undiagnosed CHD; therefore it is important for emergency physicians to have knowledge of the different clinical forms of CHD and their presentations. CHDs include a very heterogeneous group of lesions with a diverse pathophysiology and complications; however, they are represented by only a small number of signs and symptoms. The main forms of clinical presentations of CHD and their complications are as follows:

Cyanosis

Cyanosis is the appearance of a blue coloration of the skin or mucous membranes and is one of the most important physical signs of CHD and its complications. Because cyanosis depends on the absolute concentration of hemoglobin, it is more apparent in children with a high hematocrit and less so when they are anemic. If hemoglobin levels are normal, cyanosis can be detected when blood saturation values drop below 85%. There are two forms of cyanosis: central and peripheral. Central cyanosis is usually seen on the tongue and lips and occurs as a consequence of low arterial saturation due to heart, lung or neurological diseases. Peripheral cyanosis, on the other hand, results from a decrease in local blood circulation but with normal blood arterial saturation. This is frequently seen on the arms and legs in patients with heart failure, shock, diseases of blood circulation (thrombosis/embolism) and exposure to cold temperatures. All causes of central cyanosis can lead to peripheral cyanosis, but not all causes of peripheral cyanosis can lead to central cyanosis.

In patients with suspected cyanosis, the first step is to identify the patient's baseline saturation at room air. Emergency physicians should ask brief questions looking for a history (e.g. neonatal asphyxia, meconium aspiration or low Apgar score) that predisposes the patient to getting permanent pulmonary hypertension. A chest radiograph (CXR)is a good diagnostic tool that can be used to show the shape and size of the heart, estimate the flow of pulmonary circulation and detect lung pathology.

The hyperoxiatest is another simple and useful test for diagnosing the cause of cyanosis. It is performed by initially giving 100% oxygen for 10 minutes before measuring oxygen saturation with either pulse oximetry or blood gases. If the oxygen saturation does not change or the arterial oxygen pressure does not rise above 70 mmHg, it is very likely that the patient has cyanotic congenital heart disease.

However, if the oxygen saturation rises above 150 mmHg, it is very unlikely to be cyanotic congenital heart disease because these patients rarely have PaO2 values greater than 150 mmHg. When the PaO2 is between 70 and 150 mmHg, cyanotic CHD can neither be confirmed nor excluded and additional studies must be performed. In summary, a lack of response to the hyperoxia test supports the suspicion of cyanotic CHD and an urgent echocardiogram should be performed.

Heart Failure

Heart failure results from a multisystem imbalance that arises, in most cases, when the heart is no longer able to fill or to eject the blood delivered to it by the venous system. Contrary to what happens in adults where the etiology is usually ischemic, heart failure in congenital heart disease is commonly caused by volume and/or pressure overload. Anamnesis should be directed to identify feeding difficulties, sweating, poor weight gain, stridor, chest pain or syncope. Tachycardia, tachypnea, breathlessness, presence of a third heart sound, fine rales at the lung bases, hepatomegaly, soft tissue edema, oliguria, heart murmurs, distended neck veins and absent or weak femoral pulses are frequent signs and symptoms of heart failure in children. Some children with obstructive left heart diseases such as coarctation of the aorta, interrupted aortic archand hypoplastic left heart syndrome may present with cardiogenic shock to the emergency department. Often, this latter situation is incorrectly initially interpreted and treated as septic shock.

Heart Murmurs

Congenital heart disease should be considered when a heart murmur is accompanied with other signs and symptoms such as cyanosis or heart failure. Murmurs should be analyzed according to their different characteristics: timing, location, radiation, intensity, pitch and quality. Intense, diastolic and continuous murmurs are considered pathological as are all those accompanied with an abnormal physical examination.

3. Value of Additional Testing for CHD in the Emergency Department

In the face of suspected CHD, the emergency physician should order a CXR, electrocardiogram and echocardiogram. ACXR provides information about the size and the shape of the heart as well as the status of the lungs. Some CHDs may have classic findings such as the "boot shaped" heart seen in Tetralogy of Fallot and may also show signs of pulmonary hypoflow or hyperflow. Additionally, pediatric emergency physicians should always calculate the cardiothoracic index (a clinical method of expressing the size of the heart). A value greater than 50% suggests cardiomegaly. However, cardiothoracic index interpretation in young children can be difficult due to the presence of the thymus. An electrocardiogram (ECG) is useful for determining chamber hypertrophy, arrhythmias and repolarization disorders. Emergency physicians must be aware that the interpretation of pediatric ECGs and what is considered a normal ECG in a child is very different from that of an adult.

An echocardiogram is a very important tool that provides information about cardiac structure and function. However, because a pediatric echocardiogram is a unique and specialized, a physician with experience with performance and interpretation should perform it.

Chamber hypertrophy diagnosis criteria are as follows:

RIGHT ATRIAL HYPERTROPHY	Peaked P waves (P pulmonale)
LEFT ATRIAL HYPERTROPHY	Biphasic waves of lengths greater than 0.08 in infants and 0.10 in children
RIGHT VENTRICULAR HYPERTROPHY	Positive T waves in right pre-cordial leads (from V4 to V2) QRS right axis deviation greater than 120 degrees Dominant qR and R in right leads (V3 and aVR) Deep S wave in left sided leads
LEFT VENTRICULAR HYPERTROPHY	ST segment depression and inverted T waves in left sided leads Peaked R wave in V6 Deep S wave in right sided leads Deep Q wave in V5 and V6

4. Clinical Presentation and Preoperative Management of CHD in Neonates

CHD with Left Sided Obstructive Lesions and Ductal-Dependent Systemic Blood Flow

Neonates with CHD with left-sided obstructive lesions have symptoms stemming from closure of the ductus arteriosus. As a result, this leads to progressive metabolic acidosis and either congestive heart failure, cardiovascular collapse or shock. These left-right shunt lesions can be stabilized by keeping the ductus arteriosus open. This improves the cardiac output by allowing the right ventricle to support systemic blood flow. If this type of CHD is clinically suspected, prostaglandin (PGE1) infusion should be promptly started and treatment should proceed even without echocardiography confirmation [3]. This is the essential management for survival because it maintains ductal patency and balances the flow between pulmonary and systemic circulations. Peripheral organs can be affected by the resultant decrease in perfusion. Acute renal failure, necrotizing enterocolitis and intraventricular hemorrhages are common squeals of these lesions, especially if not managed properly. Clinical symptoms includes sub-acute onset of fussiness, poor feeding, pallor, respiratory distress and oliguria. If these symptoms are present, sepsis should be strongly considered and low threshold must be maintained for obtaining cultures and treating empirically with antibiotics.

To prevent excessive pulmonary blood flow, the pulmonary vascular resistance can be manipulated by adjusting the ventilation. In general, the ventilator setting should be managed as follows: titrate the FIO2 to keep systemic arterial saturation between 75- 80 %, allow enough tidal volume to obtain good chest expansion and maintain the peak inspiratory pressure> 25 cm H20 and positive end-expiratory pressure at 4-6 cm H2O. In addition, high arterial saturation and respiratory alkalosis should be avoided and the hematocrit should be kept close to 40%. Endovenous inotropics should be considered if there is clinical suspicion of excessive pulmonary blood flow.

Left-sided obstructive CHD types include coarctation of the aorta, interrupted aortic arch, critical aortic stenosis and hypoplastic left heart syndrome.

Coarctation of the Aorta in the neonate results from the acute onset obstruction of systemic blood flow leading to left ventricular pressure overload and failure with subsequent elevation of left atrial pressure and pulmonary edema. The severity of this lesion depends on the degree of the coarctation, the patency of the ductus arteriosus and the presence of associated intracardiac lesions (e.g. ventricular septal defects). Coarctation may also be associated with other complex CHDs like truncus arteriosus, double outlet right ventricle, single ventricle lesions and Shone's complex [4].

Interrupted Aortic Archmay be associated with ventricular septal defects, bicuspid aortic valve, truncus arteriosus, transposition of the great arteries, double outlet right ventricle and single ventricle complexes. Calcium levels should be closely monitored due to the frequent association with 22q11 chromosome deletion.

Critical Aortic Stenosisin neonates leads to pressure overload in the left ventricle, elevated end-diastolic pressure, elevated left atrial pressure and pulmonary edema. The left ventricle is generally dilated with poor contractility. Inadequate coronary blood flow results from tachycardia and increased left ventricular end-diastolic pressure [5].

CHD with Right-Sided Obstructive Lesions and Ductal-Dependent Pulmonary Blood Flow

Right-sided obstructive lesions usually present with central cyanosis, and pulmonary blood flow is dependent on the L-R shunt through the ductus arteriosus. The degree of cyanosis hinges on the patency of the ductus and may worsen with ductal constriction. The hyperoxia test with arterial blood gas measurement helps differentiate between a respiratory or cardiac origin. Management includes prompt infusion of PGE1 to keep the ductus arteriosus open until a Blalock-Taussig shunt can be surgically placed. In addition, ventilation management is always a primary concern in order to decrease peripheral oxygen consumption. Optimizing intravascular volume and maintaining the hematocrit around 40% improves oxygen delivery. Hyperventilation and correction of metabolic acidosis, together with pharmacological sedation and neuromuscular blockade, may help decrease peripheral vascular resistance. CHD with right-sided obstructive lesions and ductal-dependent pulmonary blood flow includes Tetralogy of Fallot with pulmonary stenosis, Tetralogy of Fallot with pulmonary atresia, Ebstein's anomaly (without atresia of either the pulmonary atresia or tricuspid valve and tricuspid atresia), critical pulmonary stenosis and pulmonary atresia with intact ventricular septum. Since some of the lesions associated with tricuspid valve atresia and pulmonary atresia with intact ventricular septum and Tetralogy of Fallot with pulmonary atresia also have single ventricle physiology, their treatments are discussed in other sections.

Transposition of the Great Arteries

In Transposition of the great arteries, the systemic and pulmonary circulations are in parallel (Graph 1: Parallel circulations). In this circumstance, most of the output of each ventricle is re-circulated back to the respective ventricle. To survive, certain anatomic sites must exist to allow for intercirculatory mixing of the pulmonary and systemic blood.

Intracardiac:

- patent foramen ovale
- atrial septal defect
- ventricular septal defect

Extracardiac:

- patent ductus arteriosus or
- bronchopulmonary collateral circulation

In patients with adequate interatrial or interventricular defects size, the level of arterial oxygen saturation is influenced primarily by the pulmonary-to-systemic blood flow ratio. A high pulmonary blood flow results in relatively high arterial oxygen saturation as long as the ventricles can adequately maintain the high output state. In situations with decreased pulmonary blood flow, an elevated pulmonary vascular resistance should be considered if the arterial oxygen saturation decreases despite adequately sized anatomic shunt sites [6, 7].

LA ⇒	LV ⇒	PA ⇒ LUNG CIRCULATION
↑↓	↑↓	↑↓
RA ⇒	RV ⇒	AO ⇒ SYSTEMIC CIRCULATION

Graph 1. Parallel circulations.

In transposition of the great arteries with an intact ventricular septum, there is inadequate mixing at the foramen ovale level which results in severe secondary hypoxemia and deficiency of oxygen supply to the tissues. An excessive right and left ventricular workload is also present. If the ductus arteriosus is closing, profound hypoxemia with pO2 < 20 mm Hg can be seen. Only a relatively small proportion of blood is exchanged by mixing between the two circulations, and as a result, only a small proportion of the effective circulation reaches the appropriate vascular bed.

To stabilize the patient, PGE1 must be started and emergent balloon atrial septostomy must be performed to enlarge the foramen ovale. In addition, hyperventilation and increased FIO2 may help to increase pulmonary blood flow. Although there is no CHD for which PGE1 is contraindicated, in cases of transposition of the great arteries with a restrictive atrial septum, cyanosis may be exacerbated by PGE1 infusion due pulmonary edema until atrial septostomy is performed [8].Congested lungs are also observed in obstructed total anomalous pulmonary venous return and emergent surgery is required to treat both of these conditions.

Single Ventricle Lesions

In this group of lesions, there is complete mixing of the systemic and venous return at the ventricular or atrial level. Therefore, the ventricular output must be divided between the two competing parallel circuits: the pulmonary and systemic arterial circulations. In single ventricle lesions, the pulmonary artery and aortic oxygen saturations are equal, and the ventricular output is the sum of the pulmonary blood flow (Qp) and the systemic blood flow (Qs). The proportion of the ventricular output that is directed to the pulmonary or systemic vascular bed depends on the amount of resistance to the flow into these circuits. The degree of obstruction to pulmonary outflow depends on the presence of the following conditions: pulmonary stenosis, pulmonary vascular resistance, pulmonary venous obstruction and left atrial pressure (obstruction to outflow through the left atrioventricular valve and atrial septum). On the other hand, the following conditions and severity determine the degree of obstruction to systemic outflow: the degree of subaortic or aortic valve stenosis, coarctation of the aorta, systemic vascular resistance and the size of the ductus arteriosus.

In some cases there is no outflow obstruction to the pulmonary and systemic circuits; therefore, before surgical procedures, ventilator and pharmacologic maneuvers are needed. The objective is to balance the ventricular output between the parallel circulations with the goal of having the systemic and pulmonary vascular beds achieve a Qp/Qs ~ 1. These maneuvers provide adequate systemic blood flow and oxygen delivery to prevent acidosis and decreases single ventricle volume overload.

$$\frac{\text{PV Sat (95-100\%)} - \text{PA 02Sat (75-80\%)} \quad 20}{\text{A02 Sat (75- 80\%)- MV O2Sat (55- 60\%)} \quad 20} = \text{------- Qp/Qs: } \sim 1$$

- PV: pulmonary venous saturation
- PA: pulmonary artery saturation
- A: aortic saturation
- MV: mixed venous saturation
- Qp/Qs: pulmonary blood flow/systemic blood flow

Patients with unbalanced single-ventricle physiology may be grouped into the following categories:

Hypoxemic patients with low pulmonary blood flow (oxygen saturation <65%):

- Severe pulmonary stenosis: The management includes elevating the blood pressure and systemic vascular resistance by increasing inotropic infusions in order to force more blood through the obstructed intracardiac pulmonary outflow. Interventional procedures, such as pulmonary valve dilation, may also be considered.
- Restrictive ductus arteriosus in lesions with ductal-dependent pulmonary blood flow
- Elevated pulmonary vascular resistance: Ventilator maneuvers are performed to decrease pulmonary vascular resistance (e.g., increased FIO2, hyperventilation-induced alkalosis, nitric oxide or iloprost). Intravenous pulmonary vasodilators are nonspecific and result in unpredictable changes in the pulmonary and systemic vascular resistances.
- Obstruction to pulmonary venous outflow causing pulmonary venous hypertension and secondary pulmonary arteriolar hypertension
- Obstructive left-sided lesions: Atrioventricular valve and restrictive atrial septal defects may require transcatheter dilation of the atrial septum [9].

Congestive heart failure in patients with excessive pulmonary blood flow:

Patients with single-ventricle physiology and high arterial oxygen saturations (>90%):are generally seen in those where the combined ventricular output is redirected into the pulmonary vascular circuit. This causes a reduction in the systemic flow, which results in inadequate tissue perfusion, metabolic acidosis, low cardiac output and shock.

Once establishment of a patent ductus arteriosus is confirmed, maneuvers to minimize systemic vascular resistance and maximize pulmonary vascular resistance should be used.

One method to increase pulmonary vascular resistance is to add supplemental inspired gases, nitrogen [10, 11] or carbon dioxide [12].This mechanism is likely due to the induction of alveolar hypoxia [13]. Other maneuvers include mechanical ventilation with pharmacological sedation and paralysis to allow permissive hypoventilation (elevate the PCO2to a goal of 40 to 50 mmHg) [14], correct metabolic acidemia, avoid excessive inotropic support (doses which favor alpha receptors), after load reduction with sodium nitroprusside and maintain the hematocrit greater than 40% to 45% (increased viscosity may also help to elevate pulmonary vascular resistance).

If a patient with unstable physiology requires intubation and pharmacological sedation to maintain adequate systemic blood flow, they should undergo urgent surgical management to achieve a more favorable physiology. This is the typical presentation of hypoplastic left heart syndrome, a left-sided obstructive lesion with ductal-dependent systemic blood flow.

Prostaglandin Administration

The initial intravenous dose of PGE1 is 0.05 mcg/kg/min. If there is no improvement, the dose should be increased to 0.1 mcg/ kg/ min. After the infant's condition has stabilized, the usual maintenance dose of PGE1 is 0.025 mcg/kg/min. Apnea, bradycardia, hypotension, fluid-electrolyte imbalances, irritability, fever and cutaneous flushing are all potential complicating side effects of PGE1.

Therefore, management of the airway is essential along with excluding the possibility of sepsis.

Apnea secondary to prostaglandin administration requires tracheal intubation. If intubation is performed, it is essential that the prostaglandin administration continue at the same dose or higher. Long-term use is associated with cortical hyperostosis, but it is a side effect that does not seem to be dose related. Monitoring in an intensive care unit is required.

Clinical Presentations and Management of Complications of CHD in Children

Attacks of Hypoxemia

Emergency physicians who work in emergency departments should have extensive knowledge of the management of attacks of hypoxemia. Children with CHD in which pulmonary blood flow is reduced may suffer from these episodes. Examples of these include Tetralogy of Fallot, tricuspid atresia and pulmonary atresia with an intact ventricular septum.

Hypoxemic attacks are surge episodes of intense cyanosis due to desaturation; the subsequent irritability and dyspnea results from an acute decrease in pulmonary blood flow. These may be of varying intensity and duration, and the most serious cases cause impaired consciousness, seizures and death. Although attacks of hypoxemia may happen at any age, the incidence seems to increase after 4 to 6 months of age and is one of several reasons for needing complete surgical repair before this age. Fortunately, the incidence of attacks of hypoxemia has decreased because many patients with cyanotic CHD undergo early surgical correction.

Pathophysiology

Until now, the exact nature of these events has been unknown. However, various mechanisms (or some combination thereof) have been described:

- Infundibulum spasm: Cyanotic attacks happen as a result of the spasmodic contraction of part of the right ventricular outflow tract called the "Infundibulum." However, this theory fails to explain why children with pulmonary atresia also experience attacks of hypoxemia. Children with this condition have an undeveloped subpulmonic infundibulum.
- Changes in systemic vascular resistance: Sudden changes in systemic vascular resistance can increase the intensity of the intracardiac right-to-left shunt.
- Sudden changes in venous return to the heart can also affect the right-to-left shunt.
- Abrupt changes in heart rate
- Alterations in sensitivity of the respiratory center

Different factors that cause patient agitation can trigger attacks of hypoxemia. Significant stressful situations, crying, invasive medical procedures and conditions such as dehydration have all been described. Because attacks of hypoxemia are more frequent in the morning, shortly after waking, it is thought that the sudden changes in $pCO2$ that occur after a lengthy sleep may explain the hypercyanosis crisis.

Infundibulum spasm and/or other mechanisms such as tachycardia increase the right-to-left shunt and cause hypoxemia and acidosis. To compensate, this creates a vicious feedback loop cycle wherein the patient begins to hyperventilate in order to increase the venous return and decrease the systemic vascular resistance, which then exacerbates the right-to-left shunt. A progressive cycle of decreased pulmonary blood flow, increased cyanosis and worsening metabolic acidosis develops from the imbalance between pulmonary and systemic circulations.

Clinical Findings

At presentation to the emergency department, these children usually have a previous diagnosis of their CHD and parents have already witnessed crises of varying intensities. Often, they tend to state that the events have been getting more severe and/or more frequent. These patients usually have different degrees of cyanosis and can adopt positional maneuvers such as squatting to improve their condition. A squatting position is often seen in children with this condition after exerting near maximal effort. The mechanism is due to compression of the femoral arteries, which results in an increased peripheral resistance and a decreased right-to-left shunt. In some patients, they may present with little or no evidence of cyanosis before the onset of the attack.

However, in the majority of cases, the cyanosis is quite obvious. Their clinical signs may range from simple crying and fussiness to a more extreme neurological status such as lethargy and even coma. Tachypnea is always seen with these attacks, however the differential diagnosis for tachypnea is long and other medical problems should be considered as well.

In children with Tetralogy of Fallot, the intensity and length of the systolic ejection murmur is closely related to the degree of infundibulum obstruction. During the spell, a previously heard heart murmur may be absent or decreased because pulmonary blood flow through the stenotic right ventricular outflow tract is reduced. There is usually only a single second heart sound due to the absence of the pulmonary component.

Attacks of hypoxemia can last from a few minutes to several hours and can be fatal. Short episodes typically end with the patient becoming weak and sleepy, however more severe crises can cause seizures, hemiparesis, brain ischemia and even coma.

Management

These patients require immediate attention in the emergency department. Appropriate positioning of the head, administration of oxygen and morphine are the first measures to take in order to reduce or terminate the attack.

Treatment is greatly based on increasing the systemic vascular resistance to decrease the right to left shunt. It is very important to keep the child calm and close to his/her parents and to avoid any painful or invasive procedures that could worsen the crisis. Sometimes it is helpful to reduce ambient light intensity and parents should be asked to keep the child in a knee-chest position in order to increase systemic vascular resistance.

Oxygen should be administered to improve saturation and raise PaO2 levels. Oxygen is administered despite the fact that this measure may prove unsuccessful due to the reduction of pulmonary blood flow during the "spell".

Even though its exact mechanism of action is unknown, administration of large doses (0.1 to 0.2 mg/kg) of subcutaneous morphine is usually used to treat the attack. In theory, morphine depresses the respiratory drive, which interferes with the hyperpnea cycle and leads to vasomotor changes. It may also be useful to administer a sedative agent like intramuscular/intranasal midazolam (0.5 mg/kg).

Ketamine may also be used to decrease agitation and increase systemic vascular resistance. Sometimes the required sedation causes respiratory depression and the patient may need to be intubated. Nevertheless, mechanical ventilation does not improve oxygenation because the problem is restriction of pulmonary blood flow.

If the crisis continues, additional measures are needed.

- Sodium bicarbonate may be administered intravenously at a dose of 2-3mEq/kg.
- Propranolol administered intravenously at a dose of 0.2 mg/kg over 4-5 minutes can produce prompt improvement. It is still unknown whether propranolol´s mechanism of action is primarily by affecting infundibular contraction, the hyperpneic ventilatory response or systemic vasomotor tone.
- IV fluids may improve the cyanosis because the ventricular outflow obstruction may be intensified in situations with depleted intravascular volume.
- Vasopressors suchphenylephrine administered intravenously at 5-20 mcg/kg/dose every 10 minutes may be used to increase systemic vascular resistance. This reduces the right-to-left shunt and subsequently improves systemic oxygenation. Vasopressor infusion requires continuous heart rate, blood pressure and oximetry monitoring.

Emergency intubation, mechanical ventilation, surgery, or extracorporeal membrane oxygenation may occasionally be needed. If patients require mechanical ventilation, it is recommended to perform rapid sequence intubation with drugs such as ketamine because it increases systemic blood pressure. Avoid drugs that cause hypotension such as benzodiazepines.

Attacks of hypoxemia should not be confused with heart failure because inotropics, diuretics and vasodilators are contraindicated in these hypoxic events. If cardiac arrhythmias occur during management, they should be promptly treated. Even though relieved with treatment, hypoxemiausually indicates that surgery will be required for definitive treatment.

To avoid future crises, physicians should warn parents to avoid triggering factors such as pain, hunger and stress as well as processes that cause vasodilatation such as fever and hot water [15].

Heart Failure: L-R Shunt Lesions

A L-R shunt cardiac lesion is an abnormal connection between the left and right side of the heart and includes atrial septal defects, ventricle septal defects, atrioventricular septal defects and patent ductus arteriosus. Of these, the most common types are ventricle septal defects, atrioventricular septal defects and patent ductus arteriosus and the definitive treatment is corrective surgery. The flow across the cardiac shunt depends on the size of the defect and the pressure difference between the two chambers on either side of the shunt. However the pressure difference is the most important factor in determining the amount of flow across the shunt. Blood will always flow from the high pressure chamber to the low pressure chamber. Therefore, in a normal heart (in the presence of a shunt), flow will be from left to right. When larger pressure-difference between the chambers, then more blood that will be shunted across the defect. . In newborns, the pulmonary vascular resistance and the right heart pressures are high resulting in a low-pressure gradient between the left and right sides of the heart and minimal flow across the defect. In these lesions, the myocardial contractility is well preserved, but cardiac failure occurs because the systemic circulation is less perfused while pulmonary circulation is overflowing with high Qp: Qs ratios greater than 1.5:1. These large shunts lesion are at risk for congestive cardiac failure with pulmonary hypertension due to the increased pulmonary blood flow and over circulation.

L-R shunt lesions symptoms and signs include murmurs as well as those consistent with congestive heart failure. Murmurs heard in shunt lesions are often generated by the turbulent blood flow across a valve. They are present when a pressure gradient develops after the neonatal pulmonary vascular resistance falls between 4- 6 weeks of age. An ASD murmur is caused by the turbulent flow over the pulmonary valve as a result of a relative pulmonary stenosis (PS). On the other hand, a large ventricular septal defect will lead to excess blood returning to the left atrium and the consequent turbulent flow through the mitral valve results in a relative mitral stenosis. This is heard as a mid-diastolic rumble. Signs of congestive heart failure include tachycardia, cardiomegaly, congested lungs sounds, hepatomegaly and peripheral edema.

Tachypnea, dyspnea and wheezing are present due to interstitial pulmonary edema with a decrease in lung compliance and increase in airway resistance. This situation causes atelectasis, ventilation/ perfusion (V/Q) mismatching, pulmonary hypertension and increases the work of breathing (recruitment of intercostal and subcostal muscles). There is a high risk for failure to thrive due to the high-energy cost of breathing. Management in stable patients involves diuretics (furosemide), digoxin and hypercaloric feedings, however surgery is ultimately required for definitive treatment.

In decompensated patients with congested lungs, intravenous diuretics should be administrated often, but oxygen therapy should be used with prudence because it will cause vasodilatation of the pulmonary circulation, which may worsen the increased pulmonary blood flow. It is recommended to maintain oxygen saturation levels at 85- 90%. If respiratory distress is present with an increased work of breathing, it may help to start with non-invasive positive pressure ventilation with a low FiO2; if the patient worsens, however, more invasive mechanical ventilation is needed. The positive pressure helps to reduce after load, alveolar edema, atelectasis and the metabolic demand. If additional inotropic support is necessary, catecholamines may be used; intravenous dobutamine (more of an inotropic than an chronotrope) infusion can also be safely administered in the emergency department. In cases of severe shock, dopamine or epinephrine may be used but preferably in an ICU setting. Lastly, it is important to optimize the hematocrit to nearly 40% and start nasogastric feeds when appropriate to ensure adequate nutritional support [16].

5. General Management of Critically Ill Children with Congenital Heart Disease in the Emergency Department

General interventions in the emergency department must be rapidly performed in patients with known (repaired or unrepaired) or suspected CHD. Initial management should include the following steps:

1. Address the ABCs (Checking the airway, breathing and circulation)
2. Administer oxygen in order to achieve their baseline level of saturation (this level can usually be provided by the parents)
3. Secure vascular access

Caution should be taken in children with Tetralogy of Fallot since pain or fear can worsen their hypoxemic attacks. If decompensated shock is present and vascular access cannot be obtained, an intraosseous line must be strongly considered.

4. Prudent initial fluid administration

Start with 5-10 mL/kg boluses unless there is concern for dehydration or hypovolemia. If one of these conditions is present, use 10-20 mL/kg boluses instead.

5. Continuous monitoring of blood pressure, heart rate and rhythm and pulse oximetry
6. Echocardiogram should be performed urgently
7. Obtain complementary studies such as CXR, ECG, blood gas, hematocrit, serum electrolytes and lactate
8. Cardiology and pediatric intensive care unit consultation

A rapid assessment should be performed to categorize the child with unrepaired or repaired CHD. After addressing the ABCs, close observation of the general appearance and color may provide useful details about the degree and distribution of the cyanosis. At baseline, these patients are often pale or cyanotic and have an increased work of breathing. Caregivers' information may help guide the physician's assessment. Oxygen saturation in a child with corrected congenital heart disease may be low in contrast with their baseline level. Supplemental oxygen administration should be titrated to meet the patient's baseline, but once this level has been reached, additional oxygen support may be harmful.

Emergency physicians should also know how to check pre-ductal and post-ductal oxygen saturations (on the right hand and left foot simultaneously). A difference of 10% or greater between the two suggests cardiac disease [17]. Often, a quick assessment of the patient can provide important details about their hydration and respiratory status. At this point parents' information must be considered, as they will likely know their child's baseline breathing condition and other important details.

Assessment of circulation must include the patient's color, central and peripheral pulses (radial and femoral pulses should be palpated and compared) and blood pressure on all four extremities. If a difference of greater than 20 mm Hg exists between the upper and lower limbs, coarctation of the aorta should be considered. Signs of congestive heart failure such as hepatomegaly, gallop rhythm and jugular venous distention must also be assessed.

When assessing for murmurs, physicians should ask themselves the following questions:

If there is a murmur:

1. Does the patient have a baseline murmur?
2. Is this murmur new?

If there is not a murmur:

3. Did the child previously have one?

Neonatal stabilization and transport:

Most neonates with congenital heart diseases need stabilization in an intensive care unit with highly trained staff. The following steps must be taken into account for stabilization:

1. Maintain the patency of the ductus arteriosus with prostaglandins if you suspect a ductal-dependent lesion. The availability of these drugs should be ensured at all emergency departments.
2. Provide proper ventilation and oxygenation; mechanical ventilation is required in cases of respiratory distress or severe cyanosis. It is advisable to keep oxygen saturation at near 80% especially in patients with heart failure. Excessive oxygen saturation can decrease vascular resistance due to pulmonary vasodilatation and can worsen the severity of symptoms.
3. Secure reliable vascular access. The umbilical vein is often useful in this case, which is typically accessible until one week of age.
4. Proper monitoring should include continuous oxygen saturation, measurement of temperature, blood pressure (ideally with an arterial catheter) and laboratory tests (calcium, blood sugar level and blood count and serum electrolytes).
5. Use inotropic agents with caution to prevent myocardial injury. Digitalis drugs are not recommended.
6. Fluid expansion and bicarbonate should be used in the presence of shock.
7. Use parenteral nutrition until shock is treated to avoid necrotizing enterocolitis.

After stabilization, neonates must be transferred for their definitive care and meticulous, thorough communication with the receiving center is necessary.

6. Management of Systemic Complications of Congenital Heart Diseases in the Emergency Department

Emergency physicians should be aware of systemic complications that may occur in patients with CHD in order to appropriately manage these children.

Cardiac Complications

Cardiac complications such as low output syndrome, postoperative heart failure and arrhythmias are usually seen in pediatric intensive care units. However, emergency department physicians should be familiar with these and be particularly attentive in children who have recently undergone surgery.

Low output syndrome is the most common postoperative complication. Patients may present with tachycardia, weak pulses, delayed capillary refill, peripheral vasoconstriction and oliguria. Invasive monitoring will show decreased central venous pressure, tachycardia, normal or low blood pressure and elevated arterial resistance. Laboratory findings typically include metabolic acidosis, high lactate levels, respiratory alkalosis, hyperkalemia and high blood urea nitrogen (BUN)/creatinine ratio. Management typically includes combination of intravenous fluids, dopamine, milrinone and epinephrine.

The most frequent arrhythmias are complete atrial-ventricular blockage, nodal rhythms and supraventricular tachycardia. In the emergency department, supraventricular tachycardia is the most frequently seen arrhythmia and emergency doctors should be familiar with its proper management.

Renal Complications

In patients with CHD, it is important to evaluate the patient for renal complications (e. g. renal failure) in the immediate post-operative period and to obtain the most recent BUN and creatinine blood values.

CHD is the most common cause of acute renal failure in infants [18]. The main causes are:

- Vascular stress of surgery (causes a reduction in renal blood flow and glomerular filtration rate, vasopressin release and shift of blood from the cortex to the medulla)
- Low cardiac output or cardiac arrest
- Medications used to improve cardiac function (inotropics medications, phosphodiesterase inhibitors)
- Mechanical circulatory support (extracorporeal circulation)
- Hypothermia (produces a decrease in renal blood flow)

The Multi-Societal Database Committee for Pediatric and Congenital Heart Disease defines acute renal dysfunction as new onset oliguria with sustained urine output < 0.5 ml/kg/h for 24 hours and/or a rise in creatinine > 1.5 times the upper limit of normal adjusted for age (or twice the most recent preoperative values) and eventual recovery of renal function without needing dialysis [19]. On the other hand, acute renal failure is defined by the same numerical parameters but without recovery and with eventual need for dialysis or hemofiltration. Renal dysfunction is relatively frequent and transitory in the immediate postoperative period and is managed in intensive care units [20]. Clinical management includes adequate hemodynamic control, proper fluid balance and diuretics; dialysis is performed only if necessary.

Hematological Complications

There is a long list of hematological complications for children who have undergone surgery for CHD. The most frequent disorders are anaphylactic reactions to blood products or antifibrinolytic drugs, cold agglutinin reactions, prothrombotic and/or hemorrhagic reactions and sickle cell crises [21].

The use of extracorporeal circulation or cardiopulmonary bypass and heparin increases the risk of bleeding in patients who have recently undergone surgery. Pediatric intensive care units must monitor the coagulation status because oftentimes these patients need administration of flesh-frozen plasma, platelets and/or packed red blood cells. Coagulation disorders are more common in children younger than 6 months since they often have a relative decreasing coagulation factors, thrombocytopenia and increased bleeding and activated partial thromboplastin times.

After some procedures, such as the Glenn or Fontan procedures, patients will need to continue with anticoagulation therapy. Emergency physicians should always ask about these procedures and the use of anticoagulation drugs like heparin, warfarin or aspirin because children may present with signs and symptoms of intracranial hypertension secondary to intracranial hemorrhage. The patient must be closely observed for neurological signs, arterial hypertension, vomiting, blurred vision, anisocoria and even a coma state.

Infectious Complications

Children who have undergone surgery for CHD may have complications such us wound infection, mediastinitis, pneumonia, endocarditis or sepsis. If any of these infectious complications are present, patients must be admitted for further evaluation and immediate therapy. Sometimes children may present with fever without a known source after surgery of CHD. In this case, if surgery was recent, hospital admission is advisable and a meticulous investigation for the source of infection initiated. Patients with wound infections may have fever, chest pain and obvious signs of swollen, with or without drainage. The emergency physician must take into account the type of procedure, predisposing factors (conditions which suppress immunity) and the patient's general appearance. The pathogen involved with specific infections will depend on the epidemiological characteristics of each institution. In all cases it is necessary to obtain blood and wound cultures. The type of antibiotic to use varies and is specific to each particular case.

The true incidence of pediatric endocarditis is unknown. In Argentina, at Hospital Nacional de Pediatría Juan P. Garrahan, the incidence is approximately 4.9/10,000 admissions/year [22].

Among patients with underlying heart conditions, CHD represents the highest percentage of children presenting with infectious endocarditis. CHD is a predisposing factor for endocarditis and, in adults, the incidence increased from 4.2% in 1992 to 9.5% in 2002.

CHD that could most easily be complicated by the development of endocarditis are ventricular septal defects, patent ductusarteriosus, abnormalities of the aortic valve and Tetralogy of Fallot. Cyanotic conditions and partially repaired shunts are at highest risk. Although complete repair of ventricular/atrial septal defects and patent ductus arteriosus almost completely removes the risk of endocarditis six months after the procedure,21%-50% of children with infectious endocarditis have had a history of cardiovascular surgery (with or without vascular implants, patches or prosthetic valves) [22]. In summary, the clinical presentation of endocarditis in children is often non-specific, and emergency physicians should always keep this condition in mind if the patient has underlying CHD.

Signs and symptoms of endocarditis	%
Fever	87%
Hepatomegaly	62%

Hematuria	41%
Dyspnea	38%
Splenomegaly	37%
Embolism (brain-spleen-kidney-lung)	24%
New heart murmur	35%
Heart failure	30%
Petechiae	27%
Vomiting	6%
Arthritis	5%
Septic shock	3%

Extracted and modified from Paganini Hugo R. Pediatric Infectious Diseases. First Edition, Ed 2007 Scientific American, Cap 72. P. 483.

The mortality rate in children with CHD is approximately 12.8%.

The recommended diagnostics tests include blood cultures, urinalysis and culture, complete blood count, BUN and creatinine levels, CXR, C-reactive protein, erythrocyte sedimentation rate, electrocardiogram and echocardiogram. However, laboratory findings are non-specific and results such as anemia, leukocytosis, hemolysis, elevated C-reactive protein and erythrocyte sedimentation rate, hematuria and proteinuria may or may not be present. Blood cultures are the most important tests for diagnosis. They must be obtained in the emergency department at the time of presentation. It is advisable to obtain adequate blood volume: 1-3 ml for infants and 5-7 ml for children. The decision whether to use antibiotic therapy in the emergency department will depend on the patient's clinical condition. It is not usually necessary to start antibiotic treatment in the emergency department unless the patient appears seriously ill.

After recent surgery, children with high fever and signs of wound infection may also present with acute mediastinitis. These patients may have pain or instability of the sternum; occasionally, mediastinitis may present as septic shock without localizing signs. After the patient is stabilized and antibiotic treatment initiated, a computed tomography of the chest may help clarify the diagnosis.

Pulmonary Complications

Pulmonary complications of CHD such as primary or secondary respiratory arrest or ventilator-associated pneumonias are sometimes seen in the pediatric intensive care unit post-operatively. Other pulmonary complications include atelectasis, pneumothorax, bronchospasm, pleural effusion and chylothorax. Signs and symptoms such as dyspnea, fever, hypoventilation, hypoxemia and respiratory acidosis will suggest these conditions. In patients with symptoms or signs of pulmonary complications, a CXR, arterial blood gases, blood cultures and complete blood counts should be obtained. Antibiotics, pleural effusion drainage and parenteral nutrition may be part of the treatment, depending on the situation. In cases of respiratory distress and respiratory acidosis, mechanical ventilation must be considered early, before further descompensation.

Neurological Complications

Neurological complications of CHD are uncommon, however surgeries that require cardiopulmonary bypass, deep hypothermia and patients who have intracardiac shunts carry a higher risk. The main complications are ischemic or hemorrhagic stroke and seizures. In the emergency department, a magnetic resonance imaging or computed tomography should be ordered if stroke is suspected.

Arrhythmias

In the presence of an arrhythmia in a patient with CHD, the ABCs must be rapidly addressed, venous access secured, and immediate ECG performed. The key features of ECG analysis in this situation are to determine whether a sinus rhythm is present, with regular, narrow QRS complexes, with each complex preceded by a P wave and each complex upright in lead I and aVF. Brady arrhythmias or congenital complete heart block may be associated with CHDs (in particular, with corrected transposition of the great arteries, Ebstein's malformation, and other similar lesions) or related to a surgical procedure, but may also occur in a structurally normal heart. A diagnosis of complete heart block with a low cardiac output needs emergent medical treatment with isoproterenol, and urgent insertion of a pacemaker may be necessary.

Conclusion

CHD are not preventable diseases and require adequate clinical support. The only way to currently improve the prognosis lies in early diagnosis and this is essential to the successful treatment of these patients. Pediatric intensive care units and emergency departments have a vital role in the care of these patients.

Acknowledgment

Our special acknowledgment to Professor Nathan Kuppermann, MD, MPH, Principal Investigator, PRIME node, Pediatric Emergency Care Applied Research Network (PECARN) and Chair of the U.C. Davis Hospital Emergency Department for the review of our chapter.

References

[1] Fyler DC: Report of the New England Regional Infant Cardiac Program. *Pediatrics* 65:377–390, 1980.

[2] Fyler DC, Rothman KJ, Parisi-Buckley L, et al: The determinants of five year survival of infants with critical congenital heart disease. *Cardiovasc. Clin. 11*:393–405, 1981.

[3] Leoni F, Huhta JC, Douglas J, et al: Effect of prostaglandin on early surgical mortality in obstructive lesions of the systemic circulation. *Br. Heart J.* 52:654–659, 1984.

[4] Shone JD, Sellars RD, Anderson RC, et al: The developmental complex of parachute mitral valve, supravalvar ring of the left atrium, subaortic stenosis, and coarctation of the aorta. *Am. J. Cardiol.* 11:714–725, 1963.

[5] Rychik J, Murdison KA, Chin AJ, et al: Surgical management of severe aortic outflow obstruction in lesions other than hypoplastic left heart syndrome: Use of pulmonary artery to aorta anastomosis. *J. Am. Coll. Cardiol.* 18:809–816, 1991.

[6] Mair DD, Ritter DG: Factors influencing intercirculatory mixing in patients with complete transposition of the great arteries. *Am. J. Cardiol.* 30:653–658, 1972.

[7] Mair DD, Ritter DG: Factors influencing systemic arterial oxygen saturation in complete transposition of the great arteries. *Am. J. Cardiol.* 31:742–748, 1973.

[8] Penny DJ, Shekerdemian LS. Management of the neonate with symptomatic congenital heart disease. *Arch. Dis. Child Fetal. Neonatal. Ed* 2001; 84:F141-5.

[9] Grady R M, Canter CE, Bridges ND: Transcatheter ASD creation in infants with left heart obstruction [abstract]. *J. Am. Coll. Cardiol.* 26:484A, 1994.

[10] Shime N, Hashimoto S, Hiramatsu N, et al. Hypoxic gas therapy using nitrogen in the preoperative management of neonates with hypoplastic left heart syndrome. *Pediatr. Crit. Care Med.* 2000; 1: 38–41.

[11] Day RW, Barton AP, Pysher TJ. Pulmonary vascular resistance of children treated with nitrogen during early infancy. *Ann. Thorac. Surg.* 1998; 65: 1400–1404.

[12] Jobes DR, Nicolson SC, Steven JM, et al. Carbon dioxide prevents pulmonary overcirculation in hypoplastic left heart syndrome. *Ann. Thorac. Surg.* 1992; 54: 150–151.

[13] Tabbutt S, Ramamoorthy C, Montenegro LM, et al. Impact of inspired gas mixtures on preoperative infants with hypoplastic left heart syndrome during controlled ventilation. *Circulation.* 2001 Sep 18;104(12 Suppl 1):I159-64.

[14] Chang AC, Zucker HA, Hickey PR, et al: Pulmonary vascular resistance in infants after cardiac surgery: Role of carbon dioxide and hydrogen ion. *Crit .Care Med.* 23:568–574, 1995.

[15] John M. Costello, Melvin C. Almodovar. Emergency care for infants and children with acute cardiac disease. *Clin. Ped. Emerg. Med.* 8:145-155. 2007.

[16] Alsoufi B, Karamlou T, McCrindle BW, et al. Management options in neonates and infants with critical left ventricular outflow tract obstruction. *European Journal of Cardio-thoracic Surgery* 31 (2007) 1013—1021.

[17] .Szlam S, Dejanovich B, Ramirez R, et al. Clinical Pediatric Emergency Medicine, Volume 13 (2) Elsevier - Jun 1, 2012.

[18] Moghal NE, Brocklebank JT, Meadow SR. A review of acute renal failure in children: incidence, etiology and outcome. *Clin. Nephrol.* 1998; 49: 91-95.

[19] Welke KF, Dearani J, Ghanayem NS, et al. Renal complications associated with the treatment of patients with congenital cardiac disease: consensus definitions from the multi-societal Database Committee for Pediatric and Congenital heart disease. *Cardiol. Young* 2008; 18(suppl. 2): 222-225).

[20] Ruza Tarrio F. y col. Tratado de Cuidados Intensivos Pediátricos. Tercera Edición. Vol I. *Capitel. Edic. Cap.* 22: 393-422.

[21] Checchia PA, Karamlou T, Maruszewki B, et al. Hematologic and infectious complications associated with the treatment of patients with congenital cardiac disease: consensus definitions from the multi-societal Database Committee for Pediatric and Congenital heart disease. *Cardiol. Young* 2008; 18 (suppl. 2): 226-233.
[22] Paganini Hugo R. Pediatric Infectious Diseases. First Edition, Ed 2007 Scientific American, *Cap.* 72. P. 483. (spanish book).

Editors' Contact Information

Dr. Raúl Cayré, M.D., Ph.D.
Cardiological Research Institute
"Prof. Dr. Alberto C. Taquini"
University of Buenos Aires and National Council of Research
Science and Technology, ININCA.UBA.CONICET
Marcelo T. de Alvear 2270
CP112AAJ, Buenos Aires, Argentina
Phone/fax:+54 +11 45083836.
E-mail: raulcayre@gmail.com

Prof. José Milei. M.D., Ph.D.
Cardiological Research Institute
"Prof. Dr. Alberto C. Taquini"
University of Buenos Aires and National Council of Research
Science and Technology, ININCA.UBA.CONICET
Marcelo T. de Alvear 2270
CP1122AAJ, Buenos Aires, Argentina
Phone/fax:+54 + 11 45083836
E-mail: ininca@fmed.uba.ar

Index

B

C

D

E

I

J

K

L

M

N

O

P

Q

R

S

T